Pallidal Surgery for the Treatment of Parkinson's Disease and Movement Disorders

Pallidal Surgery for the Treatment of Parkinson's Disease and Movement Disorders

Editors

Joachim K. Krauss, M.D.
Department of Neurosurgery
University Hospital of Berne
Berne, Switzerland
and Department of Neurosurgery
Baylor College of Medicine
Houston, Texas

Robert G. Grossman, M.D.
Department of Neurosurgery
Baylor College of Medicine
Houston, Texas

Joseph Jankovic, M.D.
Department of Neurology
Baylor College of Medicine
Houston, Texas

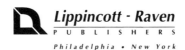

Lippincott · Raven
PUBLISHERS
Philadelphia • New York

Acquisitions Editor: Elizabeth Greenspan
Developmental Editor: Susan Rhyner
Manufacturing Manager: Kevin Watt
Supervising Editor: Liane Carita
Production Service: Bermedica Production, Ltd.
Cover Designer: OX & Company, Inc.
Indexer: Bermedica Production, Ltd.
Compositor: Circle Graphics
Printer: Maple Press

Printed in the United States of America

9 8 7 6 5 4 3 2 1

Library of Congress Cataloging-in-Publication Data

Pallidal surgery for the treatment of Parkinson's disease and movement
  disorders / [edited by] Joachim K. Krauss, Robert G. Grossman,
Joseph Jankovic.
      p.   cm.
  Includes bibliographical references and index.
  ISBN 0–7817–1225–4
  1. Globus pallidus—Surgery.   2. Parkinson's disease—Surgery.
3. Movement disorders—Surgery.   I. Krauss, Joachim K.
II. Grossman, Robert G.   III. Jankovic, Joseph.
  [DNLM: 1. Parkinson Disease—surgery.   2. Globus Pallidus—
surgery.   3. Movement Disorders—surgery.   WL 359 P167 1998]
RD594.P24   1998
617.4′81—dc21
DNLM/DLC
for Library of Congress   98-19196
                                                                              CIP

To our families, for their support and encouragement

Contents

Contributors

Roger L. Albin, M.D. *Associate Professor of Neurology, Neuroscience Laboratory Building, Director, Neuroscience Research, Geriatrics Research Education and Clinical Center, University of Michigan, 1103 East Huron, Ann Arbor, Michigan 48104*

Ron L. Alterman, M.D. *Assistant Professor of Neurosurgery, Department of Neurosurgery, The Pennsylvania Hospital, 301 South 8th Street, 2nd Floor, Duncan Building, Philadelphia, Pennsylvania 19107*

Angelo Antonini, M.D. *Movement Disorders Center, Department of Neurology, North Shore University Hospital, 444 Community Drive, Suite 206, Manhasset, New York 11030*

Roy A. E. Bakay, M.D. *Professor and Vice-Chairman, Section of Neurosurgery, Suite 2200, The Emory Clinic, 1365 Clifton Road, Atlanta, Georgia 30322*

J. M. Brotchie, M.D. *School of Biological Sciences, Division of Neuroscience, University of Manchester, 1.124 Stopford Building, Oxford Road, Manchester M13 9PT, United Kingdom*

Kim J. Burchiel, M.D. *Professor and Chairman, Department of Neurosurgery, Oregon Health Sciences University, Portland, Oregon 97201-3098*

A. R. Crossman, Ph.D., D.SC. *Professor of Anatomy, Chairman, Division of Neuroscience, School of Biological Sciences, University of Manchester, 1.124 Stopford Building, Oxford Road, Manchester M13 9PT, United Kingdom*

Janice L. Duff, R.N. *Clinical Research Associate, Division of Neurology, The Toronto Hospital, Movement Disorders Centre, 399 Bathurst Street, MP 11-306, Toronto, Ontario M5T 2S8, Canada*

David Eidelberg, M.D. *Professor of Neurology, New York University School of Medicine; Movement Disorders Center, North Shore University Hospital, 444 Community Drive, Suite 206, Manhasset, New York 11030*

Mel H. Epstein, M.D. *Professor and Chairman, Department of Neurosurgery, Rhode Island Hospital, 2 Deadley Street, MOB 555, Providence, Rhode Island 02905*

Jacques Favre, M.D. *Chef de Clinicque, Department of Neurosurgery, Centre Hospitalier Universitaire Vaudois, Lausanne, Switzerland*

Joseph H. Friedman, M.D. *Department of Neurosurgery, Rhode Island Hospital, 2 Deadley Street, MOB 555, Providence, Rhode Island 02905*

Gerhard M. Friehs, M.D. *Assistant Professor of Neurosurgery, Department of Neurosurgery, Rhode Island Hospital, 2 Deadley Street, MOB 555, Providence, Rhode Island 02905*

Monique L. Giroux, M.D. *Fellow in Movement Disorders and Functional, Neuroimaging, Department of Neurology, Emory University, WMB Suite 6000, 1639 Pierce Drive, Atlanta, Georgia 30322*

Robert G. Grossman, M.D. *Professor and Chairman, Department of Neurosurgery, Baylor College of Medicine, 6560 Fannin, Suite 944, Houston, Texas 77030*

William D. Hutchison, Ph.D.   *Assistant Professor of Surgery and Physiology, Division of Neurosurgery, The Toronto Hospital, Western Division EW6-528, 399 Bathurst Street, Toronto, Ontario M5T 2S8, Canada*

Joseph Jankovic, M.D.   *Professor of Neurology, Director, Parkinson's Disease Center and Movement Disorders Clinic, Department of Neurology, Baylor College of Medicine, 6550 Fannin, Suite 1801, Houston, Texas 77030-3498*

Patrick J. Kelly, M.D.   *Professor and Chairman, Department of Neurological Surgery, New York University Medical Center, 530 First Avenue, Suite 7A, New York, New York 10016*

William Koller, M.D., Ph.D.   *Professor and Chairman, Department of Neurology, Kansas University Medical Center, 3901 Rainbow Boulevard, Kansas City, Kansas 66160-7383*

Joachim K. Krauss, M.D.   *Director of Functional and Stereotactic Neurosurgery, Department of Neurosurgery, University Hospital of Berne, 3010 Berne, Switzerland; and Adjunct Associate Professor, Department of Neurosurgery, Baylor College of Medicine, 6560 Fannin, Suite 944, Houton, Texas 77030*

Eugene C. Lai, M.D., Ph.D.   *Associate Professor of Neurology, Department of Neurology, Baylor College of Medicine, 6550 Fannin, Suite 1801, Houston, Texas 77030*

Lauri V. Laitinen, M.D., Ph.D.   *Associate Professor of Neurosurgery, Emeritus, Dano, FIN-22340, Geta Aland, Finland*

Anthony E. Lang, M.D., F.R.C.P.C   *Division of Neurology, Toronto Western Hospital, 399 Bathurst Street, MP11-306, Toronto, Ontario M5T 2S8, Canada*

Frederick A. Lenz, M.D., Ph.D., F.R.C.S.(C)   *Associate Professor of Neurosurgery, Department of Neurosurgery, Johns Hopkins Hospital, 600 N. Wolfe Street, Meyer 7-113, Baltimore, Maryland 21287*

Andres M. Lozano, M.D., Ph.D., F.R.C.S.(C)   *Associate Professor of Surgery, Division of Neurosurgery, University of Toronto, The Toronto Hospital, Western Division, 399 Bathurst Street, Toronto, Ontario M5T 2S8, Canada*

Allen S. Mandir, M.D., Ph.D.   *Instructor, Department of Neurology, Johns Hopkins Hospital, 600 N. Wolfe Street, Pathology 210, Baltimore, Maryland 21287*

Erwin B. Montgomery, Jr., M.D.   *Professor of Neurology, Department of Neurology, Cleveland Clinic Foundation, 9500 Euclid Avenue, Cleveland, Ohio 44195*

Georg Norén, M.D., Ph.D.   *Associate Professor, Clinical Neurosciences, Department of Neurosurgery, Rhode Island Hospital, 2 Deadley Street, MOB 555, Providence, Rhode Island 02905*

William G. Ondo, M.D.   *Assistant Professor of Neurology, Department of Neurology, Baylor College of Medicine, 6550 Fannin, #1801, Houston, Texas 77030-3498*

Averell S. Overby, Dr. P.H., R.T.   *Associate Professor, School of Physical Therapy, Ohio University, Convocation Center 175, Athens, Ohio 47501*

Richard D. Penn, M.D.   *Professor of Neurosurgery, Rush-Presbyterian Hospital, 1725 West Harrison Street, Suite 755, Chicago, Illinois 60612*

Gayle M. Rettig, Ph.D.   *Assistant Professor, Department of Neurosurgery, Baylor College of Medicine, 6560 Fannin, Suite 944, Scurlock Tower, Houston, Texas 77030*

Philip A. Starr, M.D., Ph.D. *Instructor, Emory University School of Medicine, 1365 Clifton Road, Atlanta, Georgia 30322*

Jamal M. Taha, M.D. *Assistant Professor/Director of Functional, Neurosurgery, Department of Neurosurgery, University of Cincinnati, 231 Bethesda Avenue, M.L. 0515, Cincinnati, Ohio 45219-0515*

Ronald Tasker, M.D., F.R.C.S.(C) *Professor Emeritus of Surgery, Division of Neurosurgery, The Toronto Hospital, 399 Bathurst Street, MP 11-306, Toronto, Ontario M5T 2S8, Canada*

Jerrold L. Vitek, M.D., Ph.D. *Associate Professor of Neurology, Department of Neurology, Emory University, WMB Suite 6000, 1639 Pierce Drive, Atlanta, Georgia 30322*

Deborah Roberts-Warrior, MS, PT *School of Physical Therapy, Texas Women's University, 1130 M.D. Anderson Boulevard, Houston, Texas 77030*

Steven B. Wilkinson, M.D. *Associate Professor of Neurological Surgery, Department of Surgery, Division of Neurosurgery, Kansas University Medical Center, 3901 Rainbow Boulevard, Kansas City, Kansas 66160*

Foreword

The introduction of stereotactic surgery by Spiegel and Wycis in 1947 had a fundamental impact on the surgical treatment of movement disorders. In the following years, the techniques were refined and indications were elaborated in various centers all over the world. The globus pallidus was the first target which was established for the treatment of Parkinson's disease and other movement disorders.

When I with Traugott Riechert and Rolf Hassler performed the first motor thalamotomy in a patient with Parkinson's disease in Freiburg in 1952, we intended to offer a method that was more effective for the treatment of parkinsonian tremor. None of us would ever have thought that thalamotomy would push pallidotomy to the background within only a few years. For me, pallidotomy was always an effective tool. Over the years, I have performed more than 500 pallidotomies, and I also had the opportunity to observe the benefit after several years.

The globus pallidus is back as target for the surgical treatment of movement disorders. Pallidal surgery nowadays differs in many aspects from pallidal surgery as performed 40 years ago. Technical developments and innovations have contributed to make this method safer and more efficacious. When my friend Lauri Laitinen reintroduced pallidotomy a few years ago, I was somewhat skeptical, initially, like most of us. But, thanks to the hard work of different groups of neurosurgeons and neurologists, and new insights in the pathophysiology of movement disorders, pallidal surgery has been reestablished within a short period. Many questions remain to be answered. Some of these questions are the same we asked decades ago, while today there are also other questions and entirely new problems.

Functional stereotactic surgery has had a renaissance within the past few years that I would not ever have imagined. I congratulate Joachim K. Krauss, Robert G. Grossman, and Joseph Jankovic, having realized this comprehensive monograph on pallidal surgery together with a well-selected group of colleagues. This volume is a benchmark for all who are interested in the surgical treatment of movement disorders.

Fritz Mundinger

Preface

Pallidal surgery reemerged from oblivion, only a few years ago, and since then it has had a major impact on the treatment of Parkinson's disease and movement disorders. Pallidotomy was first introduced in the 1950s, but its effects on movement disorders have not been fully appreciated until recently. Although the mechanism is not yet completely understood, several well-designed clinical studies have provided evidence that pallidal surgery improves both hyperkinetic and hypokinetic movement disorders. In experienced hands pallidal surgery has been shown to be safe and effective. Nevertheless, many issues remain to be clarified. The interest in pallidal surgery is reflected by the number of publications within the past few years.

The primary objective of *Pallidal Surgery for the Treatment of Parkinson's Disease and Movement Disorders* is to present a critical review of the current knowledge on pallidal surgery. This book is clinically oriented, but we included comprehensive reviews on the basic principles of basal ganglia function. Much progress has been made in understanding normal and pathologic conditions which has furthered the development of movement disorders surgery. Furthermore, the renaissance of movement disorders surgery has stimulated interest in the study of the basal ganglia circuitry. Whether or not pallidal surgery will remain the mainstay in movement disorders surgery over the next few years remains to be seen. Future studies will undoubtedly pursue ablative procedures or deep brain stimulation of other targets, such as the subthalamic nucleus. Pallidal surgery is an evolving issue. Periodic updates on the progress in the expanding field of functional neurosurgery of movement disorders will be needed in the future.

Treatment of Parkinson's disease and other movement disorders requires a true multidisciplinary approach. Independent evaluation of surgical results is necessary for objective appreciation of its effects. Therefore, the close cooperation between neurosurgeons, neurologists, neurophysiologists, and neurobiologists is critical for future advances in movement disorders surgery.

We are indebted to the distinguished group of international authors who have contributed their pioneering experience to this volume. We also appreciate the timely manner with which this book has been produced and we express our deepest thanks to Elizabeth Greenspan and Susan Rhyner from Lippincott–Raven Publishers. We hope that this book will be helpful for all clinicians, neurosurgeons, and other health care professionals as well as basic scientists who are interested in improving the care of patients with Parkinson's disease and other movement disorders.

Joachim K. Krauss
Robert G. Grossman
Joseph Jankovic

Pallidal Surgery for the Treatment of Parkinson's Disease and Movement Disorders

Pallidal Surgery for the Treatment of Parkinson's Disease and Movement Disorders, edited by
J. K. Krauss, R. G. Grossman, and J. Jankovic.
Lippincott-Raven Publishers, Philadelphia © 1998.

1

Historical Review of Pallidal Surgery for Treatment of Parkinsonism and other Movement Disorders

*†Joachim K. Krauss and †Robert G. Grossman

*Department of Neurosurgery, Inselspital, University of Berne, Switzerland; and
†Department of Neurosurgery, Baylor College of Medicine, Houston, Texas 77030, USA

It may therefore be predicted that in the long run the stereotaxic treatment of Parkinsonism will be supplementary to treatment with L-dopa but not replaced by it . . . (56).

The development of functional stereotactic surgery was a major step in the history of neurosurgery. The techniques initially were envisioned as a tool for psychosurgery. One of the first applications of this new method, however, involved a pallidotomy in a patient with Huntington's disease. The history of the introduction of this procedure, its almost complete abandonment after somewhat more than a decade, and its recent rediscovery is most unusual. Upon reviewing this history we discover that many contemporary concepts and questions have been brought up previously. Much of this knowledge has been forgotten, and work in progress has not been finished with the decline of functional stereotactic neurosurgery during the 1970s.

At the time functional stereotactic surgery was introduced in clinical practice, during the late 1940s and the early 1950s, medical progress had slowed during the depression of the post-World War II era. Elective neurosurgical procedures during that period often were accompanied by high mortality and morbidity rates, and the development of new methods frequently was a matter of trial and error. Several factors contributed to the uprise of pallidotomies and thalamotomies during the 1950s. In particular, the need for more accu-

rate methods for accomplishing psychosurgical procedures, which were performed relatively frequently during the 1940s, had stimulated the development of stereotactic techniques (122). There was growing interest in the treatment of disabling movement disorders with prolonged life expectancy. Surgical treatment for movement disorders had evolved over the first half of the century, but the results were rather unsatisfactory. The basal ganglia only recently had been considered to be involved in motor control.

Before the basal ganglia became recognized as a target for surgical treatment of movement disorders, various operations on the peripheral and central nervous systems and on other organs were performed (59,65,84,101). Such surgical manipulations included thyroidectomy, frontal leukotomy, and dentatectomy. To alleviate hemiballism even limb amputations were recommended. Lesions in the sensory system were made by posterior rhizotomy, posterior or anterolateral cordotomy, sympathetic ramisectomy, and ganglionectomy. Many procedures directly targeted the motor system and involved excision of the motor cortex, ablation or undercutting of the premotor cortex, and destruction of the pyramidal tract at various levels (e.g., by subcortical pyramidotomy, mesencephalic pedunculotomy, or high cervical cordotomy). In general, alleviation of the movement disorder was achieved only at the cost of hemiparesis. Other side effects, such as delayed appearance of spasticity, were frequent; and long-term relief was rare in patients with preserved motor function.

Scientific communication between countries of the Western world was slow and limited during the post-World War II era. Concepts and innovations of functional stereotactic surgery were elaborated in various countries sometimes almost in parallel. Most early investigators designed and built their own systems, as standard systems were not commercially available. English was not yet unanimously accepted as the scientific language, and many scientists preferred to publish results in their own language, particularly French and German authors. This practice renders it sometimes difficult to write the history of pallidotomy giving proper credit always to the right persons. Among the leaders of the new development were Ernest Spiegel and Henry Wycis from Temple University in Philadelphia; Lars Leksell from Lund, Sweden; Jean Talairach from Paris, France; Traugott Riechert, Rolf Hassler, and Fritz Mundinger from Freiburg, Germany; John Gillingham from Edinburgh, UK; Claude Bertrand from Montreal, Canada; and Hirotaro Narabayashi from Tokyo, Japan. Irving Cooper from New York, although heavily criticized by many of his contemporaries, became one of the most popular figures in movement disorder surgery. Remarkably, Gazi Yasargil from Zürich, Switzerland was engaged in functional stereotactic surgery together with Krayenbühl during the late 1950s before he became one of the leading innovators in microneurosurgery.

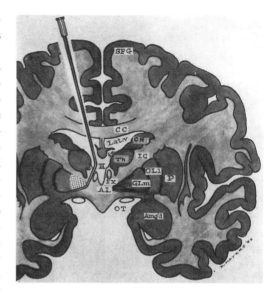

FIG. 1-1. Meyers' transventricular approach for ansotomy as performed between 1939 and 1949. (*From* ref. 84, with permission.)

BASAL GANGLIA SURGERY FOR MOVEMENT DISORDERS

Basal Ganglia

Basal ganglia surgery for treatment of movement disorders was pioneered by Russell Meyers during the 1940s (83,84). Earlier it was generally thought that such an approach would be impossible because it might result in enduring coma. Among others, Dandy had hypothesized that vegetative centers and the center of consciousness were located in the basal ganglia (30). Meyer's first patient was a 26-year-old woman suffering from parkinsonian tremors. After unsuccessfully "separating the motor from the premotor cortex" Meyers extirpated the head of the caudate nucleus via a transventricular approach in 1939. Postoperatively, the patient was free of tremor and without evidence of concomitant hemiparesis. Within the following years Meyers continued to refine his approach to the basal ganglia, targeting the putamen, the ansa lenticularis, and the pallidum (Fig. 1-1). In several instances he also placed lesions in the internal capsule. By 1949 he had operated on 58 patients suffering from various movement disorders including parkinsonian syndromes, choreoathetosis, hemiballism, and cervical dystonia. Postoperative improvement was achieved in 60% of his patients, but the operative mortality was as high as 12%. Similar results were reported by others, such as Browder, who had combined section of the anterior internal capsule with extirpation of the head of the caudate (16).

Pallidum

Meyers' series of basal ganglia operations included four procedures where he extirpated the "oral pole of the globus pallidus" (84). In 1950

Fénelon in France reported on a new method to treat parkinsonism (36): He lesioned the pallidum and the pallidofugal pathways via a temporal approach. Shortly thereafter, this method was modified by Guiot and Brion, who performed subfrontal and transsylvian approaches to insert a lesion-making electrode into the pallidum via the anterior perforate substance (46). There was a slight reduction of mortality with these techniques. Overall improvement was achieved in about 50% to 70% of patients.

DEVELOPMENT OF STEREOTACTIC PALLIDOTOMY

Stereotactic Surgery

The main principle of stereotactic surgery defining the three-dimensional position of a structure in the intracranial cavity by three variables in a cartesian coordinate system may be traced back as far as Leonardo da Vinci. Leonardo depicted the position of the third ventricle, which was thought to be the seat of the "sensus communis," on three intersecting axes (65).

The first stereotactic frame was constructed in 1908 by the neurosurgeon Horsley and the mathematician Clarke for use in animal studies to investigate cerebellar physiology (60). With this system it was possible to localize cerebral structures with reference to skull landmarks. It was not until 1947, however, that this technique was applied to humans. When Spiegel (Fig. 1-2) and colleagues introduced their new instrument, the stereoencephalotome, they used radiographic studies, including pneumoencephalography, to define internal landmarks such as the pineal calcification or the foramen of Monro for reference of the coordinates (124). Stimulated by the work of Spiegel and Wycis, neurosurgeons and neuroscientists all over the world developed their own stereotactic systems during the early 1950s, including Leksell in Sweden, Talairach in France, and Riechert in Germany (74,108,109,129).

The first stereotactic atlases were published within the next few years (111,121,129). In general, these atlases gave stereotactic coordinates referring to structures that border the third ventricle. The anterior commissure–posterior com-

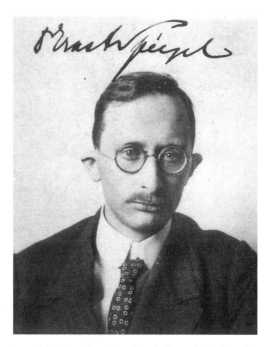

FIG. 1-2. Dr. Ernest Spiegel, Temple University, Philadelphia.

missure (AC-PC) line was established as the reference line most frequently used. Alternatively, coordinates were referenced to the foramen of Monro (FM)–PC line (56). Stereotactic target calculation initially relied completely on pneumencephalography. This method, however, often was uncomfortable for the patient and contributed to additional operative morbidity. At least 7% of patients developed transient cognitive and mental disturbances, such as confusion or restlessness (105). During the early 1960s positive contrast ventriculography became routine in functional stereotactic surgery and almost replaced pneumencephalography (101,105). Ventriculographic target determination requires adjustment of x-ray distortion for both anteroposterior and lateral films. To keep distortion to a minimum many surgeons used special setups in their operative rooms with a long distance between the x-ray tube and the x-ray plate (105). Until recently, ventriculography was considered the gold standard for target determination in functional stereotactic surgery. Only during the past few years has it been recognized that target calculation based on computed tomography or magnetic resonance imaging equals or may even be superior to ventriculography (3,49). Electrophysiological methods consisting of recording and stimulation at the target sites were soon added to the repertoire of functional stereotactic surgery during the 1950s (19,12,52,54,91).

The stereotactic atlas of Schaltenbrand and Wahren was published in 1977 (112). Coordinates, in particular for pallidal targets, differed slightly from those given in the earlier edition, the Schaltenbrand-Bailey atlas (111). Because of small demand, the Schaltenbrand-Wahren atlas was sold at 20% of its original price during the late 1980s.

First Stereotactic Pallidotomies

The first stereotactic pallidotomies were performed by Spiegel and Wycis in 1948 in patients with Huntington's disease (122). In the first patient, the primary goal was to diminish the reaction to "afferent stimuli and emotional reactions . . . able to accentuate choreic and athetotic movements" by lesioning the dorsomedial thalamic nuclei. On September 12, 1948, a 53-year-old man was operated on "by means of the stereotaxic method" and "extensive electrolytic lesions were placed in the left dorsomedial nucleus of the thalamus," and "one droplet of alcohol was injected in the region of the right globus pallidus at the level of the anterior commissure" (122). Postoperatively, alleviation of choreic movements on the left side but not on the right side was noted. Shortly thereafter pallidal lesions exclusively were made in another patient with Huntington's disease. This 68-year-old man suffered from bilateral choreic movements and underwent several subsequent operations. During the first procedure electrolytic lesions were placed in the left dorsomedial thalamus and the anterior tip of the right pallidum. The second procedure involved the lateral part of the right pallidum only. The left-sided choreic movements ceased after this operation. The third step involved targeting the contralateral pallidum and resulted in almost complete abolition of the right-sided hyperkinesias. Transient hemiparesis was noted after the second and third procedures. Spiegel and Wycis at that time explicitly tried to spare the medial part of the pallidum because they considered such a lesion to be dangerous with regard to the pyramidal tract.

Stereotactic pallidotomy as a treatment option for parkinsonism was reported during the early 1950s. Spiegel and Wycis initially were somewhat hesitant to adopt their new method for treatment of parkinsonian symptoms. They feared that pallidal lesions, according to the doctrines of Foerster, might even induce hypokinesia and rigidity instead of relieving it (118). Narabayashi performed his first pallidotomies for treatment of athetosis and parkinsonism in Japan in 1951 (Narabayashi, personal communication). Early experiences were soon reported by Riechert and colleagues (52,109), Guiot and Brion (46), Narabayashi and Okuma (95), and Spiegel and Wycis (120). Guiot and Brion considered stereotactic pallidotomy initially as an alternative for patients they considered poor candidates for their open subfrontal approaches: "*sujets trop agés, forms avancées, mauvaise résistance générale*" (46).

The development of stereotactic pallidotomy for treatment of Parkinson's disease erroneously has been attributed to Cooper. Numerous authors have cited earlier publications repeating the same plot. According to this story, in 1952 Cooper accidentally severed the anterior choroidal artery while performing a pedunculotomy on a patient with parkinsonian tremor. The patient's tremor was much alleviated postoperatively, and it was concluded that it was secondary to ischemia of the pallidum, which is partly supplied by the anterior choroidal artery. This result led Cooper to clip the artery in a series of patients to treat parkinsonian tremor (24). The mortality associated with the procedure was 13%. The story goes that Cooper then considered targeting the pallidum directly. Apparently, he started to perform chemopallidectomy in the United States in 1954. It is unclear why he ignored the work of the Philadelphia group or if he was aware of the work of the French and German pioneers of functional stereotactic surgery.

PALLIDOTOMY DURING THE 1950s AND 1960s

After pallidotomy had been shown to be effective for treating various movement disorders and parkinsonian syndromes, this method was adopted and modified by neurosurgeons all over the world. It was estimated that by 1965 more than 25,000 functional stereotactic procedures for parkinsonism had been performed worldwide (119). These activities resulted in a multitude of scientific publications (1,2,4,7–12,19–23,25–28, 32,34,40–43,46–48,51–57,61,70,75–77,85–107, 110,115–118,120–123,127–135,137,138). For several reasons, however, it is difficult nowadays to evaluate and compare the results obtained in different centers. We give a noninclusive overview in the following sections.

Operative Techniques

Various techniques to create the pallidal lesions were used during the early years of the heyday of functional stereotactic surgery (65,101). Electrolytic lesioning was the first method used by Spiegel and Wycis and subsequently by many others (65,122). The extent of these electrolytic lesions, however, was difficult to control mainly because of the fluctuations of direct (DC) currents. Later, electrical lesioning was completely replaced by high-frequency coagulation. Leksell and colleagues used a special bipolar electrode that consisted of a pair of electrodes inserted in parallel with uninsulated 10-mm tips set 8 mm apart (Fig. 1-3) (127). Some investigators applied reversible test lesions before the final lesion was made to ensure proper localization. Chemical le-

sions were produced by injecting alcohol or procaine oil at the target (26,96). Bertrand popularized the use of a small leukotome to produce a spherical lesion (7,10). Other techniques included cryogenic lesion-making, the use of inflatable balloons, induction heating by exposing small implanted metal rods to electromagnetic fields, the application of ultrasound, and the implantation of radioactive isotopes such as iridium-192 or yttrium-90 (84,101,105).

Many authors performed intraoperative test stimulations via the lesion-making electrode to verify the target and delineate responses from adjacent structures (105). It was found that pallidal stimulation could either suppress or intensify a patient's tremor depending on the frequency of the stimulus. Furthermore, nonmotor effects were recorded (Fig. 1-4). Riechert noted that at high voltages patients often expressed "a sensation of constriction in the chest combined with a feeling of anxiety" sometimes "associated with a feeling of impending death" (105). Some investigators used recording techniques to further delineate the pallidal target. Bertrand and colleagues performed "depth electroencephalography" with a "triple lead electrode" (12). With this technique they compared the signals obtained by each of the three contacts seeking "beta and theta rhythms which seem to arise from the cells of the globus."

It is important to know that Cooper and many of his disciples performed pallidotomy without using stereotactic techniques in strictu sensu

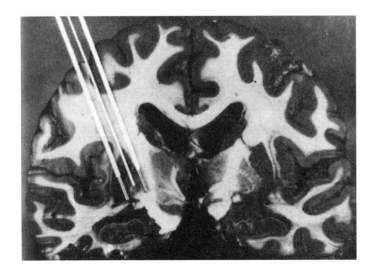

FIG. 1-3. Leksell's method of pallidotomy. The pallidal lesion was made with a special bipolar electrode set consisting of a pair of electrodes with 10-mm uninsulated tips set 8 mm apart. (*From* ref. 127, with permission.)

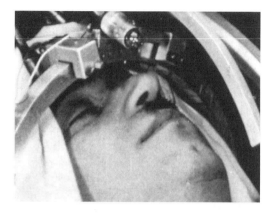

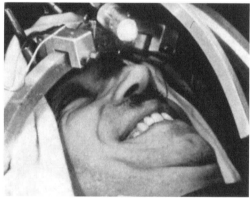

FIG. 1-4. Sequences of a film during electrical stimulation of the anterior pallidum in a patient with torsion dystonia. At stimulation with 50 Hz the patients consistently started to laugh. (*From* ref. 54, with permission.)

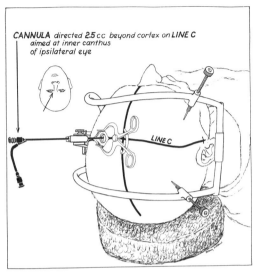

FIG. 1-5. Cooper's nonstereotactic approach for chemopallidectomy and chemothalamectomy. (*From* ref. 21, with permission.)

(19–29,100,128). Cooper did not work with a stereotactic frame during the 1950s (Fig. 1-5). In 1956 Cooper and Poloukhine stated that "one can place a lesion in the globus pallidus without the aid of a complicated stereotactic instrument" (28). Cooper did not use reference points related to structures of the third ventricle but osseous reference points of the skull to place the targeting instrument "free hand." Later, Cooper worked with an instrument similar to a frame, the "chemopallidectomy guide," which was used as a cannula holder. An alcoholic solution, Etapolin, "a mixture of 8% celloidin and 95% ethanol" often mixed with Pantopaque was injected into the target area "under roentgenographic control." Later, a "physiologic test, simply and quickly" was introduced before the lesion was made; it consisted of observing the effect of the insufflation of a balloon at the tip of the inserted cannula. The catheter could be left in place to reinject the alcoholic solution and gradually increase the lesion size. Occasionally the solution was injected via two cannulas spaced 1 cm apart. As might be assumed, the accuracy of such a procedure was questionable. Indeed, it was accepted that with this method "some of the neighboring structures" were "destroyed by the injection in at least some cases." Many of his peers, among them Spiegel, Hassler, and Levy, openly criticized Cooper's methods and regarded chemopallidectomy as inappropriate (56,77,118). Later, Cooper preferentially applied cryosurgical lesions. This method, however, was also deemed unreliable by others (118). In addition to the disadvantage of inserting a relatively thick cannula into the brain, the size of the lesion produced by this method was regarded as unpredictable.

Evaluation of Historical Series on Pallidotomy

During the 1950s there were no commonly accepted rating scales to evaluate parkinsonian symptoms and the associated disability. Many investigators used their own scales to compare the preoperative condition of the patient with the postoperative status. Moreover, many investigators limited their descriptions to the notion of whether the target symptom was influenced by surgery and if it was alleviated or abolished. Taking into account that additional lesions sometimes were placed in the internal capsule, abolition occasionally also meant that the tremor was replaced by paresis. Although some investigators developed more elaborated rating scales for single symptoms, it was uncommon during these days to consider functional disability or quality of life as an outcome measure. It must be kept in mind that common scales, such as the Schwab and England scale or the Webster scale, gained wider acceptance only during the late 1960s (114,136). Most studies on operative results from the 1950s were also limited by short-term follow-up and combining early with late postoperative results among the various patients.

Another problem with evaluating historic studies on the effects of pallidotomy on parkinsonism is the fact that at that time no proper criteria for the differential diagnosis of parkinsonian syndromes were available. During the 1950s there were still many patients suffering from postencephalitic parkinsonism due to encephalitis lethargica during the 1920s. Other parkinsonian syndromes, such as supranuclear palsy, were yet to be described. This entity was not recognized until the landmark report of Steele et al. in 1964 (125). In addition, definition of idiopathic Parkinson's disease was quite different from today's concepts. Svennilson et al., for example, stated that with parkinsonism "it is generally accepted that the majority of cases are either inflammatory or secondary to vascular disease" (127). Many investigators were aware of the diagnostic problems and limitations. It was noted that "precision in diagnosis is impossible" (127). Others, rather arbitrarily, classified their patients as having idiopathic Parkinson's disease or postencephalitic parkinsonism without commenting on the differentiating criteria. The heterogeneity of parkinsonian syndromes is nicely demonstrated by a list summarizing the probable etiology in a series of 422 parkinsonian patients by Mundinger and

Riechert in 1961: "hereditary parkinsonism, 8 patients; presumably hereditary parkinsonism, 2 patients; postencephalitic parkinsonism (Economo), 70 patients; probable postencephalitic parkinsonism, 55 patients; arteriosclerotic parkinsonism, 34 patients; parkinsonism due to malaria, 24 patients; parkinsonism due to lues, 4 patients; parkinsonism after intoxications, 7 patients; parkinsonism of unclear etiology, 218 patients" (87). It should be noted here that the accuracy of the clinical diagnosis of idiopathic Parkinson's disease still continues to be a challenge in some cases today (62).

A comparison of contemporary and historic series is rendered useless particularly with regard to the concept of levodopa response as a diagnostic feature of Parkinson's disease. Whereas levodopa nonresponders are generally excluded from pallidotomy nowadays, their proportion may have been high in some historical series, which also may have had an impact considering the controversial reports on the improvement of bradykinetic symptoms.

In some reports the results of thalamotomy and pallidotomy for treatment of parkinsonism were not described separately for each procedure (23,75). In other instances surgery for "double-lesions" in the thalamus and the pallidum (Fig. 1-6) were performed on the same side simultaneously (34). Several surgeons also combined lesioning of the pallidum with capsular lesions, particularly in the posterior limb of the internal capsule (42). Although such lesions may have involved pallidal outflow pathways and were not associated with hemiparesis in some series, lesioning of corticospinal tract fibers in others cannot be excluded. Some neurosurgeons even *intended* to produce postoperative hemiparesis. Obrador and Dierssen, for example, stated that "a certain postoperative degree of the so-called pyramidal tract syndrome seems to be, in our experience, a favorable factor, and, in fact, we aimed to obtain some slight pyramidal involvement" (98). Such points of view were strongly opposed by others such as Spiegel and Riechert (105, 118).

Statistical analysis of medical data was not usually performed during the 1950s. Even simple statistical procedures were not appreciated. Most

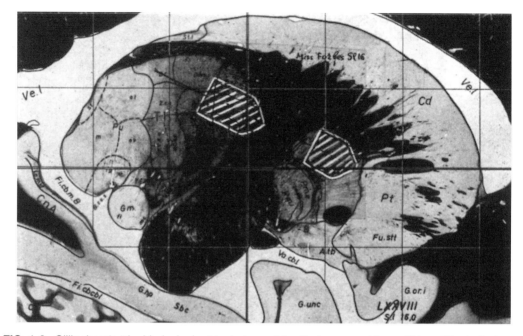

FIG. 1-6. Gillingham's "double-lesioning" technique of the thalamus and the pallidum. The trajectory is plotted on a sagittal section of the Schaltenbrand-Bailey atlas, 16 mm from the midline. (*From* ref. 42, with permission.)

often the results were purely descriptive, often even without quantification.

Where Was the Target Located Within the Pallidum?

It is commonly thought that during the first decade of pallidotomy the target within the pallidum was generally located in the anterodorsal part of the medial pallidum. Review of the historic data, however, reveals that there was no consensus on where the lesion was best placed within the pallidum, a point that was well recognized. It was also debated whether the best results would be achieved by pallidotomy, pallidoansotomy, or ansotomy alone (76,84,137). In 1959 Levy reported a study on the variety of the pallidal target with regard to the foramen of Monro–posterior commissure (FM-PC) line (76). Levy at that time was a stipendiate of the Swiss Academy of Science, studying under the guidance of Riechert in Freiburg. This comparative study considered not only the target coordinates

but also the technique of lesion-making and the axis of the instrument within the pallidum (i.e., the angle of the trajectory in relation to the FM-PC line) (Fig. 1-7). Thus the pallidal targets of various investigators were depicted graphically including those for the groups of Riechert, Hassler, and Mundinger; Talairach; Spiegel and Wycis; Guiot and Brion; Leksell; Rémond; Bertrand; and Cooper. This study shows that some groups primarily targeted the medial pallidum (Riechert; Talairach; Spiegel) or the medial and lateral pallidum (Guiot; Leksell; Bertrand). Although the lesion did not include the ventral pallidum in some of the groups, there were remarkable exceptions. Rémond et al., for example, who reported their method in 1958 in French in the *Revue Neurologique,* located their target in the posteroventral lateral portion of the medial pallidum (103). Bertrand and colleagues, as early as in 1958, stated that anterior pallidal lesions did not affect parkinsonian tremor and rigidity and that including the pallidofugal pathways yielded more beneficial results (12). Interestingly

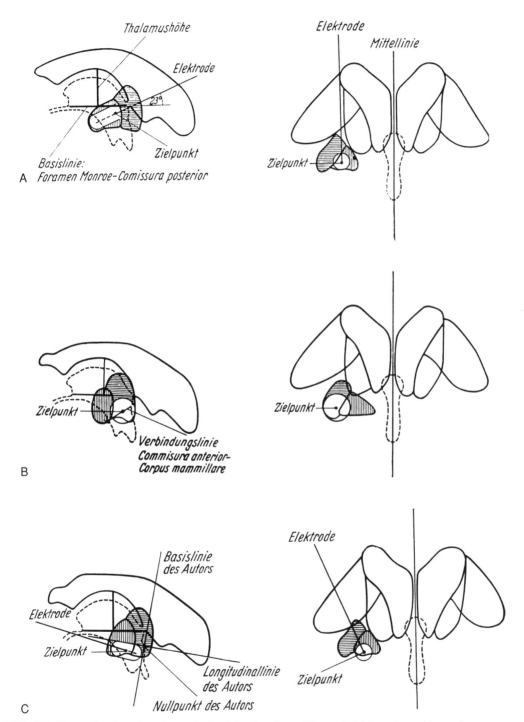

FIG. 1-7. Examples from Levy's analysis of the location of the pallidal target used by various neuro-surgeons during the 1950s. **A:** Riechert and Hassler. **B:** Guiot and Brion. **C:** Rémond. The medial pallidum is depicted by longitudinal bars, the lateral pallidum by horizontal bars against the outlines of the ventricles. The target area corresponds to the white dots, respectively. Sagittal sections are on the left and coronal sections on the right. (*From* ref. 76, with permission.)

they also thought that lesioning the pallidal outflow to the brainstem, in particular that of the pal-
lidorubral and pallidoreticular pathways, was
pivotal for postoperative success. Levy did not
compare clinical outcome with regard to the various targets, but he suggested that this should be
done in the future. When Svennilson et al. published their results using Leksell's method in
1960, they described the lesion to be "on the
postero-medial aspect of the medial nucleus of
the pallidum" (127). Whether their lesion was indeed more posterior and more ventral than the
target of some other neurosurgeons may be debated. With regard to Leksell's lesion-making
technique, these lesions were quite large and definitely destroyed portions of the lateral and medial pallidum, including the central and dorsal
areas. Interestingly, at about the same time,
Spiegel and Wycis had considered the location of
the pallidal target to be more posterior (Gildenberg, personal communication).

Pathophysiological Models
and Parkinsonian Target Symptoms

Pathophysiological models for parkinsonism became more elaborated during the 1950s. Often
the observations during surgery were incorporated into these models, or they stimulated the
formulation of new hypotheses. Pallidothalamic
pathways were already well known, while the
subthalamic nucleus, in general, was not incorporated into the functional circuits (Fig. 1-8).
Nevertheless, Hassler and Riechert hypothesized
that via "descending pathways to the subthalamic
nucleus, reticular formation and the red nucleus"
a change in "the dynamic equilibrium in the anterior horn cells" might be induced (54). These
authors also suggested a somatotopic organization of pallidal cells, with the leg represented
more caudally and the arm in central areas (Fig.
1-9). Some investigators tried to explain parkinsonian symptoms on the basis of specific pathomechanisms, whereas others worked with rather
holistic concepts. The latter approach is best exemplified by Meyers' illustrative rotating disk
model (Fig. 1-10) (84).

Pallidotomy was considered to be most effective treatment for parkinsonian rigidity, as the

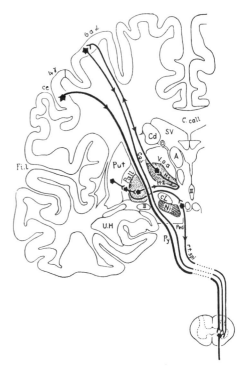

FIG. 1-8. Early simplified model of pallidal motor pathways in the basal ganglia circuitry. (*From* ref. 53, with permission.)

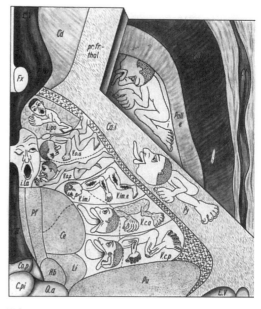

FIG. 1-9. Pallidal and thalamic homunculi. (*From* ref. 56, with permission.)

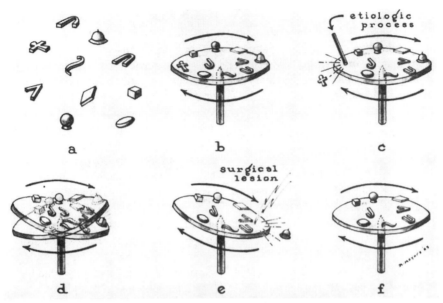

FIG. 1-10. Meyers' rotating disc model offered a holistic approach to explain the occurrence of movement disorders and their treatment by surgical lesioning. (*From* ref. 84, with permission.)

pallidum was thought to be directly involved in the generation of rigidity. It was hypothesized that rigidity was secondary to "increased plastic tonicization of the motor system" when "pallidal function is no longer damped" (77). Narabayashi concluded that the pallidum was "the higher center of gamma function" with the lower center located in the brainstem (91).

Bradykinetic and akinetic symptoms in general were not regarded as indications for functional stereotactic surgery. The terms akinesia, hypokinesia, and bradykinesia were not used consistently during the 1950s. Some investigators tried to differentiate such symptoms, but the terms were often used interchangeably. Bradykinesia was not yet fully recognized as an independent symptom of parkinsonism by many investigators. Housepian and Pool brought attention to the fact that bradykinesia may exist as a symptom by itself after surgery (61). It was also thought that a negative motor symptom could not be improved by a lesion. This is exemplified by the quote of Hassler et al., who noted that "for theoretical reasons alone, one could hardly expect an improvement of akinesia by a stereotaxic operation" (56). Consequently, they considered pallidotomy to be

not effective for alleviation of hypokinetic symptoms. They also thought akinesia occasionally was even increased by pallidotomy, at least temporarily. Pathophysiological models of parkinsonism could not explain the occurrence of parkinsonian akinesia. Hypokinetic symptoms were thought not to result from basal ganglia dysfunction but from impaired "conduction from the nigra cells to the anterior horn motor apparatus" (56). Despite the theoretical difficulty of explaining the phenomenon, it was occasionally noted that akinetic symptoms were ameliorated by pallidotomy. This effect, however, then was mostly attributed to "the relaxation of the muscular hypertonia" (i.e., secondary to the relief of rigidity) (77). The paper of Svennilson et al. is one of the few exceptions that clearly outlines the amelioration of bradykinesia (127).

Tremor, it was explained, results from "a disturbance in the postural mechanism of the cerebellum and the brainstem" (77). The postoperative improvement after placing pallidal or thalamic lesions was thought to be due to "restoring the equilibrium between motor cortex, cerebellum and brainstem at a new level" or as "interrupting the tonicizing influence of the motor cortex on the brainstem when it is no longer under cerebellar control" (77). It was commonly thought that pallidotomy was effective treatment for tremor, but that its efficacy could not be predicted and that large lesions were necessary to achieve persisting alleviation of tremor.

Results and Side Effects of Pallidotomy for Parkinsonism

A multitude of clinical studies on the outcome of parkinsonism after pallidotomy were reported from the late 1950s until the mid-1960s (1,2, 8–10,19,21,23,25–28,32,34,40–42,46,47, 51–57, 61,70,75–77,85–88,91,95–103,105,106,115–117,118,120,123,127,128,132,134,135,137). The strength of many of these studies, however, is limited because of the lack of long-term follow-up and objective evaluation of outcome. Overall in parkinsonian patients, abolition or reduction of rigidity was reported in about 50% to 90% after pallidotomy in various series and alleviation of tremor in about 45% to 85%. Operative mortality, in general, ranged from 1% to 8%; and permanent complications were reported in about 3% to 20% of patients. We review here some of the most important series, series with large case numbers, and studies that had a pivotal impact on the further development of treatment or were otherwise remarkable in that they presented more detail.

Narabayashi and colleagues were among the first to report intermediate-term follow-up results of pallidotomy for parkinsonism (95,96). In their early series of 26 patients they used a procaine "oil-and-wax" mixture injected stereotactically into the pallidum to produce the lesion. One of the twenty-six patients died. The most frequent side effect was transient hemiparesis. On follow-up ranging from 18 to 32 months Narabayashi found no difference in outcome between patients with Parkinson's disease and postencephalitic parkinsonism. He observed alleviation of rigidity and tremor, but at that time he thought that the latter was secondary to diminished rigidity. Interestingly, in a later publication Narabayashi described bilateral amelioration of autonomic syndromes such as hyperhydrosis, hypersalivation, and facial seborrhea after unilateral pallidotomy (91).

Spiegel et al. summarized their experience with 71 pallidotomies performed on 50 parkinsonian patients in 1958, with follow-up examinations ranging between 1 and 6 years (123). The report included nine patients who had undergone staged bilateral procedures. Rigidity was described as "definitely" reduced in 72% of patients. Marked reduction or abolition of tremor was achieved in 45% of patients and moderate reduction in 33%. In six cases recurrence of tremor was noted within a few months postoperatively. Interestingly, in the five patients who underwent reoperation very good results were achieved after the lesion was placed more posteriorly. The mortality was 2.8%, and operative morbidity included transient "hemiplegia" (13%), transient facial weakness (8%), transient "monoplegia" (4%), and permanent "hemiplegia" (4%).

In 1966 Mundinger and Riechert reported the results of 1679 functional stereotactic operations for parkinsonism (up to 1964) including more than 600 pallidotomies (88). They compared the immediate postoperative outcome for various parkinsonian symptoms after pallidotomy versus thalamotomy. Rigidity was abolished in 56% after unilateral pallidotomy and in 48% after unilateral thalamotomy; it was markedly alleviated in 35% of each group, respectively, moderately improved in 7.5% and 15.0%, and unchanged in 2% and 2%. For tremor the early postoperative ratios (unilateral pallidotomy/unilateral thalamotomy) were as follows: abolition 27%/42%, marked improvement 36%/43%, moderate improvement 29%/13%, unchanged 8%/2%. Operative mortality was reduced from 2.7% during the early 1950s to 0.5% during the mid-1960s, yielding a mean mortality of 0.9% (86–88). Permanent side effects included hemiparesis in 0.8% of the patients and partial visual field loss in about 1%. According to the dissertation of Arntz, transient mild mental alterations were observed in 35% of the patients after pallidotomy (5). This side effect may have been at least partially related to the pneumencephalography, which had been used for target localization (105). Patients who underwent ipsilateral pallidotomy and thalamotomy had a 50% chance of developing transient mild mental disturbances. Long-term evaluation (after a mean of 2.1 ± 1.8 years) demonstrated that rigidity recurred in only 9% after pallidal lesions but in 21% after thalamic lesions. On the other hand, tremor recurred in 30% after pallidotomy but in only 12% after thalamotomy (5). In many instances long-term alleviation was also noted for posture, propulsion, and gait disturbance (86,88). The results were clearly better when temperature-controlled high-frequency coagulation was performed routinely (45).

Less favorable results were reported by Van Manen, who used a different electrocoagulation technique (134). He placed as many as 30 lesions in a patient during one operative procedure but with rather short coagulation times. In a series of 43 patients, 4 died, yielding an operative mortality rate of 9.3% with the technique used. There were also many complications in the survivors, including severe postoperative speech disturbances in 14 patients.

Cooper summarized the results of his chemopallidectomies on various occasions with increasing case numbers, but he never presented a detailed analysis (19,21,23,25–28). He claimed that rigidity was "relieved" in 80% to 85% of his patients and tremor in 75% to 85%, with a mortality rate of about 2% and an incidence of persistent "hemiparesis or other neurologic complication" of 3%. Later, however, when he favored thalamotomy he stated that "tremor was relieved in only 60%" after pallidotomy; and he then reported somewhat varying figures for postoperative mental disturbance (8%) and speech disorders (10%).

Other authors reported much poorer results of pallidotomy using Cooper's technique. In 1960 Taarnhoj et al. reported an exemplary series of 118 parkinsonian patients who had undergone chemopallidectomy without stereotactic localization (128). Thirteen patients were operated on bilaterally. The postoperative follow-up ranged from 1 to 26 months (mean 10 months). Of the 118 patients, 10 (8%) died during the immediate postoperative phase. Postoperative complications were frequent. "Severe depression in the level of consciousness" was observed in 43 patients, of whom only 24 recovered completely. Contralateral appendicular paresis was noted in 25 patients. The weakness diminished in most cases, but it was permanent in five. Other side effects included mutism and increased preoperative symptoms such as "negativism, stubbornness, inactivity and inability to initiate movements." Taarnhoj et al. pointed out the difficulty of evaluating the surgical results when taking into account only the alleviation of the cardinal symptoms tremor and rigidity, as had been done in many previous series: "In some of our patients who obtained complete control of tremor marked postoperative mental changes or hemiplegia have created a much more serious problem than the tremor did." Immediately postoperatively there was amelioration of tremor in 88% of their patients, of rigidity in 76%, and of gait disturbance in 51%. Overall, they thought that 53% of their patients had benefited from the procedure; the condition was unchanged in 15% and worsened in 19%.

Some side effects that are only rarely reported nowadays were observed more frequently in some series of the 1950s. For example, increased speech disturbances after pallidotomy were described with varying frequency (79). It had been estimated that speech disturbances ranging from "dysphonia, aphasia to mutism" occurred in as many as 7% to 20% of patients in Cooper's series (79). Probably the high incidence of such complications can be explained by the relatively low accuracy associated with placing the pallidal lesion.

Many studies excluded patients over age 65 (42). Risk factors that were thought to predict a higher complication rate were old age, cerebral atrophy, and advanced disease (42,127,137). Riechert noted that although the postoperative improvement of symptoms was equally good in different age groups the functional benefit was much better in younger patients (106).

Although postoperative changes of other parkinsonian symptoms were only rarely studied systematically, in general no alleviation of hypophonia, festination, sialorrhea, or oculogyric crises was reported after unilateral procedures (40). Bilateral pallidotomy, on the other hand, occasionally appeared to ameliorate oculogyric crises (41). Other positive effects described after pallidotomy included a "return of the sense of well-being" and weight gain in patients who previously had lost weight (40).

The important study of Svennilson et al. was almost neglected when it was reported in 1960 (127). It is one of the few studies that applied a more rigid scientific protocol for evaluating postoperative results. Two independent observers rated the change of parkinsonian symptoms and functional disability. The study included 81 parkinsonian patients who underwent pallidotomy between 1951 and 1957 using Leksell's technique. Bilateral procedures were done in only three cases. The postoperative improvement of parkinsonian symptoms was quantified and was presented in diagrams. A "significant and lasting" relief of rigidity was achieved in 79% of the patients. In contrast to many other previously reported studies, "lasting remission" of tremor was obtained in a high proportion of patients (i.e., 82%). Most remarkably, Svennilson et al. noted that "the most obvious gain was improved mobility, in terms of strength, range, speed and precision," and they further commented that "the effect was largely confined to the contralateral limbs, but it was also evident in the gait and in mobility of the trunk." Furthermore, they noted that "painful muscular spasms and cramps" were abolished by the operation. They concluded that "tremor, hypokinesia and rigidity are relieved to an equal extent by operation." Side effects usually were mild and transient. In 54% of the patients mild contralateral weakness was noted directly after the operation and was confined to the face in all but three patients. Postoperative cognitive deficits were clearly more frequent in patients with cerebral atrophy.

Bilateral Pallidotomy for Parkinsonism

With regard to the problems of proper evaluation of the historic series on unilateral pallidotomy, it is even more difficult to review the results of bilateral pallidotomy. In many studies data are summarized regardless of whether patients underwent bilateral pallidotomy, bilateral thalamotomy, or pallidotomy on one side and thalamotomy on the other (32). The reported results of bilateral pallidotomy performed either simultaneously or in stages have been inconsistent (1,42,50,99,102,123,128). Some investigators thought that the benefit after treatment of the second side in patients undergoing staged bilateral pallidotomy was comparatively less than after the first operation. In one series of 13 patients who underwent bilateral pallidotomy using Cooper's technique, 2 patients died; the general condition was described as worse postoperatively in 4, unchanged in 2, and improved in only 5 (128). The nature and number of postoperative complications differed considerably among series (99). In general, it was assumed that the proportional risk after bilateral pallidotomy was higher than just the added risk of two simultaneous or subsequent procedures. In particular, postoperative "mental disorders and hallucinations" were described (50,77,132). Hassler discouraged the use of bilateral pallidotomy because of a relatively high incidence of a lack of spontaneity postoperatively (51). Riechert raised the question of whether bilateral basal ganglia lesions should be placed at all in symmetrical structures (106). On the other hand, Krayenbühl et al. reported a higher incidence of speech disturbances and mental alterations after combined thalamotomy and contralateral pallidotomy than after bilateral thalamotomy (70).

Few investigators described consistently positive results with bilateral pallidotomy. In 1962 Orthner and colleagues reported in detail 18 patients in whom they had performed staged bilateral pallidotomy with a mean interval of 12 months using a modification of Riechert's technique (99). Their primary target was the ansa lenticularis, and they explicitly tried to spare the anterodorsal pallidum by making the lesions small. The mean postoperative follow-up was 2.1 years. In 14 cases the rigidity was markedly alleviated. They also noted fewer oculogyric crises in two patients and relief of compulsions, obsessions, and anxiety. The morbidity was low, and there were no instances in which vegetative symptoms (e.g., drooling) worsened. A "certain loss of spontaneity" was seen in five patients but was thought not to be the direct consequence of the procedure. The authors hypothesized that apathy was more likely to result when the lesion affected the "oral region" of the pallidum bilaterally and was less likely when the lesion was restricted to the "posterior half of the pallidum."

Pallidotomy for Treatment of Other Movement Disorders

The effect of pallidotomy on movement disorders other than parkinsonism often was reported anecdotally. Similar to the reports on parkinsonism, some series summarized postoperative results regardless of whether pallidotomy or thalamotomy had been performed. There were numerous descriptive case reports and case series (4,11, 19,20,22,43,47,53,69,86,89–94,98,104, 105,110,118,122,123,130,131,133,135,138).

Narabayashi presented the results of pallidotomy for treatment of choreoathetotic movements in children with cerebral palsy as early as in 1952 (92). He later noted that after a follow-up ranging from 6 to 78 months marked improvement was achieved in 21% of the patients, moderate improvement in 41%, and mild amelioration in 27% (93). Rather disappointing treatment results for choreoathetosis were reported by others (133). Yasargil brought attention to the problem that the operative procedure was more complicated because general anesthesia was frequently necessary in these patients (138). Some authors thought that pallidal lesions were not sufficient to alleviate choreoathetotic movement disorders and recommended additional lesioning of motor fibers (12).

Cooper reported the benefit of chemopallidectomy for a variety of movement disorders including choreoathetosis, dystonia, and hemiballism. He claimed that alleviation of involuntary movements had been obtained in 20 of 30 patients and illustrated impressive case reports with preoperative and postoperative photographs (19,22).

Spiegel et al. described a reduction of choreic movements in four patients with Huntington's disease after pallidotomy (123). The operation was not effective in a patient with "electric chorea" and in one with senile chorea. They also reported a reduction of involuntary movements in a patient with "posthemiplegic athetosis," "definite improvement" in two patients with "double athetosis" who were operated on contralateral to the more affected side, and slight reduction of athetotic movements in two patients with cerebral palsy. Pallidotomy was also effective in two patients with dystonia musculorum deformans, eliminating dystonic postures in one patient with a follow-up of 2 years and yielding mild improvement for 1 year in another patient.

By 1969 Mundinger et al. had performed 309 functional stereotactic procedures for movement disorders other than Parkinson's disease (89). In 65 instances the target was the medial pallidum. Follow-up varied but extended to years in several cases. When the results for pallidal lesions were compared with those for thalamic or "subthalamic" lesions in 80 patients with "torsion dystonia" operated on between 1950 and 1968, it was judged that postoperative benefit was achieved in 62% of patients after pallidotomy (with "fair to medium" outcome in 21% and "good" outcome in 41%) and in 75% of patients after thalamotomy ("fair to medium" outcome in 20% and "good" outcome in 55%). A similar shift to better results was described in 67 patients with choreoathetotic syndromes: overall improvement in 29% after pallidotomy ("fair to medium" 29%, "good" 0%) and in 51% after thalamotomy ("fair to medium" 33%, "good" 18%).

As mentioned above, reduced choreatic movements contralateral to the side of the pallidotomy was described occasionally (53,123). Nevertheless, it was concluded that pallidotomy was rarely indicated in patients with Huntington's disease (86). Although alleviation of the movement disorder was achieved, functional benefit was limited because of progression of the underlying disease and the cognitive impairment with advanced disease. Similar considerations excluded most patients with Wilson's disease as candidates for functional stereotactic surgery (86).

Pallidotomy was performed in several patients with hemiballism (69). Different targets within the pallidum were chosen: anterior pole (130), medial pallidum (4,20,69,89,110,138), and lateral pallidum (131). Pallidotomy was highly effective in almost all patients, but in those reported in the early literature it remains unclear as to whether and to what degree postoperative hemiparesis was present (43,47,135). According to current models of the functional organization of the basal ganglia, it is difficult to explain the effect that lesions of the medial pallidum would have on hemiballism.

Pallidotomy was performed infrequently for treatment of cervical dystonia (11,90). During the 1950s Mundinger et al. had performed pallidotomy in seven patients with cervical dystonia. Although good improvement was observed in 40% of these patients postoperatively, no long-term benefit was achieved. Bertrand and colleagues thought that pallidal lesions were beneficial for cervical dystonia when combined with thalamic lesions (11).

Pathoanatomical Investigation of Pallidal Lesions

Relatively few autopsy data of patients with movement disorders who had undergone pallidotomy have been reported, and only rarely clinicopathological correlations were made (48, 56,117). In 1979 Hassler et al. described in detail the autopsy findings of 17 parkinsonian patients (56). They demonstrated only minor deviations of the lesion from the planned target: 1.2 mm for the sagittal coordinate, 1.6 mm for the axial coordinate, and 1.1 mm for the vertical coordinate. Several of these patients had undergone pallidotomy alone or in combination with thalamotomy. Most often the lesion extended into the lateral pallidum. The size of the pallidal lesion generally did not correlate with alleviation of tremor. In fact, in one patient "complete destruction of the ansa lenticularis in addition to that of the pallidum" was reported not to have abolished tremor.

Hanich and Maloney autopsied the brains of 15 parkinsonian patients who had been operated on by combined ipsilateral pallidotomy and thalamotomy by Gillingham (48). In general, the lesions correlated close with the planned target. Again, pallidal lesions frequently extended into the lateral pallidum. Most notably, no correlations were found between lesion size and clinical results.

Smith reviewed the autopsies of 17 patients with Parkinson's disease who were operated on by Walsh in the United Kingdom (117). Three methods were used for lesion-making, including Cooper's balloon method and monopolar and bipolar electrocoagulation. Lesions produced with the balloon method were large. It was concluded that lesioning was more accurate with monopolar than with bipolar coagulation.

ABANDONING PALLIDOTOMY

It is remarkable that the eclipse of pallidotomy occurred at the time the paper of Svennilson et al. was published and when a more posterior and inferior target within the medial pallidum was considered advantageous by other surgeons as well.

Thalamotomy

One of the main reasons for abandoning pallidotomy was the increasing popularity of thalamotomy. The motor thalamus [i.e., the ventrolateral (VL) thalamus] was first considered a target for the treatment of movement disorders by Hassler based on his anatomic and physiological studies. The first VL thalamotomy was performed in 1952 in Freiburg on a patient with Parkinson's disease. The operation was done by Mundinger; and the results were published 2 years later, in 1954, by Hassler and Riechert in German in *Der Nervenarzt* (52). Similar to the issue of pallidotomy, Cooper has been incorrectly credited also for the development of stereotactic motor thalamotomy. According to this attribution, which has been cited repeatedly, Cooper introduced thalamotomy after he inadvertently misplaced a pallidal lesion in the thalamus (84). This "remarkable act of surgical serependity," which occurred in 1955, was said to be due to an error "in trigonometric calculations" of one of Cooper's associates (101). Though not a novel concept, Cooper's subsequent switch from pallidotomy to thalamotomy definitely helped to propagate the latter as an effective method for treating parkinsonian tremor. It was demonstrated that, particularly with regard to tremor, better and more long-lasting effects were achieved with thalamotomy. According to Mundinger and Riechert, abolition or marked alleviation of tremor was seen in 62% of their patients after unilateral pallidotomy and in 85% after unilateral thalamotomy (88).

Introduction of Levodopa

Medical treatment of parkinsonism during the 1950s had relied mainly on anticholinergic drugs and had played only a minor role in the overall treatment of the disease. The scenario changed rapidly when the effects of levodopa were described. Dopaminergic deficits in parkinsonism were first considered by Carlsson and colleagues (18). First attempts to replace dopamine in the form of D,L-dopa were made as early as in 1961 by Birkmayer and Hornykiewicz (13). Therapy with D,L-dopa, however, was limited because it produced severe vomiting. Several years later Cotzias and others introduced levodopa into clinical medicine (29). Levodopa was better tolerated and was shown to be more efficacious. Subsequently, the number of neurosurgical procedures performed for treatment of movement disorders dropped rapidly (39). It is said that Cooper's yearly case load dropped from 700 to 25 cases (65). Hauser et al. estimated that in 1992 fewer than 100 thalamotomies for parkinsonian tremor were performed in the United States (58).

Pallidal Lesions and Akinesia

With regard to the beneficial effect of levodopa on parkinsonian akinesia, such symptoms became universally recognized as a basic feature of Parkinson's disease. The origin of akinesia, however, remained obscure. Hypokinetic symptoms were thought to result from degeneration within distinct areas of the basal ganglia (81). In addition to degeneration of nigrostriatal pathways and afferent sensory striatal pathways, "a variable degeneration of the striatal pathway via the globus pallidus" was also suspected to be involved (81). Furthermore, based on histopathological studies it was concluded that exogenous pallidal lesions might be associated with the occurrence of akinesia (66). During the 1980s many clinicians believed that from a theoretical point of view pallidotomy influenced akinesia, if at all, only by making it worse.

Pallidotomy: Almost Forgotten

Pallidotomy was almost completely forgotten during the 1970s and mid-1980s. Neurological and neurosurgical textbooks generally did not refer to this treatment modality except when reviewing historical facts. When the comprehensive textbook *Stereotaxy of the Human Brain,* which accompanied the atlas of Schaltenbrand

and Wahren, was published in 1982 pallidotomy was not even listed in the index (113).

It is interesting to note that rare instances of the continued use of pallidotomy were reported. These reports remained essentially unnoticed. Burzaco from the Fundacion Jimenez Diaz in Madrid, for example, described the results of pallidotomy performed between 1962 and 1984 in 37 patients with various movement disorders other than Parkinson's disease (17). He observed satisfactory results with pallidotomy particularly for dystonic movement disorders and thought the results more favorable than with thalamotomy. In 1987 Blond and colleagues, who were associated with Talairach at that time, reported the results of lesioning both the ventroposterolateral thalamus and the internal pallidum by stereotactic implantation of radioactive yttrium-90 in 12 patients with dyskinesias due to cerebral palsy (14). Abolition or alleviation of the dyskinesias was achieved in 73%. These authors mentioned that between 1968 and 1983 such "bifocal" lesions had also been performed in 60 patients with Parkinson's disease.

REVIVAL OF PALLIDAL SURGERY

The reinterest in surgical treatment of movement disorders has been stimulated by a variety of events and developments (44,58,68). After its enthusiastic initial perception, the limitations and side effects of levodopa therapy became more and more evident. It was recognized that many patients experienced a relative loss of efficacy over the years, and that disabling motor fluctuations and levodopa-induced dyskinesias occurred. Increasing attention was focused on surgery for Parkinson's disease when the prospects of neurotransplantation were viewed with great expectation. After Madrazo and colleagues reported their results of autologous transplantation of adrenal medullary tissue to the striatum for treatment of Parkinson's disease in 1987 (80), many centers worldwide adopted grafting operations. Although adrenal medullary tissue grafting was later largely deemed ineffective, public attention increased when neurotransplantation was performed with fetal mesencephalic tissue (38).

Along with the need for better documentation and evaluation of postoperative results, rating scales became more elaborated. Modified versions of the Core Assessment Program for Intracerebral Transplantations (CAPIT) protocol were rapidly accepted by the neurosurgical community to judge postoperative changes on and off levodopa medication with the Unified Parkinson's Disease Rating Scale (UPDRS) (73). Another pivotal impetus for the revival of pallidotomy was the development of pathophysiological models that helped us better understand the mechanisms of basal ganglia surgery (6,15,31, 37,82). One of the crucial points of the new models of basal ganglia organization and the pathomechanisms of Parkinson's disease was the conclusion that parkinsonian bradykinesia, the classic "negative symptom," was not due to reduced basal ganglia activity as assumed previously but to overinhibition by increased inhibitory activity of the medial segment of the globus pallidum. This concept had a significant impact on the selection of patients subsequently submitted to pallidotomy. Furthermore, refinements of methods and techniques in neurosurgery, neuroradiology, and neurophysiology contributed to the renaissance of movement disorder surgery.

Laitinen's Rediscovery of Pallidotomy

The rediscovery of pallidotomy to treat Parkinson's disease was initiated by Lauri Laitinen, neurosurgeon at the Sophiahemmet Hospital in Stockholm, Sweden during the mid-1980s (71,72). After personal discussions with the late Lars Leksell, Laitinen was stimulated to attempt surgical treatment of parkinsonian bradykinesia by reintroducing posteroventral pallidotomy. The first patient was operated on in 1985, and by 1990 Laitinen and coworkers had gathered experience in 38 parkinsonian patients. Thirty-four patients underwent unilateral pallidotomy, and four patients had a bilateral pallidal procedure.

Laitinen et al. introduced some technical modifications to Leksell's original method. The target was localized with stereotactic computed tomography instead of ventriculography, and electrical stimulation and lesions were made with a monopolar, instead of a bipolar, electrode. Using a monopolar electrode Laitinen redefined the pallidal target, for which he chose the following coordinates: 2 to 3 mm rostral to the midcommissural point and 3 to 6 mm below and 18 to 21 mm lateral to the intercommissural line. The target was confirmed by applying electrical stimulation, observing threshold responses of the adjacent optic tract and internal capsule, and impedance measurements. The results were evaluated with general rating scales, considering the "degree of dysfunction" of the corresponding symptom.

The publication of Laitinen's results in 1992 (72) had a major impact on the reintroduction of pallidotomy in particular and on the further development of functional stereotactic surgery for treatment of movement disorders in general. Notably, bradykinesia and rigidity were alleviated in 35 of the 38 patients (92%); and benefit was reported for tremor, pain, levodopa-induced dyskinesias, gait, and speech in most of the patients at a mean follow-up of 28 months. The most common side effect was homonymous hemianopsia, which occurred after 6 of the 42 pallidotomies (14%). Laitinen stated that he intended to place the lesion in the lateral part of the posteroventral pallidum. Interestingly, he later moved his target farther laterally, stimulating an important controversy regarding where the ideal pallidal lesion should be located.

Renaissance of Pallidotomy

The reintroduction of pallidotomy in the United States dates back to the early 1990s. After Laitinen had presented his preliminary data at international meetings, the procedure was pioneered by Dogali and colleagues in New York and DeLong and Bakay and colleagues in Atlanta. According to Dogali and Beric, the first "modern" pallidotomy in the United States was performed in December 1991 at the Department of Neurosurgery, Hospital for Joint Diseases–New York University Medical Center (Dogali and Beric, personal communication).

Dogali was encouraged to regard targets other than the thalamus for functional stereotactic surgery on movement disorders after reading reports on the experimental studies of the Atlanta group. He initially considered the possibility of placing lesions in the subthalamic nucleus in

Parkinson's disease patients and discussed the issue with Ransohoff. However, as a neurosurgeon who had actively participated in the first wave of functional stereotactic surgery for treatment of movement disorders, Ransohoff strongly opposed using the subthalamic nucleus as a target because he was aware of the feared side effect of hemiballism. Instead, he suggested targeting the pallidum. After Dogali visited Laitinen in Sweden in 1991 the first patient in New York underwent pallidotomy in the presence of Laitinen and Tasker. Soon thereafter, by February 1992, the New York group included microelectrode recording as a routine part of the procedure (126). Patient evaluation included a prospective protocol to assess patients off and on levodopa according to the UPDRS. The results of the first 18 patients with a 1-year follow-up were reported in 1995 (33).

Based on their vast experience with animal studies, the Atlanta group refined techniques for intraoperative microelectrode recording. The concept of mapping the pallidum and tailoring the lesion was further elaborated. Subsequently, professionals from all over the world visited this center to become acquainted with and learn their operative techniques. Microelectrode recording rapidly became accepted as a helpful technique for intraoperative delineation of the final target (63).

The positive results of pallidotomy were soon confirmed by neurosurgical centers in Toronto, Loma Linda, Houston, and other places (64,78). Most preliminary reports described promising results, in particular with regard to bradykinesia and levodopa-induced dyskinesias. Within the next few years the interest in pallidotomy rapidly spread throughout the United States (67). The procedure initially classified as "investigational" was soon approved by health insurance carriers in most states in 1995 and 1996. At that time pallidotomy still played only a minor role in most European countries despite the pioneering work of Laitinen. In October 1995 a 3-day meeting with the title "Pallidotomy . . . Where Are We?" was held in Irvine, California, attended by more than 200 participants. The experience achieved within the relatively short period of 3 years was reviewed; and it became obvious that further

prospective studies, in particular with regard to long-term outcome, were needed before the procedure could be considered routine. A questionnaire about the current practice of pallidotomy was circulated to all participants of the meeting. This survey, which presented a noninclusive sample of 28 centers performing pallidotomy in North America, yielded interesting insights into the methodology used and the opinions on indications for pallidotomy (35). According to the survey 1015 patients had undergone 1219 pallidotomies in the 28 participating centers, but it was estimated that at least twice as many centers were active in North America. The survey also demonstrated how rapidly pallidotomy had been readopted.

Techniques for deep brain stimulation have recently been introduced to pallidal surgery. It remains to be seen whether contemporary pallidal surgery based on improved and refined techniques will maintain this time a firm place in the therapeutic armamentarium of the treatment of Parkinson's disease and other movement disorders.

REFERENCES

1. Alajouanine T, Houdart R, Remond A, Morin J. Resultats cliniques de la coagulation pallidolenticulaire dans la maladie de Parkinson. *Rev Neurol(Paris)* 1958; 99:385–394.
2. Alberts WW, Feinstein B, Levin G, Wright EW, Darland MG, Scott EL. Stereotaxic surgery for parkinsonism. *J Neurosurg* 1965;23:174–183.
3. Alterman RL, Kall BA, Cohen H, Kelly PJ. Stereotactic ventrolateral thalamotomy: is ventriculography necessary? *Neurosurgery* 1995;37:717–722.
4. Andy OJ. Diencephalic coagulation in the treatment of hemiballismus. *Confin Neurol* 1962;22:346-350.
5. Arntz K. Symptomatologische Auswertung des Parkinsonsyndroms nach Encephalitis, Arteriosklerose, Malaria, Intoxikation und Lues und der postoperativen und Langzeitergebnisse nach stereotaktischen Hirnoperationen. Inaugural dissertation, Albert-Ludwigs-Universität, Freiburg, 1961.
6. Bergman H, Wichmann T, De Long MR. Reversal of experimental parkinsonism by lesions of the subthalamic nucleus. *Science* 1990;249:1436–1438.
7. Bertrand CM. A pneumotaxic technique for producing localized cerebral lesions and its use in the treatment of Parkinson's disease. *J Neurosurg* 1958;15:251–264.
8. Bertrand C, Martinez N. Localization of lesions, mostly with regard to tremor and rigidity. *Confin Neurol* 1962; 22:274–282.
9. Bertrand C, Martinez N, Gauthier C. Surgical treatment of parkinsonism: the use of a pneumotaxic guide with recording and stimulation. *Can Med Assoc J* 1960; 82:921–923.

10. Bertrand C, Martinèz SN, Poirier L, Gauthier C. Experimental studies and surgical treatment of extrapyramidal diseases. In: Fields WS, ed. *Pathogenesis and treatment of parkinsonism*. Springfield, IL: Charles C Thomas Publisher, 1958;299–315.

11. Bertrand CM, Molina-Negro P, Martinez SN. Combined stereotactic and peripheral surgical approach for spasmodic torticollis. *Appl Neurophysiol* 1978; 41:122–133.

12. Bertrand C, Poirier L, Martinez N, Gauthier C. Pneumotaxic localization, recording, stimulation, and section of basal brain structures in dyskinesia. *Neurology* 1958;8:783–786.

13. Birkmayer W, Hornykiewicz O. Der L-Dioxyphenylalanin (L-Dopa)-Effekt bei der Parkinson-Akinese. *Wien Klin Wochenschr* 1961;73:787–788.

14. Blond S, Musolino A, Munari C, et al. Intérets de la destruction stéréotaxique bifocale en cas de dyskinésies chez des patients ayant une infirmité motrice d'origine cérébrale. *Neurochirurgie* 1987;33:455–461.

15. Brotchie JM, Mitchell IJ, Sambrook MA, Crossman AR. Alleviation of parkinsonism by antagonism of excitatory amino acid transmission in the medial segment of the globus pallidus in rat and primate. *Mov Disord* 1991;6:133–138.

16. Browder Y. Section of the fibers to the anterior limb of the internal capsule in parkinsonism. *Am J Surg* 1948; 75:264–268.

17. Burzaco J. Stereotactic pallidotomy in extrapyramidal disorders. *Appl Neurophysiol* 1985;48:283–287.

18. Carlsson A, Lindqvist M, Magnusson T. 3,4-Dihydroxyphenylalanine and 5-hydroxytryptophan as reserpine antagonists. *Nature* 1957;180:1200–1201.

19. Cooper IS. An investigation of neurosurgical alleviation of parkinsonism, chorea, athetosis and dystonia. *Ann Intern Med* 1956;5:381–392.

20. Cooper IS. Hemiballismus and hemichorea. In: Cooper IS, ed. *Involuntary movement disorders*. New York: Hoeber, 1969;293–315.

21. Cooper IS. *Parkinsonism: its medical and surgical therapy*. Springfield, IL: Charles C Thomas Publisher, 1961.

22. Cooper IS. Relief of juvenile involuntary movement disorders by chemopallidectomy. *JAMA* 1957; 164:1297–1301.

23. Cooper IS. Results of 1,000 consecutive basal ganglia operations for parkinsonism. *Ann Intern Med* 1960; 52:483–499.

24. Cooper IS. Surgical occlusion of the anterior choroidal artery in parkinsonism. *Surg Gynecol Obstet* 1954; 99:207–219.

25. Cooper IS. Surgical treatment of parkinsonism. *Annu Rev Med* 1965;16:309–330.

26. Cooper IS, Bravo G. Chemopallidectomy and chemothalamectomy. *J Neurosurg* 1958;15:244–250.

27. Cooper IS, Bravo GJ. Implications of a five-year study of 700 basal ganglia operations. *Neurology* 1958; 8:701–707.

28. Cooper IS, Poloukhine N. The globus pallidus as a surgical target. *J Am Geriat Soc* 1956;4:1182–1213.

29. Cotzias GC, Van Woert MH, Schiffer LM. Aromatic amino acids and modification of parkinsonism. *N Engl J Med* 1967;276:374–379.

30. Dandy WE. Changes in our conceptions of localization of certain functions in the brain. *Am J Physiol* 1930; 93:643–647.

31. De Long MR, Crutcher MD, Georgopoulos AP. Primate globus pallidus and subthalamic nucleus: functional organization. *J Neurophysiol* 1985;53:530–543.

32. Dierssen G, Obrador S. The problem of bilateral lesions in stereotaxic surgery. *Confin Neurol* 1967;29:181–185.

33. Dogali M, Fazzini E, Kolodny E, et al. Stereotactic ventral pallidotomy for Parkinson's disease. *Neurology* 1995;45:753–761.

34. Fager CA. Effectiveness of stereoencephalotomy in treatment of Parkinson's disease. *JAMA* 1962;179: 703–707.

35. Favre J, Taha JM, Nguyen TT, Gildenberg PL, Burchiel KJ. Pallidotomy: a survey of current practice in North America. *Neurosurgery* 1996;39:883–892.

36. Fénelon F. Essais de traitement neurochirurgical du syndrome parkisonien par intervention directe sur les voies extrapyramidales immédiatement sousstriopallidales (ou lenticulaires). *Rev Neurol* 1950;83:437–440.

37. Filion M, Tremblay L. Abnormal spontaneous activity of globus pallidus neurons in monkeys with MPTP-induced parkinsonism. *Brain Res* 1991;547:142–151.

38. Freeman TB, Olanow CW, Hauser RA, et al. Bilateral fetal nigral transplantation into the postcommissural putamen in Parkinson's disease. *Ann Neurol* 1995; 38:379–388.

39. Gildenberg PL. Whatever happened to stereotactic surgery? *Neurosurgery* 1987;20:983–987.

40. Gillingham FJ. Parkinsonism. *J Chronic Dis* 1961; 13:215–220.

41. Gillingham FJ, Kalyanaraman S, Donaldson AA. Bilateral stereotaxic lesions in the management of parkinsonism and the dyskinesias. *BMJ* 1964;2;656–659.

42. Gillingham FJ, Watson WS, Donaldson AA, Naughton JAL. The surgical treatment of parkinsonism. *BMJ* 1960;2:1395–1402.

43. Gioino GG, Dierssen G, Cooper IS. The effect of subcortical lesions on production and alleviation of hemiballic or hemichoreic movements. *J Neurol Sci* 1966;3:10–36.

44. Goetz CG, De Long MR, Penn RD, Bakay RAE. Neurosurgical horizons in Parkinson's disease. *Neurology* 1993;43:1–7.

45. Gross I. Klinische Vergleichsuntersuchungen zwischen der konventionellen und der frequenzreinen, temperaturkontrollierten Hochfrequenzkoagulation zur stereotaktischen subkortikalen Ausschaltung. Inaugural dissertation, Albert-Ludwigs-Universität, Freiburg, 1964.

46. Guiot G, Brion S. Traitement des mouvements anormaux par la coagulation pallidale: technique et résultats. *Rev Neurol* 1953;89:578–580.

47. Gurny J, Kaplan AD, Lambre J, et al. Treatment of Parkinson's disease and other extrapyramidal disorders by chemopallidectomy using Fenelon's technique. In: van Bogaert L, Radermecker J, eds. *Proceedings of the 1st International Congress of Neurological Science*, London: Pergamon Press, 1957;116–118.

48. Hanich A, Maloney AFJ. Localization of stereotaxic lesions in the treatment of parkinsonism: a clinico-pathological comparison. *J Neurosurg* 1969;31:393–399.

49. Hariz MI, Bergenheim AT. A comparative study on ventriculographic and computerized tomography-guided determinations of brain targets in functional stereotaxis. *J Neurosurg* 1990;73:565–571.

50. Hartmann von Monakow K. Halluzinosen nach doppelseitiger stereotaktischer Operation bei Parkinson-Kranken. *Arch Psychiatry* 1959;199:477–486.

51. Hassler R. Gezielte Operationen gegen extrapyramidale Bewegungsstörungen. In: Schaltenbrand G, Bailey P, eds. *Einführung in die stereotaktischen Operationen.* Stuttgart: Thieme Medical Publishers, 1977;472–488.

52. Hassler R, Riechert T. Indikationen und Lokalisationsmethode der gezielten Hirnoperationen. *Nervenarzt* 1954;25:441–447.

53. Hassler R, Riechert T. Über die Symptomatik und operative Behandlung der extrapyramidalen Bewegungsstörungen. *Med Klin* 1958;53:817–824.

54. Hassler R, Riechert T. Wirkungen der Reizungen und Koagulationen in den Stammganglien bei stereotaktischen Hirnoperationen. *Nervenarzt* 1961;32:97–109.

55. Hassler R, Mundinger F, Riechert T. Correlations between clinical and autoptic findings in stereotactic operations of parkinsonism. *Confin Neurol* 1965; 26:282–290.

56. Hassler R, Mundinger F, Riechert T. The future of therapy in parkinsonism. In: Hassler R, Mundinger F, Riechert T, eds. *Stereotaxis in Parkinson syndrome.* New York: Springer-Verlag 1979.

57. Hassler R, Riechert T, Mundinger F, Umbach W, Ganglberger JA. Physiological observations in stereotaxic operations in extrapyramidal motor disturbances. *Brain* 1960;83:337–354.

58. Hauser RA, Freeman TB, Olanow CW. Surgical therapies for Parkinson's disease. In: Kurlan R, ed. *Treatment of movement disorders.* Philadelphia: Lippincott-Raven Publishers, 1995;57–93.

59. Horsley V. Remarks on the surgery of the central nervous system. *BMJ* 1890;21:125–132.

60. Horsley V, Clarke RH. The structure and function of the cerebellum examined by a new method. *Brain* 1908;31:45–124.

61. Housepian EM, Pool JL. An evaluation of pallido-ansal surgery. In: Fields WS, ed. *Pathogenesis and treatment of parkinsonism.* Springfield, IL Charles C Thomas Publisher, 1958;317–324.

62. Hughes AJ, Daniel SE, Kilford L, Lees AJ. The accuracy of clinical diagnosis of idiopathic Parkinson's disease: a clinicopathological study. *J Neurol Neurosurg Psychiatry* 1992;55:181–184.

63. Hutchison WD, Lozano AM, Davis KD, Saint-Cyr JA, Lang AE, Dostrovsky JO. Differential neuronal activity in segments of globus pallidus in Parkinson's disease patients. *Neuroreport* 1994;5:1533–1537.

64. Iacono RP, Shima F, Lonser RR, Kuniyoshi S, Maeda G, Yamada S. The results, indications, and physiology of posteroventral pallidotomy for patients with Parkinson's disease. *Neurosurgery* 1995;36:1118–1127.

65. Iskandar BJ, Nashold BS. History of functional neurosurgery. *Neurosurg Clin North Am* 1995;6:1–25.

66. Jellinger K. Exogenous lesions of the pallidum. In: Vinken PJ, Bruyn GW, Klawans HL, eds. *Handbook of clinical neurology.* Amsterdam: Elsevier Science, 1986:465–492.

67. Kelly PJ. Pallidotomy in Parkinson's disease. *Neurosurgery* 1995;36:1154–1157.

68. Krauss JK, Jankovic J. Surgical treatment of Parkinson's disease. *Am Fam Physician* 1996;54:1621–1629.

69. Krauss JK, Mundinger F. Functional stereotactic surgery for hemiballism. *J Neurosurg* 1996;85:278–286.

70. Krayenbühl H, Wyss OAM, Yasargil MG. Bilateral thalamotomy and pallidotomy as treatment for bilateral parkinsonism. *J Neurosurg* 1961;18:429–444.

71. Laitinen LV. Pallidotomy for Parkinson's disease. *Neurosurg Clin North Am* 1995;6:105–112.

72. Laitinen LV, Bergenheim AT, Hariz MI. Leksell's posteroventral pallidotomy in the treatment of Parkinson's disease. *J Neurosurg* 1992;76:53–61.

73. Langston JW, Widner H, Goetz CG, et al. Core assessment program for intracerebral transplantations (CAPIT). *Mov Disord* 1992;7:2–13.

74. Leksell L. A stereotaxic apparatus for intracerebral surgery. *Acta Chir Scand* 1949;99:229–233.

75. Levin G, Feinstein B, Kreul EJ, Alberts WW, Wright EW. Stereotaxic surgery for parkinsonism. *J Neurosurg* 1961;18:210–216.

76. Levy A. Die Pallidotomie beim Parkinsonsyndrom. Eine vergleichende anatomoradiologische Studie. *Arch Psychiatr Nervenkr* 1959;199:487–507.

77. Levy A. Stereotaxic brain operations in Parkinson's syndrome and related motor disturbances: comparison of lesions in the pallidum and thalamus with those in the internal capsule. *Confin Neurol* 1967;[suppl]: 1–70.

78. Lozano AM, Lang AE, Galvez-Jimenez N, et al. Effect of GPi pallidotomy on motor function in Parkinson's disease. *Lancet* 1995;346:1383–1387.

79. Luchsinger R, Siegfried J, Kohenof M, Dubois C. Klinische und experimentell-phonetische Untersuchungen der Sprache vor und nach stereotaktischen Operationen bei Parkinson-Patienten. *Folia Phoniatr* 1966; 18:197–217.

80. Madrazo I, Druker-Colin R, Diaz V, Martinez-Mata J, Torres C, Becerril JJ. Open microsurgical autograft of adrenal medulla to right caudate nucleus in two patients with intractable Parkinson's disease. *N Engl J Med* 1987;316:831–834.

81. Markham CH. Essay on akinesia. In: Siegfried J, ed. *Parkinson's disease,* vol 2. Bern: Huber, 1973:207–212.

82. Marsden CD, Obeso JA. The functions of the basal ganglia and the paradox of stereotaxic surgery in Parkinson's disease. *Brain* 1994;117:877–897.

83. Meyers R. Surgical experiments in the therapy of certain extrapyramidal diseases: a current evaluation. *Acta Psychiatr Neurol* 1951;67:1–42.

84. Meyers R. The surgery of the hyperkinetic disorders. In: Vinken PJ, Bruyn GW, eds. *Handbook of clinical neurology,* vol 6. Amsterdam: North Holland Publishers, 1968:844–878.

85. Mundinger F. 30 Jahre stereotaktische Hirnoperationen beim Parkinsonismus (Ergebnisse im Vergleich pallido-thalamo-subthalamischer Ausschaltungen und Indikationen). In: Gänshirt H, Berlit P, Haack G, eds. *Pathophysiologie, Klinik und Therapie des Parkinsonismus.* Basel: Editiones Roche, 1983:331–357.

86. Mundinger F, Riechert T. Die stereotaktischen Hirnoperationen zur Behandlung extrapyramidaler Bewegungsstörungen (Parkinsonismus und Hyperkinesen) und ihre Resultate. *Fortschr Neurol Psychiatr* 1963; 31:1–66, 69–120.

87. Mundinger F, Riechert T. Ergebnisse der stereotaktischen Hirnoperationen bei extrapyramidalen Bewegungsstörungen auf Grund postoperativer und Langzeituntersuchungen. *Dtsch Z Nervenheilkd* 1961; 182:542–576.

88. Mundinger F, Riechert T. Indikation und Langzeitergebnisse von 1400 uni- und bilateralen stereotaktischen Eingriffen beim Parkinsonsyndrom. *Wien Z Nervenheilkd* 1966;23:147–177.

89. Mundinger F, Riechert T, Disselhoff J. Long term results of stereotaxic operations on extrapyramidal

hyperkinesia (excluding parkinsonism). *Confin Neurol* 1970;32:71–78.

90. Mundinger F, Riechert T, Disselhoff J. Long-term results of stereotactic treatment of spasmodic torticollis. *Confin Neurol* 1972;34:41–46.

91. Narabayashi H. Neurophysiological ideas on pallidotomy and ventrolateral thalamotomy for hyperkinesias. *Confin Neurol* 1962;22:291–303.

92. Narabayashi H. Procaine oil blocking of pallidum in cases of athetose double. *Psychiatr Neurol Jpn* 1952; 54:672–677.

93. Narabayashi H. Results of stereotaxic surgery in cerebral palsy. *Confin Neurol* 1965;26:342–345.

94. Narabayashi H. Stereotaxic surgery for athetosis of the spastic state of cerebral palsy. *Confin Neurol* 1962; 22:364–367.

95. Narabayashi H, Okuma T. Procaine oil blocking of the globus pallidus for the treatment of rigidity and tremor of parkinsonism. *Proc Jpn Acad* 1953;29:134–137.

96. Narabayashi H, Okuma T, Shikiba S. Procaine oil blocking of the globus pallidus. *Arch Neurol Psychiatry* 1956;75:36–48.

97. Obrador S. A simplified neurosurgical technique for approaching and damaging the region of the globus pallidus in Parkinson's disease. *J Neurol Neurosurg Psychiatry* 1957;20:47–49.

98. Obrador S, Dierssen G. Results and complications following one hundred subcortical lesions performed in Parkinson's disease and other hyperkinesias. *Acta Neurochir (Wien)* 1959;7:206–215.

99. Orthner H, Roeder F, Leitzke G. Erfahrungen mit stereotaktischen Eingriffen. IV. Mitteilung: Ueber den Dauereffekt der doppelseitigen Pallidotomie beim Parkinsonsyndrom. *Acta Neurochir (Wien)* 1962;10:572–629.

100. Paxton HD, Dow RS. Two year's experience with chemopallidectomy. *JAMA* 1958;168:755–757.

101. Redfern RM. History of stereotactic surgery for Parkinson's disease. *Br J Neurosurg* 1989;3:271–304.

102. Reichenbach W, Markwalder H. Ueber stereotaktische Hirnoperationen mit besonderer Berücksichtigung des Parkinsonismus. *Schweiz Med Wochenschr* 1958;88:797–801.

103. Rémond A, Houdart R, Lecasble R, Dandey M, Aubert P. Recherches sur l'approche stéréotaxique des structures pallidales et sur l'exploration de leurs voies d'abord. *Rev Neurol (Paris)* 1958;99:355–384.

104. Riechert T. Long-term follow-up of results of stereotaxic treatment in extrapyramidal disorders. *Confin Neurol* 1962;22:356–363.

105. Riechert T. *Stereotactic brain operations.* Bern: Huber, 1980.

106. Riechert T. Stereotaxic operations for extrapyramidal motor disturbances with particular regard to age groups. *Confin Neurol* 1965;26:213–217.

107. Riechert T. The stereotactic technique and its application in extrapyramidal hyperkinesia. *Confin Neurol* 1972;34:325–330.

108. Riechert T, Mundinger F. Beschreibung und Anwendung eines Zielgerätes für stereotaktische Hirnoperationen (II. Modell). *Acta Neurochir (Wien)* 1956;3:308–337.

109. Riechert T, Wolff M. Die technische Durchführung von gezielten Hirnoperationen. *Arch Psychiatr Z Neurol* 1953;190:297–316.

110. Roeder F, Orthner H. Erfahrungen mit stereotaktischen Eingriffen. I. Zur Pathogenese und Therapie extrapyra

midalmotorischer Bewegungsstörungen; erfolgreiche Behandlung eines Falles von schwerem Hemiballismus mit gezielter Elektrokoagulation des Globus pallidus. *Dtsch Z Nervenheilkd* 1956;175:419–434.

111. Schaltenbrand G, Bailey P. *Introduction to stereotaxis with an atlas of the human brain.* Stuttgart: Thieme, 1959.

112. Schaltenbrand G, Wahren P. *Atlas for stereotaxy of the human brain.* Stuttgart: Thieme, 1977.

113. Schaltenbrand G, Walker AE. *Stereotaxy of the human brain,* 2nd ed. New York: Thieme Medical Publishers, 1982.

114. Schwab RS. Progression and prognosis in Parkinson's disease. *J Nerv Ment Dis* 1960;130:556–566.

115. Selby G. Stereotactic surgery for the relief of Parkinson's disease. Part 1. A critical review. *J Neurol Sci* 1967;5:315–342.

116. Selby G. Stereotactic surgery for the relief of Parkinson's disease. Part 2. An analysis of the results in a series of 303 patients (413 operations). *J Neurol Sci* 1967;5:343–375.

117. Smith MC. Pathological findings subsequent to stereotactic lesions. *J Neurosurg* 1966;[suppl II]:443–445.

118. Spiegel EA. Development of stereoencephalotomy for extrapyramidal diseases. *J Neurosurg* 1966;[suppl II]: 433–439.

119. Spiegel EA. Methodological problems in stereoencephalotomy. *Confin Neurol* 1965;26:125–132.

120. Spiegel EA, Wycis HT. Ansotomy in paralysis agitans. *Arch Neurol* 1954;71:598–614.

121. Spiegel EA, Wycis HT. *Stereoencephalotomy. Part I.* Orlando: Grune & Stratton, 1952.

122. Spiegel EA, Wycis HT. Thalamotomy and pallidotomy for treatment of choreic movements. *Acta Neurochir (Wien)* 1952;2:417–422.

123. Spiegel EA, Wycis HT, Baird HW. Long-range effects of electro-pallidoansotomy in extrapyramidal and convulsive disorders. *Neurology* 1958;8:734–740.

124. Spiegel EA, Wycis HT, Marks M, Lee AJ. Stereotaxic apparatus for operations on the human brain. *Science* 1947;106:349–350.

125. Steele JC, Richardson JC, Olszewski J. Progressive supranuclear palsy: a heterogeneous degeneration involving the brain stem, basal ganglia and cerebellum, with vertical gaze and pseudobulbar palsy, nuchal dystonia and dementia. *Arch Neurol* 1964;10:333–359.

126. Sterio D, Beric A, Dogali M, Fazzini E, Alfaro G, Devinsky O. Neurophysiological properties of pallidal neurons in Parkinson's disease. *Ann Neurol* 1994;35:586–591.

127. Svennilson E, Torvik A, Lowe R, Leksell L. Treatment of parkinsonism by stereotactic thermolesions in the pallidal region. *Acta Psychiatr Neurol Scand* 1960; 35:358–377.

128. Taarnhoj P, Arnois DC, Donahue LA. Chemopallidectomy as a treatment for Parkinson's disease. *J Neurosurg* 1960;17:459–468.

129. Talairach J, David M, Tournoux P, Corredor H, Kvasina T. *Atlas d'anatomie stéréotaxique.* Paris: Masson & Cie, 1957.

130. Talairach J, Paillas JE, David M. Dyskinésie de type hémiballique traitée par cortectomie frontale limitée, puis par coagulation de l'anse lenticulaire et de la portion interne du globus pallidus. *Rev Neurol (Paris)* 1950;83:440–451.

131. Tsubokawa T, Moriyasu N. Lateral pallidotomy for relief of ballistic movement: its basic evidences and clinical application. *Confin Neurol* 1975;7:10–15.

132. Umbach W, Riechert T. Bewusstseinsstörungen unter dem Bild akinetisch-mutistischer Verhaltensweisen nach stereotaktischen Ausschaltungen in den Stammganglien. *Arch Psychiatry* 1963;204:96–112.

133. Van Manen J. Indications for stereotaxic operations in cerebral palsy. *Confin Neurol* 1965;26:254–257.

134. Van Manen J. Résultats de interventions stéréotaxiques pour le syndrome parkinsonien. *Neurochirurgie* 1960; 6:260–263.

135. Velasco-Suarez MM. Pallidotomy in the treatment of some dyskinesias. In: van Bogaert L, Radermecker J, eds. *Proceedings of the 1st International Congress of Neurological Science.* London: Pergamon Press, 1957:151–159.

136. Webster DD. Critical analysis of the disability in Parkinson's disease. *Mod Treat* 1968;5:257–282.

137. Wycis HT, Spiegel EA. Long range results of pallido-ansotomy in paralysis agitans and parkinsonism. In: Fields WS, ed. *Pathogenesis and treatment of parkinsonism.* Springfield, IL: Charles C Thomas Publisher, 1958;294–298.

138. Yasargil MG. Die Ergebnisse der stereotaktischen Operationen bei Hyperkinesien. *Schweiz Med Wochenschr* 1962;92:1550–1565.

Pallidal Surgery for the Treatment of Parkinson's Disease and Movement Disorders, edited by
J. K. Krauss, R. G. Grossman, and J. Jankovic.
Lippincott-Raven Publishers, Philadelphia © 1998.

2

Primate Models for the Study of Basal Ganglia Physiology and Dysfunction

A. R. Crossman and J. M. Brotchie

*Division of Neuroscience, School of Biological Sciences, University of Manchester,
Manchester M13 9PT, United Kingdom*

It has been known for more than a century that the basal ganglia are concerned with the control of movement and that basal ganglia pathology in humans is associated with movement disorders. With a few spectacular exceptions, however, human clinicopathological, correlative studies have contributed relatively little to elucidation of the central nervous mechanisms that mediate disorders of movement in basal ganglia disease in terms of the activity of specific brain pathways, transmitters, and receptors. Much more informative have been experimental studies in animals, where attempts have been made to replicate human neuropathology or other precipitating factors and then to study the underlying mechanisms using a variety of analytical techniques.

The model for this type of approach remains the pioneering work of Whittier, Mettler, and colleagues, who studied the neuronal mechanisms of ballism in primates almost half a century ago (29,85,86). Since that time, a number of important animal models of basal ganglia disease have been developed, including Parkinson's disease, Huntington's disease, L-dopa-induced dyskinesia, dystonia, and tardive dyskinesia. Some of these models have proved to be highly informative and have provided insight into how basal ganglia mechanisms become disturbed and how specific brain structures and pathways contribute to the mediation of abnormal movement. This has led to the development of two simple, but robust and commonly accepted, conceptual models of the neural mechanisms underlying parkinsonian akinesia on the one hand and abnormal involuntary movements (dyskinesias) on the other (Figs. 2-1, 2-2, 2-3).

These disorders appear to represent two diametrically opposed mechanisms, at either end of the pathophysiological spectrum. They also appear to be generic constructs, in that the core mechanisms proposed for dyskinesias seem to apply to a variety of dyskinetic manifestations (chorea, ballism, L-dopa-induced dyskinesia) with widely differing etiologies. The development and analysis of these animal models has led directly to tangible benefits for patients suffering from basal ganglia disorders. Nowhere is this more clearly demonstrated than in the current resurgence of interest in the application of refined neurosurgical interventions to treat Parkinson's disease and the dyskinetic complications of long-term treatment. Thus both pallidal surgery and subthalamic stimulation (10) derive their scientific rationales directly from studies on the *N*-methyl-4-phenyl-1,2,3,6-tetrahydropyridine (MPTP) primate model of Parkinson's disease.

The purpose of this chapter is to review primate models of basal ganglia dysfunction and describe their contribution to our understanding of the neural mechanisms underlying disorders of movement, particularly insofar as they have relevance to the use of pallidal surgery. Not all models have contributed in equal measure. The following account is therefore highly selective in

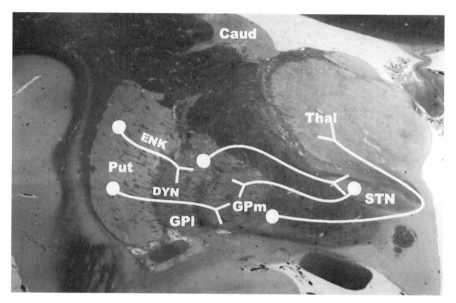

FIG. 2-1. Section through the human forebrain showing the principal components of the basal ganglia and their interconnections. *Caud,* caudate nucleus; *DYN,* dynorphin-containing pathway; *ENK,* enkephalin-containing pathway; *GPl,* lateral segment of globus pallidus; *GPm,* medial segment of globus pallidus; *Put,* putamen; *STN,* subthalamic nucleus; *Thal,* thalamus.

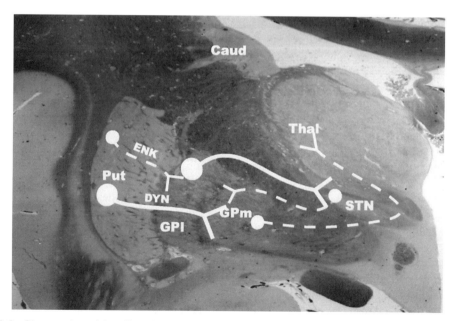

FIG. 2-2. Changes in activity of basal ganglia pathways associated with dyskinesia. Thickened lines represent increased activity; interrupted lines represent decreased activity. See Fig. 2-1 for abbreviations.

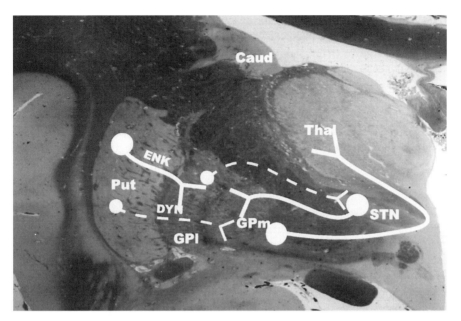

FIG. 2-3. Changes in activity of basal ganglia pathways associated with parkinsonism. See Fig. 2-1 for abbreviations.

terms of the models described, concentrating on those that have contributed most to the current state of knowledge. Most studies of direct relevance to the development of pallidotomy for the treatment of movement disorders have been performed in primates and so form the focus of the present review. A more widely ranging review of the breadth of activity in this field has been published elsewhere (34).

FUNCTIONAL ANATOMY OF THE BASAL GANGLIA

The core structures of the basal ganglia concerned with the control of movement (35) constitute the corpus striatum, which consists of the striatum (or neostriatum) and globus pallidus (Fig. 2-1). Often the subthalamic nucleus (STN), substantia nigra (SN), and ventral thalamic nuclei are included in a working definition because of their close anatomical and functional association with the basal ganglia.

The striatum consists of the caudate nucleus and the putamen, incompletely separated by the internal capsule. In many ways they are best regarded as a single entity, as they share much in terms of internal organization and connections. An important difference for present purposes, however, is that the motor regions of the frontal cortex project specifically to the putamen, which is thus often regarded as the more overtly "motor" part of the striatum. The striatum is often regarded as the "input center" of the basal ganglia on the grounds that most of the afferent connections to the basal ganglia from extrinsic sources are directed there. These include the dopaminergic nigrostriatal pathway, from the pars compacta of the substantia nigra (SNc), an extensive glutamatergic corticostriatal projection from widespread areas of the cerebral cortex, and a projection from the intralaminar nuclei of the thalamus. The striatonigral pathway assumes particular importance clinically because of its importance in Parkinson's disease.

The transmitter dopamine appears to have a dual action within the striatum, having opposite effects on the two principal striatal cell populations that give rise to its efferent projections (73,74). Thus dopamine is thought to be inhibitory to striatopallidal neurons projecting to the lateral segment of the globus pallidus and ex-citatory to neurons projecting to the medial seg-ment (see below).

The striatum contains relatively few interneu-rons. Most of the cells, the so-called medium spiny neurons, project out of the striatum to the two main target areas: the globus pallidus (GP) and substantia nigra, pars reticulata (SNr). These neurons utilize the inhibitory transmitter γ-aminobutyric acid (GABA). The globus pallidus (or pallidum) consists of two distinct portions, referred to as the lateral, or external, segment (GPl, GPe) and the medial, or internal, segment (GPm, GPi). These structures have different af-ferent and efferent connections, which assume central importance in current theories of basal ganglia function and dysfunction. The medial segment of the globus pallidus is regarded (to-gether with the pars reticulata of the substantia nigra) as the principal "output center" of the basal ganglia, as most of the fibers projecting to distant levels of the neuraxis originate there. The GPm appears to contain few, if any, interneu-rons. The principal afferent connection is from the striatum. This is called the "direct pathway" because it directly controls the activity of medial pallidal output cells. The neurons of the direct pathway synthesize the peptides substance P and dynorphin, by which they can be distinguished immunocytochemically. By far the largest effer-ent projection from the GPm is directed to the thalamus, the fibers ending predominantly in ventral tier nuclei (ventral anterior and ventral lateral nuclei) and the intralaminar nuclei. The ventral anterior and ventral lateral nuclei in turn project to motor regions of the cerebral cortex, especially to the premotor and supplementary motor areas of the frontal lobe. In addition, the medial pallidal segment sends a relatively small projection caudally, ending in the pedunculo-pontine nucleus (nucleus tegmenti pedunculo-pontinus) of the caudal midbrain. Medial pallidal efferent fibers are GABAergic.

The lateral segment of the globus pallidus, like the medial segment, receives a major GABA-ergic projection from the striatum. This is the ori-gin of the "indirect pathway," as it is thought to influence the activity of medial pallidal output cells via the intermediary of the subthalamic nu-cleus. The lateral pallidal segment sends a major projection across the internal capsule to the sub-thalamic nucleus and establishes intrapallidal connections from lateral to medial segments. Both of these pathways are GABAergic and therefore inhibitory. The subthalamic nucleus also receives input from the cerebral cortex and intralaminar thalamic nuclei. Its major efferent projections are directed to the output centers of the basal ganglia, globus pallidus, and substantia nigra, pars reticulata. These projections are exci-tatory and mediated by an amino acid, probably glutamate. Electrophysiological and pathophys-iological studies have shown that these pathways have an important role in exciting basal ganglia output neurons, which when disrupted have a profound influence on motor behavior.

Current conceptual models of the function and dysfunction of the basal ganglia concentrate on the core interconnections outlined above. Many other afferent and efferent pathways are known to exist, but their functional role in physiology and patho-physiology is far from clear. The basal ganglia connections outlined above are considered to con-stitute one of several parallel circuits that inter-connect striatal, thalamic, and cortical levels (2).

Stated briefly, activity in the indirect pathway, transmitted through the GP1–STN–GPm–tha-lamic–cortical circuit, is thought to be responsi-ble for inhibiting unwanted or inappropriate movement/behavior. Activity in the direct path-way, on the other hand, is thought to facilitate and reinforce intended, behaviorally relevant motor behavior. The way in which the principal interconnections of basal ganglia nuclei interact has been deduced from a variety of experimental studies and, to a lesser extent, from the study of human postmortem material. The models have been challenged in a number of minor ways over recent years but remain essentially intact as the most parsimonious and self-consistent models of how the basal ganglia work and how movement disorders such as parkinsonism and dyskinesias are mediated.

BALLISM

Ballism is often referred to as ballismus or, when occurring unilaterally, hemiballism or hemiballismus. It is a vigorous, forceful, hyperkinetic movement disorder, sometimes producing flailing movements because of the involvement of the proximal limb and associated axial musculature (7). Ballism is unique. It is the only abnormal involuntary movement disorder produced by a single, small lesion in a specific brain nucleus. Although human cases of ballism have been reported to occur following lesions in many disparate brain structures, the classic review of the literature by Whittier (84) firmly established that this movement disorder is almost invariably associated with a lesion of the subthalamic nucleus.

The first animal model of a human basal ganglia disorder to be subjected to systematic functional analysis was ballism in the macaque monkey, produced by a lesion of the subthalamic nucleus. This has proved to be an instructive model, and it provided the first real insights of modern times into the roles of specific basal ganglia structures in mediating dyskinesia.

Lesion of the Subthalamic Nucleus and Analytic Surgery

The Columbia University group demonstrated that it was possible to replicate the human condition in monkeys by electrothermal coagulation of the subthalamic nucleus (29,86). The dyskinesia thus produced also exhibited characteristics of chorea and athetosis. It was dubbed "subthalamic dyskinesia" and "choreoid hyperkinesia"; it appeared, when severe, to be "the simian equivalent of ballism." The authors concluded that a least 20% of the nucleus had to be destroyed to induce dyskinesia, although in some instances it was achieved by lesser lesions when they also involved the connections of the subthalamic nucleus, notably the subthalamic fasciculus by which subthalamopallidal fibers traverse the internal capsule.

This model of human dyskinesia, and subsequently developed variations based on pharmacological manipulation of the STN, have proved to be extraordinarily informative of the neural mechanisms underlying dyskinesia. In a series of studies, Mettler's team attempted the systematic analysis of pathways that mediated

dyskinesia by investigating the effects of subsequent, or secondary, lesions. The source of activity that drives ballism has never been identified. Martin (57) speculated, on the basis of careful clinical observations in humans, that it might be driven by vestibular input, but this point has never been tested by direct experimentation. It has, however, been shown that ballism is not dependent on afferent input from the affected limbs or on spinal proprioceptive pathways, as it is not abolished by dorsal rhizotomy (section of the dorsal roots of spinal nerves) (81) or dorsal column lesions (25). More positive data were obtained when lesions were placed in the output pathways of the STN. The subthalamic nucleus has two major efferent targets, namely the globus pallidus and the substantia nigra, pars reticulata (27,70), both of which project to thalamic and brainstem motor areas.

The main achievement of secondary lesion studies was the demonstration that dyskinesia was mediated through pallidal rather than nigral efferent pathways. Thus lesions of the substantia nigra did not ameliorate ballism (82), but it was completely abolished by lesions of the globus pallidus (29,86). The globus pallidus consists of two distinct segments (medial and lateral) each with different efferent projections. Because the lateral segment projects principally to the subthalamic nucleus, which was the site of the provocative lesion, the ameliorating effect of pallidal lesions was reasonably interpreted as being due specifically to involvement of the medial segment. These data are in concordance with an extensive human surgical literature that describes the beneficial effects on various dyskinesias, including ballism, of lesions placed in the globus pallidus or its efferent projection system to the thalamus (e.g., ref. 32). The medial globus pallidus projects to a number of nuclei within the lateral thalamic complex, principally to the ventral lateral and ventral anterior nuclei and to the centromedian nucleus of the intralaminar group. It also sends a smaller number of fibers to the brainstem nucleus tegmenti pedunculopontinus. The placement of secondary lesions in the thalamic territories of pallidal efferents demonstrated that ballism in monkeys was ameliorated by lesioning the ventral thalamic area (29), which, once again, is in accordance with an extensive human surgical literature on thalamic surgery for movement disorders (e.g., refs. 32,58). Lesion of the intralaminar nuclei, including the centromedian nucleus, was without lasting effect (28).

Ventral thalamic nuclei represent the principal route by which basal ganglia mechanisms gain access to the motor regions of the cerebral cortex, principally to the premotor and supplementary motor cortices (4,77). Ablation of the premotor cortex in the monkey was without effect on ballism; but when lesions were extended to include the primary motor cortex dyskinesia was abolished, although it was accompanied by a contralateral hemiparesis (26). Similar observations were made in humans during the early days of neurosurgical procedures for dyskinesias, including ballism (3,20). On the presumption that abnormal activity mediating ballism was conveyed to lower motor neurons by descending corticospinal fibers or corticobulbar fibers, with a relay in brainstem nuclei, lesions of the brainstem and spinal cord were made in animals exhibiting ballism. The only brainstem nucleus studied in this way was the red nucleus, lesions of which were reported to reduce the intensity of dyskinesia without affecting its basic pattern (24). Transection of spinal white matter tracts showed that dyskinesia was abolished only by destruction of the dorsal portion of the lateral funiculus (through which run the corticospinal and rubrospinal tracts); but it was associated, like extensive cortical lesions, with concomitant hemiparesis (25). Lesions of the ventral part of the lateral funiculus (carrying the medullary reticulospinal tracts and lateral vestibulospinal tracts) or the ventral funiculus (carrying the pontine reticulospinal tracts and medial longitudinal fasciculus) had no such effect.

In summary, this unique series of systematic studies of experimental ballism provided the best evidence available that abnormal activity sustaining dyskinesia following subthalamic lesion was channeled through the medial globus pallidus, ventral thalamus, cerebral cortex, and corticospinal tract.

Pharmacological Manipulation of the Subthalamic Nucleus and 2-Deoxyglucose Uptake Studies

Up to about the mid-1980s it was generally believed that the subthalamic nucleus exerted an inhibitory influence on the globus pallidus, using GABA as its transmitter. Ballism was therefore regarded as a "release phenomenon" whereby the globus pallidus was relieved of subthalamic inhibition and was thus responsible for the generation of abnormal activity. Furthermore, the subthalamic nucleus and its bizarre syndrome were something of a neurological curiosity, warranting a few lines at most in standard texts. After all, ballism is rare, and the subthalamic nucleus was unconnected with any other neurological disturbance. As a result of research, however, the physiological function of the subthalamic nucleus has been completely revised, and it has been discovered to occupy a pivotal role in basal ganglia function, being implicated in several forms of dyskinesia and, most surprisingly, in Parkinson's disease.

The next step in understanding the pathophysiological mechanisms of dyskinesias depended on the development of new primate models and new analytical techniques. This era also provided enlightening information on the functional relation between apparently different forms of dyskinesia.

First it was demonstrated that ballism could be induced in a reversible fashion in primates by direct intracerebral injection of the GABA antagonist bicuculline, which was injected into the subthalamic nucleus through an indwelling cannula (38,39). This action appears to induce depolarization blockade of subthalamic neurons, temporarily mimicking a subthalamic lesion. An extensive series of injections in the ventral diencephalon, internal capsule, and globus pallidus showed conclusively that the site of action was the subthalamic nucleus (39). As with subthalamic nucleus lesions, the dyskinesia was sometimes of a vigorous, flailing nature characteristic of classic ballism, and sometimes it was more restricted, to the body part affected, predominating in the distal extremities and being of a choreic nature.

This model was subjected to functional analysis using the 2-deoxyglucose (2-DG) uptake technique (68). 2-DG is an analogue of glucose that is taken up by cells using the same transport mechanism as for glucose. It is phosphorylated by hexokinase, but the product is not a substrate for further metabolism and thus accumulates within the cell (80). Following a period of altered physiological activity of neurons, the regional accumulation of 2-DG, as visualized autoradiographically, can be used as an index of neuronal functional activity. Experimental evidence, gained from studying the hypothalamo-hypophyseal system of the rat under conditions of known physiological perturbation, indicates that changes in 2-DG accumulation reflect changes in the activity of nerve terminals, where metabolic demand is most sensitive to electrical activity, because of the large surface/volume ratio (59,78).

2-Deoxyglucose analysis in the presence of ballism revealed a dramatic reduction in the accumulation in both segments of the globus pallidus and in the substantia nigra, pars reticulata, the main output targets of the subthalamic nucleus (68). This finding was interpreted as indicating a reduction in the activity of subthalamo-pallidal and subthalamonigral terminals and was entirely consistent with the concept of reduced STN activity in ballism. Contrary to expectation, however, decreased 2-DG uptake was also found in the ventral anterior and ventral lateral thalamus, suggesting a concomitant reduction in neuronal activity in the pallidothalamic pathway. This interpretation was supported by a simultaneous decrease in 2-DG uptake in the pedunculopontine nucleus, the brainstem target of medial pallidal efferents. These results provided the first physiological evidence, in a behavioral model, that the subthalamic nucleus in fact exerts an excitatory, rather than an inhibitory, influence on the output of the basal ganglia. This point was also demonstrated in single-cell electrophysiological recording studies (48,69). The transmitter involved in subthalamopallidal transmission was identified as glutamic acid by a number of converging lines of evidence. Immunocytochemical studies demonstrated glutamate immunoreactivity in subthalamic neuronal perikarya (79), and electrophysiological experiments showed that glutamate receptor antagonism blocked subthalamopallidal transmission (69). In neurochemical studies a high-affinity transmitter uptake system for glutamate was identified in the pallidum, which was specifically depleted by subthalamic nucleus lesions (18).

The apparent paradox of decreased subthalamic excitation of the globus pallidus in ballism and the well established ability of pallidal lesions to abolish dyskinesia clearly indicated that the simplistic notion of decreased pallidal activity per se as being the central mechanism in dyskinesia was naïve. It was concluded that it must be the precise temporal pattern of abnormal medial pallidal activity that sustains dyskinesia (68).

CHOREA

The term chorea describes an abnormal involuntary movement disorder characterized by "excessive, spontaneous movements, irregularly timed, nonrepetitive, randomly distributed, and abrupt in character" (7). It commonly involves the distal parts of the extremities and the orofacial musculature. The archetypal form occurs with Huntington's disease. This inherited, neurodegenerative condition is distinguished neuropathologically by progressive atrophic changes in the basal ganglia and cerebral cortex. The striatum bears the brunt of the disease, becoming greatly reduced in size, with massive loss of efferent projection neurons, which normally contribute to the striatopallidal and striatonigral pathways. One of the most important landmarks in Huntington's disease research was the discovery of a profound loss of GABA, the transmitter utilized by striatal efferent fibers, and enzymic markers of GABA metabolism (e.g., glutamate decarboxylase) from the basal ganglia in the postmortem Huntington's brain (14,15,60).

GABA Antagonism in the Lateral Pallidal Segment and 2-DG Uptake Studies

It was subsequently shown that chorea could be produced experimentally in primates by localized blockade of GABA transmission in the globus pallidus via intracerebral injection of GABA antagonists through an indwelling cannula (39,47). The site of action was identified as the lateral pallidal segment. This observation found resonance with the results of more detailed, human neuropathological studies, which examined the status of peptide neuromodulators in the basal ganglia of patients with Huntington's disease.

Here it was found that enkephalin, which is co-localized with GABA in the striatopallidal projection to the lateral pallidal segment (the origin of the indirect pathway) was depleted relatively early in disease progression, when chorea is often most prominent (1,76). In contrast, substance P, which is co-localized with GABA in the direct pathway to the medial pallidal segment, was relatively preserved (9), although it too declined during later stages of the disease.

Both animal and human data therefore suggested that loss of the indirect striatopallidal projection to the lateral pallidal segment was particularly important in the generation of chorea. An explanation of how this could be so was provided by 2-DG metabolic mapping studies in monkeys with experimental chorea (66). These studies showed that when chorea was elicited by blockade of striatopallidal transmission in the GPl, there was an increase in 2-DG accumulation by the ipsilateral subthalamic nucleus. By analyzing the pattern of 2-DG uptake change in the STN in relation to the topographical organization of the pallidosubthalamic pathway, which projects from the lateral pallidal segment to the subthalamic nucleus, it was concluded that the 2-DG change in STN was due to overactivity of the pallidosubthalamic pathway induced by loss of striatopallidal inhibition. At the same time, these experiments showed that there was a decrease in 2-DG accumulation by the medial globus pallidus, consistent with a decrease in subthalamopallidal activity. This could be accounted for by the inhibition of subthalamic nucleus neurons by an overactive GABAergic pallidosubthalamic pathway, which in turn would lead to abnormal underactivity of the medial pallidal segment.

These studies were important for two reasons. First, they provided a possible mechanism for the choreiform movements of Huntington's disease. Second, they provided a functional link between chorea and ballism. The distinction or unity of these conditions had been a matter of long-standing debate that was unresolvable without information on the neural mechanisms by which they are mediated. The experimental data presented above clearly suggested that the two are mediated by a common neural mechanism, a central feature of which is abnormal underactivity of both the subthalamic nucleus and the medial globus pallidus (65).

Physical similarities between the expression of chorea and ballism have been noted by many observers. The proposed mechanism could easily explain why ballism (associated with focal destruction of a small nucleus influencing the whole of the basal ganglia output) is a gross disorder, affecting the whole of one side of the body, whereas chorea (associated with slow, progressive degeneration of the striatum) is a more variable disorder in terms of regional distribution, amplitude, and forcefulness.

Glutamate Antagonism in the Medial Pallidal Segment

If both chorea and ballism are due to underactivity of the subthalamopallidal pathway (in chorea due to physiological inhibition of the STN by an overactive GPl and in ballism due to direct lesion of the STN), it should be possible to induce dyskinesia by pharmacological blockade of glutamatergic subthalamopallidal transmission in the medial pallidal segment. This was shown to be the case in experiments where a glutamate antagonist was injected directly into the GPm in the monkey through an implanted cannula (75). An important observation from these behavioral studies in primates was that essentially the same form of dyskinesia was produced by: (a) blockade of GABA transmission by the striatopallidal pathway in GPl; (b) depolarization blockade of STN neurons; and (c) blockade of glutamate transmission by the subthalamopallidal pathway in the GPm. This reinforced the view that ballism and chores are, in a qualitative sense, mediated by common neural mechanisms that include abnormal underactivity of the STN and GPm.

A problem with this simplistic model of underactive STN and GPm in dyskinesia is that, although subthalamic nucleus lesions readily induce dyskinesia, lesions of the globus pallidus never do. There is good evidence for this in both humans and experimental primates. In contrast, pallidal lesions abolish ballism, although pallidotomy was not performed in the primate model of chorea. However, pallidotomy, thalamotomy, and motor cortical lesions have all been reported to ameliorate the dyskinesia of Huntington's disease in humans (32).

Any concept of the mechanism underlying dyskinesia must therefore accommodate the facts that: (a) GPm neurons are underactive in dyskinesia; and (b) GPm sustains dyskinesias, and lesions of GPm lead to their alleviation. These points reemphasize the notion that abnormal temporal and spatial patterns of GPm activity must be important in the generation of choreiform movements, and that these abnormal patterns can be induced by any mechanism that compromises the effect of excitatory subthalamic input on medial pallidal neurons.

MPTP-INDUCED PARKINSONISM

Parkinson's disease is the most common movement disorder associated with basal ganglia dysfunction. It is characterized by the classic triad of akinesia/bradykinesia, rigidity, and tremor, although the clinical manifestation of these symptoms varies considerably among patients. The central neuropathological change is progressive degeneration of the dopaminergic neurons of the pars compacta of the substantia nigra, which project to the striatum in the nigrostriatal tract. The demonstration that dopamine was severely depleted from the striatum in the brains of parkinsonian patients led directly to the rational introduction of the use of L-dihydroxyphenylalanine (L-dopa) therapy, whereby dopaminergic function is restored by administration of its immediate metabolic precursor. This has been the mainstay of parkinsonian treatment for more than 30 years.

A number of animal models of Parkinson's disease have been developed, the most notable being the use of 6-hydroxydopamine (6-OHDA) to lesion the nigrostriatal pathway experimentally in the rat (83). The 6-OHDA model has yielded much valuable information on striatal function and has been a common test-bed for potential antiparkinsonian agents. The discovery that the neurotoxin MPTP produced parkinsonism in humans, however (40,54), heralded the beginning of a new era in Parkinson's disease research. In a series of clinical observations and experimental studies that comprise a remarkable tale of forensic neuroscience, it was shown that accidental MPTP self-administration in drug abusers induced a clinical condition virtually indistinguishable from idiopathic Parkinson's disease (40,52–54) that was L-dopa-responsive. One patient's brain was examined postmortem and revealed the characteristic loss of pigmented cells from the substantia nigra (40). Soon afterward it was demonstrated that a similar condition could be induced in monkeys (21,22,30) accompanied by nigral pathology (22,30,55) and lesions in other catecholamine cell groups commonly involved in human Parkinson's disease, such as the ventral tegmental area and the locus ceruleus (36,64). The MPTP primate model is, without doubt, the best available animal model of Parkinson's disease in humans. Its use has provided many new insights into the neural mechanisms mediating parkinsonian symptoms and has led directly to advances in the treatment of humans.

In particular, 2-DG uptake studies and single-unit recording in MPTP primates have revealed the changes in activity of specific basal ganglia pathways that follow nigral dopaminergic lesions. 2-DG studies revealed that there is a large increase in metabolic activity in the lateral segment of the globus pallidus following induction of MPTP-induced parkinsonism (36,37,62,63), suggesting abnormal overactivity of the "indirect" striatopallidal projection to the GPl due to loss of inhibitory dopaminergic innervation. This situation would cause excessive inhibition of lateral pallidal neurons, which project heavily to the subthalamic nucleus. Such a conclusion is entirely consistent with one of the most remarkable findings of the 2-DG experiments, namely a marked reduction in 2-DG accumulation by the STN in MPTP-induced parkinsonism (36,37,62,63).

The most parsimonious explanation of this observation is that the subthalamic nucleus is relieved of inhibition by the GPl, which would lead to abnormal levels of STN overactivity. Because of the excitatory nature of the subthalamopallidal projection, this situation would in turn cause overactivity of medial pallidal segment neurons. Regional 2-DG uptake findings supported this reasoning, as increases in 2-DG uptake were found in the ventral lateral and ventral anterior thalamic regions and in the pedunculopontine nucleus, the main targets of medial pallidal efferents.

These studies shed light particularly on two important aspects of the pathophysiology of parkinsonism. First, they demonstrated that parkinsonism is associated with abnormal overactivity of the medial segment of the globus pallidus. In elegant single-unit recording studies in MPTP monkeys, it was demonstrated that GPm neurons exhibit abnormal patterning of spontaneous activity and abnormally enhanced responsiveness (41,44). Second, the 2-DG studies provided evidence, for the first time, that the STN is involved in the pathophysiology of parkinsonism (36,62). Overactivity of the STN was confirmed in single-unit recording studies (13). The potential importance of these findings for the treatment of human disease was demonstrated in experiments where the blockade of overactive subthalamopallidal transmission, by direct injection of a glutamate antagonist into the GPm, was found to alleviate parkinsonism completely in the MPTP monkey (19,45). These findings provided the essential experimental background for recent developments in the neurosurgical treatment of Parkinson's disease in humans by posteroventral pallidotomy (8,42,49) and subthalamic nucleus stimulation (10,11).

Evidence from MPTP primates clearly indicates that the medial pallidum is abnormally overactive in parkinsonism and that reversal of this overactivity can alleviate parkinsonism. Although it may seem logical to suppose that destructive lesions of the GPm would be effective, this procedure does not appear to have been performed in experimental primates prior to its current application in humans in a number of centers worldwide. The resurgence of interest in this procedure and the rapid expansion of its application to humans appears to have been due to the suddenly widespread recognition of previously overlooked contemporary reports of the beneficial effects of pallidal surgery on human

Parkinson's disease (50,51). The best operative technique, the optimal size and location of lesions, and the long-term outcome of pallidal surgery are still the subjects of some controversy, which will be partly resolved by ongoing longitudinal studies. It does appear, however, that the effect of pallidotomy on the primary akinesia of Parkinson's disease is not as marked as initially hoped, and patients continue to require antiparkinsonian drug therapy after pallidotomy. The procedure does have a profound beneficial effect on L-dopa-induced dyskinesia (see below), which is greatly reduced or abolished after pallidotomy. This is of great advantage to patients, as dyskinesias often limit the usefulness of dopaminergic drugs and after pallidotomy the benefit of L-dopa can be redeemed. Experience with pallidotomy in humans does seem to some extent at variance with experimental studies, where complete reversal of akinesia has been reported to result from pharmacological blockade of subthalamopallidal transmission in the GPm (19,45). Possible explanations may lie in the qualitative difference between blockade of excitation and neuronal destruction or in the extent to which the entirety of pallidal outflow is affected by each procedure.

The possible use of subthalamic nucleus manipulation to treat human Parkinson's disease has also received considerable interest because (a) it is known that the subthalamic nucleus is abnormally overactive in parkinsonism, and (b) it has been shown in the MPTP primate model that subthalamic nucleus lesion alleviates parkinsonian motor disability. This is a remarkable phenomenon in which well placed lesions, even when unilateral, can transform an animal with severe parkinsonism into one with no discernible parkinsonian features and no future requirement for L-dopa treatment (5,6,12). The effect is apparent immediately on recovery from anesthesia and has been documented, with no loss of efficacy, for more than 1 year. There has been relatively little interest shown in applying this discovery to the treatment of human Parkinson's disease, probably because of caution on the part of neurosurgeons aware of the targeting problem with such a small nucleus, the close proximity of the hypothalamus and internal capsule, and the infamous association of the STN with ballism.

Nevertheless, a small number of subthalamotomies have been reported in humans with encouraging results (71). Dramatic improvement in parkinsonian patients has been reported following STN stimulation through indwelling electrodes (10,11,56). This procedure probably causes depolarization blockade of STN neurons, mimicking the effect of a subthalamic lesion. Of particular note is the marked improvement of primary akinesia, first reported in the monkey with STN lesions.

L-DOPA-INDUCED DYSKINESIA

A number of complications may arise during long-term treatment of Parkinson's disease with L-dopa or dopamine agonists, including "wearing off," the "on–off effect," and the appearance of abnormal involuntary movements (dyskinesias) and postures (dystonia). Such complications may eventually affect up to 80% of patients and can severely limit the usefulness of drug therapy in these individuals. The development of dyskinesias depends on activation of striatal dopamine receptors, although receptor supersensitivity per se is insufficient to explain their appearance. Dyskinesias have been linked to the pulsatile mode of drug delivery and can sometimes be reduced or minimized by slow-release preparations and constant infusion techniques.

Studies on MPTP primates revealed that all of the major motor complications encountered in humans undergoing long-term L-dopa treatment could be replicated in these animals, in particular L-dopa- or dopamine agonist-induced peak dose dyskinesia and dystonia (16,17,23,31,36). This remains the best model of drug-induced dyskinesia available and has yielded much valuable information on the behavioral pharmacology of dyskinesia and the molecular basis of striatal changes induced by long-term exposure to dyskinesia-inducing agents. The cascade of events linking dopamine receptor stimulation to the appearance of dyskinesia are poorly understood. Current evidence suggests that the neuropeptides, which are co-localized with GABA in striatal projection neurons, are implicated in the process (46). As with other forms of dyskinesia, 2-DG metabolic mapping studies have provided insight into the changes in activity in specific basal ganglia pathways that accompany L-dopa-induced dyskinesia (61,67). Changes in 2-DG uptake in the globus pallidus, subthalamic nucleus, and thalamus have been demonstrated that are consistent with the hypothesis that long-term L-dopa or dopamine agonist treatment of parkinsonism induces abnormally low functional activity in the indirect striatopallidal pathway to the GPl (33). It causes disinhibition of GPl neurons, which in turn leads to physiological inhibition of the subthalamic nucleus and thus decreased activity of medial pallidal output neurons to the thalamus.

It has been proposed therefore that all forms of choreic movement disorders so far subjected to detailed analytical study share a common underlying mechanism, the central features of which are abnormal underactivity of the subthalamic nucleus and the medial pallidal segment. The effect of medial pallidal lesions has not been investigated in the primate model of L-dopa-induced dyskinesia, but it has been demonstrated that dyskinesia is completely abolished by lesions of the ventral lateral thalamus (72).

The neural mechanisms underlying L-dopa-induced dystonia are far from clear. Such evidence as is available from primate studies indicates an exacerbation of qualitatively similar changes in basal ganglia pathways as is observed with choreiform dyskinesia (61,67). Thus it is thought that dystonia is associated with abnormal underactivity of the GPm. The effect of GPm lesions on L-dopa-induced dystonia has not been investigated, but thalamic lesions do not alleviate the condition (72). The relation between L-dopa-induced dystonia and other forms of the disorder, such as idiopathic torsion dystonia, is not entirely clear, but 2-DG studies in primates and fluorodeoxyglucose positron emission tomography data in humans suggest that they may be closely related in terms of pathophysiological mechanisms (43). Pallidotomy and thalamotomy have been reported to be of benefit for various forms of dystonia in humans, including L-dopa-induced dystonia and torsion dystonia.

SUMMARY

There are a number of excellent animal models of human basal ganglia disorders, including Parkinson's disease, ballism, chorea, and L-dopa-induced dyskinesia. Largely from the study of such models, two generic constructs have been developed that describe the pathophysiological mechanisms underlying (a) parkinsonian akinesia and (b) dyskinesia in terms of changes in the activities of specific brain pathways.

Parkinsonian akinesia is thought to be caused by overactivity of the indirect, and underactivity of the direct, striatopallidal pathways following the disruption of striatal dopaminergic transmission. Both of these effects induce abnormal overactivity of the medial globus pallidus, from which basal ganglia outflow originates. The effect of the indirect pathway on the GPm is brought about by mediation of the subthalamic nucleus, which is also abnormally hyperactive in parkinsonism and activates GPm neurons via a glutamatergic subthalamopallidal projection. Counteraction of the effect of the overactive STN in experimental animals by lesioning the STN itself or pharmacological blockade of glutamatergic transmission in the GPm alleviates parkinsonian motor disability.

Dyskinesia, in contrast, involves abnormal underactivity of STN and medial pallidal neurons. It may be induced in a number of ways, such as lesion of the STN (ballism), degeneration of the indirect striatopallidal pathway (Huntington's chorea), or the long-term effect of dopamine receptor activation in the parkinsonian striatum (L-dopa-induced dyskinesia). Dystonia may also be mediated by underactivity of GPm neurons. Although dyskinesia is associated with abnormal underactivity of medial pallidal neurons, the medial pallidum sustains dyskinesia, and the integrity of the GPm is necessary for dyskinesia to occur. Thus evidence from experimental primates and humans indicates that lesioning the medial pallidum alleviates all choreiform dyskinesias. This explains why one of the most dramatic effects of posteroventral pallidotomy for Parkinson's disease is the alleviation of L-dopa-induced dyskinesia and dystonia.

REFERENCES

1. Albin RL, Qin Y, Young AB, Penney JB, Chesselet MF. Preproenkephalin messenger RNA-containing neurons in striatum of patients with symptomatic and presymptomatic Huntington's disease: an in situ hybridization study. *Ann Neurol* 1991;30:542–549.
2. Alexander GE, Crutcher MD, DeLong MR. Basal ganglia-thalamocortical circuits: parallel substrates for motor, oculomotor, "prefrontal" and "limbic" functions. *Prog Brain Res* 1990;85:119–146.
3. Alpers BJ, Jaeger R. Hemiballism and its control by ablation of the motor cortex. *Arch Neurol* 1950; 64:285–287.
4. Asanuma C, Thach WT, Jones EG. Distribution of cerebellar terminations and their relation to other afferent terminations in the ventral lateral thalamic region of the monkey. *Brain Res* 1983;286:237–265.
5. Aziz TZ, Peggs D, Agarwal E, Sambrook MA, Crossman AR. Subthalamic nucleotomy alleviates parkinsonism in the 1-methyl-4-phenyl-1,2,3,6-tetrahydropyridine (MPTP)-exposed primate. *Br J Neurosurg* 1992;6:575–582.
6. Aziz TZ, Peggs D, Sambrook MA, Crossman AR. Lesion of the subthalamic nucleus for the alleviation of 1-methyl-4-phenyl-1,2,3,6-tetrahydropyridine (MPTP)-induced parkinsonism in the primate. *Mov Disord* 1991; 6:288–292.
7. Barbeau A, Duvoisin RC, Gerstenbrand F, Lakke JP, Marsden CD, Stern G. Classification of extrapyramidal disorders; proposal for an international classification and glossary of terms. *J Neurol Sci* 1981;51:311–327.
8. Baron MS, Vitek JL, Bakay RA, et al. Treatment of advanced Parkinson's disease by posterior GPi pallidotomy: 1-year results of a pilot study. *Ann Neurol* 1996; 40:355–366.
9. Beal MF, Ellison DW, Mazurek MF, et al. A detailed examination of substance P in pathologically graded cases of Huntington's disease. *J Neurol Sci* 1988;84:51–61.
10. Benabid AL, Pollak P, Gross C, et al. Acute and long-term effects of subthalamic nucleus stimulation in Parkinson's disease. *Stereotact Funct Neurosurg* 1994; 62:76–84.
11. Benazzouz A, Gross C, Feger J, Boraud T, Bioulac B. Reversal of rigidity and improvement in motor performance by subthalamic high-frequency stimulation in MPTP-treated monkeys. *Eur J Neurosci* 1993; 5:382–389.
12. Bergman H, Wichmann T, DeLong MR. Reversal of experimental parkinsonism by lesions of the subthalamic nucleus. *Science* 1990;249:1436–1438.
13. Bergman H, Wichmann T, Karmon B, DeLong MR. The primate subthalamic nucleus. II. Neuronal activity in the MPTP model of parkinsonism. *J Neurophysiol* 1994; 72:507–520.
14. Bird ED, Iversen LL. Huntington's chorea: postmortem measurement of glutamic acid decarboxylase, choline acetyltransferase and dopamine in basal ganglia. *Brain* 1974;97:457–472.
15. Bird ED, Mackay AVP, Rayner CN, Iversen LL. Reduced glutamic-acid-decarboxylase activity of postmortem brain in Huntington's chorea. *Lancet* 1973; 1:1090–1092.
16. Blanchet PJ, Calon F, Martel JC, et al. Continuous administration decreases and pulsatile administration increases behavioral sensitivity to a novel dopamine D2

agonist (U-91356A) in MPTP-exposed monkeys. *J Pharmacol Exp Ther* 1995;272:854–859.

17. Boyce S, Clarke CE, Luquin R, et al. Induction of chorea and dystonia in parkinsonian primates. *Mov Disord* 1990;5:3–7.

18. Brotchie JM, Crossman AR. D-[³H]Aspartate and [¹⁴C]GABA uptake in the basal ganglia of rats following lesions in the subthalamic region suggest a role for excitatory amino acid but not GABA-mediated transmission in subthalamic nucleus efferents. *Exp Neurol* 1991; 113:171–181.

19. Brotchie JM, Mitchell IJ, Sambrook MA, Crossman AR. Alleviation of parkinsonism by antagonism of excitatory amino acid transmission in the medial segment of the globus pallidus in rat and primate. *Mov Disord* 1991; 6:133–138.

20. Bucy PC. Cortical extirpation in the treatment of involuntary movements. *Am J Surg* 1948;75:256–263.

21. Burns RS, Chiueh CC, Markey SP, Ebert MH, Jacobowitz DM, Kopin IJ. A primate model of parkinsonism: selective destruction of dopaminergic neurons in the pars compacta of the substantia nigra by *N*-methyl-4-phenyl-1,2,3,6-tetrahydropyridine. *Proc Natl Acad Sci USA* 1983;80:4546–4550.

22. Burns RS, Markey SP, Phillips JM, Chiueh CC. The neurotoxicity of 1-methyl-4-phenyl-1,2,3,6-tetrahydropyridine in the monkey and man. *Can J Neurol Sci* 1984;11:166–168.

23. Calon F, Goulet M, Blanchet PJ, et al. Levodopa or D2 agonist induced dyskinesia in MPTP monkeys: correlation with changes in dopamine and GABAA receptors in the striatopallidal complex. *Brain Res* 1995;680:43–52.

24. Carpenter MB, Brittin GM. Subthalamic hyperkinesia in the rhesus monkey: effects of secondary lesions in red nucleus and brachium conjunctivum. *J Neurophysiol* 1958;21:400–413.

25. Carpenter MB, Hinman A. Spinal tracts mediating subthalamic hyperkinesia: physiological effects of partial selective cordotomies upon dyskinesia in the rhesus monkey. *J Neurophysiol* 1960;23:288–304.

26. Carpenter MB, Mettler FA. Analysis of subthalamic hyperkinesia in the monkey with special reference to ablations of agranular cortex. *J Comp Neurol* 1951;95: 125–158.

27. Carpenter MB, Batton RR, Carleton SC, Keller JT. Interconnections and organization of pallidal and subthalamic nucleus neurons in the monkey. *J Comp Neurol* 1981;197:579–603.

28. Carpenter MB, Strominger NL, Weiss AH. Effects of lesions in the intralaminar thalamic nuclei upon subthalamic dyskinesia. *Arch Neurol* 1965;13:113–125.

29. Carpenter MB, Whittier JR, Mettler FA. Analysis of choreoid hyperkinesia in the rhesus monkey: surgical and pharmacological analysis of hyperkinesia resulting from lesions in the subthalamic nucleus of Luys. *J Comp Neurol* 1950;92:293–332.

30. Chiueh CC, Markey SP, Burns RS, Johannessen JN, Jacobowitz DM, Kopin IJ. Selective neurotoxic effects of *N*-methyl-4-phenyl-1,2,3,6-tetrahydropyridine (MPTP) in subhuman primates and man: a new animal model of Parkinson's disease. *Psychopharmacol Bull* 1984; 20:548–553.

31. Clarke CE, Sambrook MA, Mitchell IJ, Crossman AR. Levodopa-induced dyskinesia and response fluctuations in primates rendered parkinsonian with 1-methyl-4-

phenyl-1,2,3,6-tetrahydropyridine (MPTP). *J Neurol Sci* 1987;78:273–280.

32. Cooper IS. *Involuntary movement disorders.* New York: Hoeber, 1969.

33. Crossman AR. A hypothesis on the pathophysiological mechanisms that underlie levodopa- or dopamine agonist-induced dyskinesia in Parkinson's disease: implications for future strategies in treatment. *Mov Disord* 1990;5:100–108.

34. Crossman AR. Primate models of dyskinesia: the experimental approach to the study of basal ganglia-related involuntary movement disorders. *Neuroscience* 1987; 21:1–40.

35. Crossman AR, Neary D. *Neuroanatomy: an illustrated colour text,* 1st ed. Edinburgh: Churchill Livingstone, 1995.

36. Crossman AR, Clarke CE, Boyce S, Robertson RG, Sambrook MA. MPTP-induced parkinsonism in the monkey: neurochemical pathology, complications of treatment and pathophysiological mechanisms. *Can J Neurol Sci* 1987;14:428–435.

37. Crossman AR, Mitchell IJ, Sambrook MA. Regional brain uptake of 2-deoxyglucose in *N*-methyl-4-phenyl-1,2,3,6- tetrahydropyridine (MPTP)-induced parkinsonism in the macaque monkey. *Neuropharmacology* 1985; 24:587–591.

38. Crossman AR, Sambrook MA, Jackson A. Experimental hemiballismus in the baboon produced by injection of a gamma-aminobutyric acid antagonist into the basal ganglia. *Neurosci Lett* 1980;20:369–372.

39. Crossman AR, Sambrook MA, Jackson A. Experimental hemichorea/hemiballismus in the monkey: studies on the intracerebral site of action in a drug-induced dyskinesia. *Brain* 1984;107:579–596.

40. Davis GC, Williams AC, Markey SP, et al. Chronic parkinsonism secondary to intravenous injection of meperidine analogues. *Psychiatr Res* 1979;1:249–254.

41. DeLong MR. Primate models of movement disorders of basal ganglia origin. *Trends Neurosci* 1990;13:281–285.

42. Dogali M, Fazzini E, Kolodny E, et al. Stereotactic ventral pallidotomy for Parkinson's disease. *Neurology* 1995;45:753–761.

43. Eidelberg D, Moeller JR, Ishikawa T, et al. The metabolic topography of idiopathic torsion dystonia. *Brain* 1995;118:1473–1484.

44. Filion M, Tremblay L. Abnormal spontaneous activity of globus pallidus neurons in monkeys with MPTP-induced parkinsonism. *Brain Res* 1991;547:142–151.

45. Graham WC, Robertson RG, Sambrook MA, Crossman AR. Injection of excitatory amino acid antagonists into the medial pallidal segment of a 1-methyl-4-phenyl-1,2,3,6-tetrahydropyridine (MPTP) treated primate reverses motor symptoms of parkinsonism. *Life Sci* 1990; 47:PL91–PL97.

46. Henry B, Brotchie JM. Potential of opioid antagonists in the treatment of levodopa-induced dyskinesias in Parkinson's disease. *Drugs Aging* 1996;9:149–158.

47. Jackson A, Crossman AR. Experimental choreoathetosis produced by injection of a gamma-aminobutyric acid antagonist into the lentiform nucleus in the monkey. *Neurosci Lett* 1984;46:41–45.

48. Kita H, Kitai ST. Intracellular study of rat globus pallidus neurons: membrane properties and responses to neostriatal, subthalamic and nigral stimulation. *Brain Res* 1991;564:296–305.

49. Laitinen LV. Ventroposterolateral pallidotomy. *Stereo-tact Funct Neurosurg* 1994;62:41–52.

50. Laitinen LV, Bergenheim AT, Hariz MI. Leksell's pos-teroventral pallidotomy in the treatment of Parkinson's disease [see comments]. *J Neurosurg* 1992;76:53–61.

51. Laitinen LV, Bergenheim AT, Hariz MI. Ventroposterolateral pallidotomy can abolish all parkinsonian symptoms. *Stereotact Funct Neurosurg* 1992;58:14–21.

52. Langston JW. MPTP and Parkinson's disease. *Trends Neurosci* 1985;8:79–83.

53. Langston JW, Ballard P. Parkinsonism induced by 1-methyl-4-phenyl-1,2,3,6-tetrahydropyridine (MPTP): implications for treatment and the pathogenesis of Parkinson's disease. *Can J Neurol Sci* 1984;11:160–165.

54. Langston JW, Ballard P, Tetrud JW, Irwin I. Chronic parkinsonism in humans due to a product of meperidine-analog synthesis. *Science* 1983;219:979–980.

55. Langston JW, Forno LS, Rebert CS, Irwin I. Selective nigral toxicity after systemic administration of 1-methyl-4-phenyl-1,2,5,6-tetrahydropyridine (MPTP) in the squirrel monkey. *Brain Res* 1984;292:390–394.

56. Limousin P, Pollak P, Benazzouz A, et al. Bilateral sub-thalamic nucleus stimulation for severe Parkinson's disease. *Mov Disord* 1995;10:672–674.

57. Martin JP. *The basal ganglia and posture*. London: Pit-man Medical, 1967.

58. Martin JP, McCaul JR. Acute hemiballismus treated by ventrolateral thalamolysis. *Brain* 1959;82:105–108.

59. Mata M, Fink DJ, Gainer H, et al. Activity-dependent energy metabolism in rat posterior pituitary primarily reflects sodium pump activity. *J Neurochem* 1980; 34:213–215.

60. McGeer PL, McGeer EG. Enzymes associated with the metabolism of catecholamines, acetylcholine and GABA in human controls and patients with Parkinson's disease and Huntington's chorea. *J Neurochem* 1976;26:65–76.

61. Mitchell IJ, Boyce S, Sambrook MA, Crossman AR. A 2-deoxyglucose study of the effects of dopamine ago-nists on the parkinsonian primate brain: implications for the neural mechanisms that mediate dopamine agonist-induced dyskinesia. *Brain* 1992;115:809–824.

62. Mitchell IJ, Clarke CE, Boyce S, et al. Neural mecha-nisms underlying parkinsonian symptoms based upon re-gional uptake of 2-deoxyglucose in monkeys exposed to 1-methyl-4-phenyl-1,2,3,6-tetrahydropyridine. *Neuro-science* 1989;32:213–226.

63. Mitchell IJ, Cross AJ, Sambrook MA, Crossman AR. Neural mechanisms mediating 1-methyl-4-phenyl-1,2,3,6-tetrahydropyridine-induced parkinsonism in the mon-key: relative contributions of the striatopallidal and stri-atonigral pathways as suggested by 2-deoxyglucose up-take. *Neurosci Lett* 1986;63:61–65.

64. Mitchell IJ, Cross AJ, Sambrook MA, Crossman AR. Sites of the neurotoxic action of 1-methyl-4-phenyl-1,2,3,6-tetrahydropyridine in the macaque monkey in-clude the ventral tegmental area and the locus coeruleus. *Neurosci Lett* 1985;61:195–200.

65. Mitchell IJ, Jackson A, Sambrook MA, Crossman AR. Common neural mechanisms in experimental chorea and hemiballismus in the monkey: evidence from 2-deoxyglucose autoradiography. *Brain Res* 1985; 339:346–350.

66. Mitchell IJ, Jackson A, Sambrook MA, Crossman AR. The role of the subthalamic nucleus in experimental

chorea: evidence from 2-deoxyglucose metabolic map-ping and horseradish peroxidase tracing studies. *Brain* 1989;112:1533–1548.

67. Mitchell IJ, Luquin R, Boyce S, et al. Neural mecha-nisms of dystonia: evidence from a 2-deoxyglucose up-take study in a primate model of dopamine agonist-induced dystonia. *Mov Disord* 1990;5:49–54.

68. Mitchell IJ, Sambrook MA, Crossman AR. Subcortical changes in the regional uptake of [^{3}H]-2-deoxyglucose in the brain of the monkey during experimental chor-eiform dyskinesia elicited by injection of a gamma-aminobutyric acid antagonist into the subthalamic nu-cleus. *Brain* 1985;108:405–422.

69. Nakanishi H, Kita H, Kitai ST. Intracellular study of rat entopeduncular nucleus neurons in an in vitro slice preparation: response to subthalamic stimulation. *Brain Res* 1991;549:285–291.

70. Nauta HJW, Cole M. Efferent projections of the sub-thalamic nucleus: an autoradiographic study in monkey and cat. *J Comp Neurol* 1978;180:1–16.

71. Obeso JA, Guridi J, DeLong M. Surgery for Parkinson's disease. *J Neurol Neurosurg Psychiatry* 1997;62:2–8.

72. Page RD, Sambrook MA, Crossman AR. Thalamotomy for the alleviation of levodopa-induced dyskinesia: ex-perimental studies in the 1-methyl-4-phenyl-1,2,3,6-tetrahydropyridine-treated parkinsonian monkey. *Neu-roscience* 1993;55:147–165.

73. Penney JB, Young AB. Speculations on the functional anatomy of basal ganglia disorders. *Annu Rev Neurosci* 1983;6:73–94.

74. Penney JB, Young AB. Striatal inhomogeneities and basal ganglia function. *Mov Disord* 1986;1:3–15.

75. Robertson RG, Farmery SM, Sambrook MA, Crossman AR. Dyskinesia in the primate following injection of an excitatory amino acid antagonist into the medial segment of the globus pallidus. *Brain Res* 1989;476:317–322.

76. Sapp E, Ge P, Aizawa H, et al. Evidence for a preferen-tial loss of enkephalin immunoreactivity in the external globus pallidus in low grade Huntington's disease using high resolution image analysis. *Neuroscience* 1995; 64:397–404.

77. Schell GR, Strick PL. The origin of thalamic inputs to the arcuate premotor and supplementary motor areas. *J Neu-rosci* 1984;4:539–560.

78. Schwartz WJ, Smith CB, Davidsen L, Savaki H, Sokoloff L. Metabolic mapping of functional activity in the hypothalamo-neurohypophysial system of the rat. *Science* 1979;205:723–725.

79. Smith Y, Parent A. Neurons of the subthalamic nucleus in primates display glutamate but not GABA immunore-activity. *Brain Res* 1988;453:353–356.

80. Sokoloff L, Reivich M, Kennedy C, et al. The [^{14}C] de-oxyglucose method for the measurement of local cere-bral glucose utilization: theory, procedure, and normal values in the conscious and anesthetized albino rat. *J Neurochem* 1977;28:897–916.

81. Stein BM, Carpenter MB. Effects of dorsal rhizotomy upon subthalamic dyskinesia in the monkey. *Arch Neu-rol* 1965;13:567–583.

82. Strominger NL, Carpenter MB. Effects of lesions in the substantia nigra upon subthalamic dyskinesia in the monkey. *Neurology* 1965;15:587–594.

83. Ungerstedt U. Postsynaptic supersensitivity after 6-hydroxy-dopamine induced degeneration of the nigro-

striatal dopamine system. *Acta Physiol Scand* 1971; [Suppl 367]:69–93.

84. Whittier J R. Ballism and the subthalamic nucleus (nucleus hypothalamicus: corpus Luysi). *Arch Neurol Psychiatry* 1947;58:672–692.

85. Whittier J R, Mettler FA. Studies on the subthalamus of the rhesus monkey. I. Anatomy and fiber connections of the subthalamic nucleus of Luys. *J Comp Neurol* 1949; 90:281–317.

86. Whittier J R, Mettler FA. Studies on the subthalamus of the rhesus monkey. II. Hyperkinesia and other physiological effects of subthalamic lesions, with special reference to the subthalamic nucleus of Luys. *J Comp Neurol* 1949;90:319–372.

Pallidal Surgery for the Treatment of Parkinson's Disease and Movement Disorders, edited by J. K. Krauss, R. G. Grossman, and J. Jankovic. Lippincott-Raven Publishers, Philadelphia © 1998.

3

Pathophysiology of Parkinsonism and Dyskinesias

Roger L. Albin

Department of Neurology, University of Michigan, Geriatrics Research, Education, and Clinical Center, Ann Arbor, Michigan 48104, USA

Research since the late 1970s has added considerably to our knowledge of basal ganglia structure and function. Much of this research has been driven by a desire to improve the treatment of Parkinson's disease and related disorders. A convergence of clinical findings, data from postmortem human studies, and experiments with animal models of parkinsonism contributed to the development of a model of the pathophysiology of parkinsonism and hyperkinetic movement disorders with considerable explanatory power (2,16,20). The existence of this model contributed to the revival of interest in surgical therapies for Parkinson's disease, and the outcomes of surgical intervention have provided valuable new data to evaluate the model (see below). The model is based on four basic principles of basal ganglia organization (Table 3-1).

BASAL GANGLIA ORGANIZATION

The basal ganglia are a group of subcortical nuclei that form a functional system by virtue of dense and hierarchical interconnections. The primate basal ganglia are composed of the striatal complex, the two segments of the globus pallidus, the two portions of the substantia nigra, and the subthalamic nucleus (Fig. 3-1). The primary afferent structure of the basal ganglia is the striatal complex, which receives innervation from the neocortex and allied structures. In primates the dorsal striatum has two components, the medial caudate

and lateral putamen, separated by fibers of the internal capsule. These nuclei receive information from virtually the whole of the cortical mantle in a topographically arranged fashion. The ventral extensions of the striatal complex—the nucleus accumbens and olfactory tubercle—receive innervation from the hippocampal formation, amygdala, and primary olfactory cortex, regions thought to participate in "limbic circuits." The striatal complex also receives significant innervation from midline thalamic nuclei. The corticostriate (and allied inputs) and thalamostriate projections are excitatory and use glutamate as their primary neurotransmitter (25,72).

Approximately 90% of striatal neurons are projection neurons whose primary axonal arbors terminate outside the striatal complex. These medium spiny neurons (so called because of their size and the existence of abundant dendritic spines) receive corticostriate synapses, primarily on the heads of the spines. Striatal projection neurons innervate the internal and external segments of the globus pallidus (GPi and GPe, respectively; in most mammals the globus pallidus proper is the homologue of the external segment of the primate globus pallidus, and the entopeduncular nucleus is the homologue of the internal segment of the primate globus pallidus) and the two portions of the substantia nigra (the pars compacta and the pars reticulata; SNc and SNr). The GPi and SNr are the output stations of the basal ganglia; these structures project to the ven-

TABLE 3-1. *Basic principles of basal ganglia organization*

1. The basal ganglia form part of a corticothalamic-basal ganglionic-thalamocortical loop.
2. Striatal projection neurons are segregated into subpopulations based on the projection target, neuropeptide expression, and receptor expression.
3. Striatal projection neuron subpopulations are differentially regulated by dopaminergic afferents from the substantia nigra.
4. The subthalamic nucleus is a key modulator of basal ganglia output.

tral anterior/ventral lateral (VA/VL) and mediodorsal (MD) thalamic nuclei, with the GPi possessing additional projections to the lateral habenula, the SNr possessing additional projections to the superior colliculus, and both GPi and SNr projecting to the pedunculopontine nucleus. There are also collateral projections from the GPi and SNr to the midline thalamic nuclei.

The classic neurotransmitter of both striatal projection neurons and GPi/SNr neurons is the inhibitory amino acid Υ-aminobutyric acid (GABA). Intercalated within this basic striato-GPi/SNr-thalamic circuit are two loops intrinsic to the basal ganglia: the pallidosubthalamic circuit and the reciprocal connection between the striatum and the SNc. The GPe receives an inhibitory GABAergic input from the striatum and projects in turn primarily to the subthalamic nucleus (STN). The latter gives rise to an excitatory/glutamatergic set of inputs to the GPi, SNr, SNc, and GPe (12,66). The SNc is reciprocally connected with the striatum, giving rise to the well characterized and massive striatal dopaminergic innervation. The dopaminergic terminals of nigrostriatal neurons synapse on striatal projection neurons, most commonly on the neck of dendritic spines whose heads receive corticostriate input (71). This "triadic" arrangement of corticostriate and nigrostriatal synapses on striatal

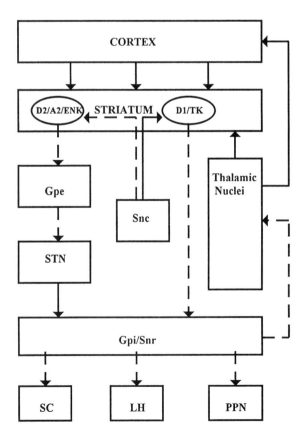

FIG. 3-1. Basal ganglia. *SC,* superior colliculus; *LH,* lateral habenula; *PPN,* pedunculopontine nucleus; *Gpi,* internal segment of the globus pallidus; *Snr,* substantia nigra pars reticulata; STN, subthalamic nucleus; *Snc,* substantia nigra pars compacta; *Gpe,* external segment of the globus pallidus; *D2,* dopamine type 2 receptors; *D1,* dopamine type 1 receptors; *A2,* adenosine type 2 receptors; *ENK,* enkephalins; *TK,* tachykinins. *Solid lines* are excitatory connections; *broken lines* are inhibitory connections.

projection neuron dendritic spines suggests the presence of complex interactions between dopaminergic and cortical inputs to striatal projection neurons. In addition, some evidence indicates the presence of presynaptic dopaminergic heteroreceptors on corticostriate terminals, and other data suggest that glutamatergic inputs can modulate dopamine release, possibly via the action of nitric oxide (26,27,45).

The VA/VL and MD thalamic nuclei are considered to be the major route through which the basal ganglia modulate motor performance, although descending projections to the brainstem could be important and are a relatively uninvestigated topic. These thalamic nuclei project to the primary motor cortex, premotor cortices, and prefrontal cortex (35). Thalamocortical neurons are excitatory and glutamatergic, and regulation of the activity of thalamocortical activation is suggested to be the means by which basal ganglia output influences motor performance. The first major principle of basal ganglia organization is to view the basal ganglia as participants in a large corticobasal ganglionic-thalamocortical loop that funnels information from the whole cortical mantle (and related areas) to a more restricted set of motor, premotor, and prefrontal cortical fields.

A second major principle of basal ganglia organization is the idea that striatal projection neurons are segregated into a series of discrete pools on the basis of their projection targets and neuropeptide content. There are thought to be largely segregated pools of striatal neurons projecting to each striatal target nucleus (GPe, GPi, SNr, SNc). These pools of striatal projection neurons are distinguished also by expression of neuropeptides. Striato-GPe neurons express enkephalins; and striato-GPi, striato-SNr, and striato-SNc neurons express tachykinins (28,32,38). There is evidence that the segregation of striatal projection neurons is more marked in primates than rodents. On the other hand, some preliminary work with sensitive tract tracing techniques in nonhuman primates has suggested that the segregation of striatal output neurons has been overstated (57). At present, the balance of the anatomic and functional evidence (see below) favors substantial segregation of striatal projection neurons. The anatomic segregation of striatal projection neurons is probably

paralleled by functional differentiation of striatal projection neurons. Alexander et al. proposed the existence of several parallel loops coursing throughout the whole corticobasal ganglionic-thalamic circuit with specialization of different groups of striatal neurons for a variety of motor and nonmotor functions (4). Although still somewhat controversial, this idea has considerable anatomic and electrophysiologic support (36). The relation of the functional specialization of striatal projection neurons to their anatomic segregation based on projection targets is not known.

A considerable body of evidence suggests that the different pools of striatal neurons are differentially regulated by striatal afferents. The most persuasive evidence comes from studies of the consequences of chronic striatal dopaminergic denervation in either unilateral 6-hydroxydopamine (6-OHDA)-lesioned rats or unilaterally N-methyl-4-phenyl-1,2,3,6-tetrahydropyridine (MPTP)-lesioned primates. Several lines of converging anatomic and functional evidence indicate that dopamine is excitatory to striato-SNr neurons while inhibiting striato-GPe neurons. For example, unilateral destruction of the nigrostriatal projection in either primates or rats results in robust increases of enkephalin synthesis in striato-GPe neurons and diminished expression of tachykinin synthesis in striato-SNr neurons (32). These reciprocal changes in neuropeptide expression are thought to reflect reciprocal changes in the activity of striato-GPe and striato-SNr neurons. Other measures of striatal output neuron activity are consistent with these inferences. For example, receptor autoradiography studies in unilateral 6-OHDA-lesioned rats of the globus pallidus (homologue of the primate GPe) and SNr GABA-A receptors also reveal reciprocal changes (54). The pallidal GABA-A receptors are down-regulated, indicating increased activity of GABAergic striatal inputs, whereas SNr GABA-A receptors are up-regulated, indicating diminished GABAergic input from the striato-SNr neurons. Similar results have been found in unilaterally MPTP-lesioned primates and direct measurement of extracellular GABA in the GPe with *in vivo* microdialysis in unilaterally MPTP-lesioned primates are consistent with the results of receptor-binding studies (64,65). It is difficult to measure the activity of defined striatal projection neurons electrophysiologically. Somewhat more indirect assays, looking at either the activity of pallidal units or determining regional basal ganglia metabolic activity with the [^{14}C]2-deoxyglucose technique are consistent with the conclusion that dopamine inhibits striato-GPe neurons while exciting striato-SNr neurons (49,50).

The basis of the differential effect of dopamine on striato-GPe and striato-SNr neurons lies probably in the differential distribution of dopamine receptors. Although initially somewhat controversial, it is now accepted generally that striato-GPe neurons express predominantly D2 receptors, and striato-GPi/SNr neurons express predominantly D1 receptors (29,74). These different dopamine receptor subtypes are known to have divergent signal transduction properties, though the mechanism(s) by which they regulate neuronal excitability are unknown. Dopamine receptors are not the only neurotransmitter receptor segregated among striatal projection neuron populations. Adenosine A2a receptors are predominantly localized on striato-GPe neurons, and some data suggest differential localization of *N*-methyl-D-aspartate (NMDA) receptors among striatal projection neurons (67,75).

Because of the prominent differential effects of dopamine on striatal projection neuron subpopulations, other striatal afferents, notably corticostriate afferents, could differentially regulate striatal projection neuron subpopulation activity. When this issue was examined, there was no evidence of large-scale segregation of glutamate receptors among striatal neuron subpopulations, although there is a suggestion of a quantitative difference in NMDA receptor expression among striatonigral and striatopallidal (GPe homologue) neurons in rats (75). Some limited functional studies have suggested a preferential relation between corticostriate projection neuron activity and striato-GPe neuron activation (9,59,76). Anatomical studies in nonhuman primates have indicated that thalamostriatal axons preferentially innervate striato-GPi/SNr projection neurons (70).

The fourth principle of basal ganglia organization stresses the importance of the subthalamic nucleus (STN) as a regulator of basal ganglia output to the thalamus. By virtue of its major excitatory inputs to the GPi and SNr, the STN is a major determinant of GPi/SNr neuron activity and basal ganglia output. The magnitude and character of STN output to its targets can have a profound effect on basal ganglia output to the thalamus and other basal ganglia targets.

These four principles of basal ganglia organization comprise the basis for a model of basal ganglia pathophysiology with considerable heuristic value. These ideas should not be regarded as dogma. Parent and Hazrati have provided a thoughtful critique of some of these ideas, particularly the notion of segregated striatal output pathways and the concept that the striatum influences STN activity via the GPe (55,56). Future studies may dismiss these ideas and provide a more accurate concept of basal ganglia organization.

PATHOPHYSIOLOGY OF PARKINSON'S DISEASE

The consequences of striatal dopaminergic denervation ramify throughout the basal ganglia (Fig. 3-2). As described above, loss of striatal dopamine innervation (idiopathic Parkinson's disease, MPTP, 6-OHDA), dopamine depletion (α-methyltyrosine, reserpine, tetrabenazine) or blockade of dopamine effect (neuroleptics, antiemetics) results in diminished striato-GPi/SNr activity and disinhibited striato-GPe neuron activity. These two effects have interesting and complementary consequences. The diminished activity of striato-GPi/SNr projection neurons reduces GABAergic inhibition of the GPi and SNr. Simultaneously, the increased activity of striato-GPe neurons inhibits GPe neurons projecting to the STN. Decreased activity of GABAergic pallidosubthalamic neurons disinhibits the STN. The now excessively active STN provides an additional excitatory input to the GPi/SNr. The end result is excessive activity of the GPi/SNr and increased inhibition of the thalamic nuclei receiving basal ganglia input. The decreased thalamocortical neuron activity results in deficient excitatory input to motor, premotor, and prefrontal cortices and may cause the motor deficits of parkinsonism.

Several relevant clinical and experimental data sets support this model. Electrophysiolog-

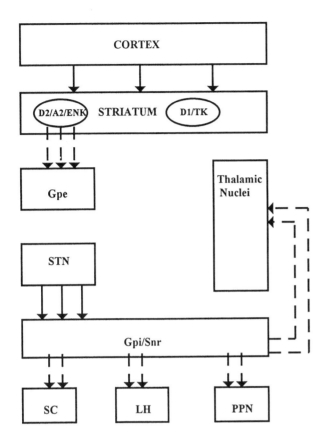

FIG. 3-2. Current model of parkinsonism. Loss of SNc input results in disinhibited striato-GPe output with diminished striato-GPi/SNr output. The result is increased excitatory drive from the STN to the GPi/SNr with diminished inhibitory input from the striatum. This is thought to result in increased inhibitory GABAergic output to basal ganglia targets and deficient thalamocortical activation. See Fig. 3-1 for explanation of abbreviations.

ical studies of unilaterally lesioned MPTP monkeys demonstrate STN and GPi overactivity (8,80). The consequences of STN or GPi lesions in both MPTP primates and human Parkinson's disease (PD) patients are consistent also with this model. Destruction of the STN in MPTP-lesioned primates produces substantial alleviation of all features of parkinsonism in these animals (5,7). Similar findings have been documented in case reports of human PD victims who have suffered infarction of the STN (68). Posteroventral GPi pallidotomy, another intervention aimed at reducing excessive basal ganglia output to the thalamus, is efficacious in ameliorating all the cardinal features of PD and is now accepted as a standard component of the therapeutic armamentarium for advanced PD (6,21,42,46). A logical extension of this approach is STN stimulation. With the correct stimulus parameters, implanted stimulators can cause depolarization blockade of neurons. Promising preliminary results have been obtained with this approach (44).

Functional neuroimaging studies support this model. Using motor paradigms that produce increased blood flow (activation) in the motor cortices, particularly the supplementary motor area, a region with prominent afferents from the basal ganglia recipient thalamic regions, several studies have documented deficient activation of the supplementary motor cortex in PD patients (60). These activation deficits are at least partially offset by treatment with dopamine agonists or after pallidotomy, consistent with this model's prediction of deficient thalamocortical excitation (13,31). In a logical extension of these studies, Davis et al. studied regional cortical blood flow in PD patients undergoing GPi stimulation (17). At high-frequency stimulation parameters that probably produce GPi neuron inactivation, there was marked clinical improvement and increased blood flow in premotor regions.

DEFICIENCIES OF THE MODEL

This model has been a success in two major ways: It has led to some interesting and testable predictions, and it has provided support for the successful revival of surgical treatment for PD. The core ideas of this model—the concept that the basal ganglia is a large recurrent corticobasal ganglionic-thalamocortical loop, the importance of the STN, the parallel output systems of striato-GPe and striato-GPi/SNr projection neurons, and the differential regulation of the dual striatal output circuits by the nigrostriatal input—seem well established. There are, not surprisingly, some major shortcomings of this model. One major defect is that it is a model of pathophysiology, not a model of basal ganglia function (47). This model is a successful example of clinicopathological correlation but is silent as to what functions are normally subserved by the basal ganglia. Unfortunately, our knowledge of normal basal ganglia functions is limited and has not advanced much beyond the ideas that the basal ganglia are involved in motor function/sensorimotor integration. This lack of knowledge about normal function is an obstacle to the development of concrete, physiologically based hypotheses concerning the bases for motor dysfunction in basal ganglia disorders. Increased understanding of normal basal ganglia functions is indispensable for generation of novel ideas about the pathophysiology of movement disorders.

Another problem with this model is that it is essentially a cartoon of basal ganglia anatomy. When formulating the ideas of the corticopallidal-thalamocortical loop and the dual parallel and opposing outputs from the striatum, some important basal ganglia afferents, efferents, and interconnections have been neglected. Because of an absence of physiological data and obvious behavioral consequences following experimental midline thalamic lesions, the thalamostriate projection is neglected in this model. Similarly, the STN receives a major projection from motor and frontal cortices, perhaps as collaterals of the corticospinal tract (1). The role of this pathway in STN function is largely unknown. The STN also receives dopaminergic innervation from the SNc, and the STN has both dopamine D1- and D2-like receptors (37,40). Stimulation of STN dopamine receptors in rats alters the activity of STN neurons and produces abnormal orofacial movements (58). In PD it is likely that dopaminergic neurons projecting to the STN are affected, as are the nigrostriatal projection, leading to the possibility that dopaminergic denervation of the STN is contributing to abnormal STN function in PD. The potential importance of these other afferents to the STN is underscored by the fact that GPe lesions do not reproduce the electrophysiological changes found in STN neurons following striatal dopamine denervation (33,48).

Several important interconnections between basal ganglia nuclei are neglected in this model. The GPe projects not only to the STN but also to the SNr and the GPi. These inhibitory GABA-ergic projections tend to synapse on neuronal somas, where even a modest degree of inhibition could have major effects on cell excitability. Rather than serving as a relay of striatal output, the GPe could well serve as an additional integrative center for processing information through the basal ganglia (14,56). The STN projections to the GPi/SNr are major features of this model, but the model neglects the recurrent STN-GPe projection. Following unilateral 6-OHDA lesions in rats, glutamic acid decarboxylase (GAD) mRNA levels become elevated, a possible corollary of *increased* GPe neuron activity (39). Lesions of the STN tend to reduce the GPe neuron GAD mRNA elevation, suggesting that elevated GPe GAD elevation is a result of increased STN excitatory input to the GPe (19).

This model neglects as well some potentially important basal ganglia outputs. The GPe sends a direct projection to the reticular nucleus of the thalamus (RTN), and it is likely that this GPe–RTN projection is physiologically important. Reticular nucleus GAD mRNA levels rise markedly in rats with 6-OHDA lesions (18,34). Collaterals of GPi and SNr neurons projecting to the VA/VL and mediodorsal thalamic nuclei project as well to the midline thalamic nuclei, offering another channel to the neocortex and a possible corollary loop back to the striatum. The GPi/SNr also project to the brainstem, notably the pedunculopontine nucleus; and this projection could have an important impact on motor function. Finally, whereas the SNr/GPi-thalamus projections have been emphasized in the regulation of motor performance, the SNr projects to the superior colliculus. In the basal ganglia literature, the role of this region in the control of eye movements, particularly saccades, has been emphasized; but the superior colliculus is a multimodal integration area that could be influencing many aspects of motor function.

The complexity of basal ganglia projections to the thalamus highlights another major defect of this model: its neglect of thalamic physiology. The VA/VL and MD nuclei in this model function as slavish relays of basal ganglia output whose only function is to invert the polarity of basal output effects. This cannot be correct. Thalamocortical projection neurons exhibit complex responses to afferent input, and thalamic nuclei contain populations of GABAergic interneurons whose behavior can markedly influence thalamocortical projection function (69). Also, the reticular nucleus of the thalamus contains GABAergic neurons and is reciprocally connected with all the other thalamic nuclei, adding another level of complexity to the regulation of thalamocortical projection neuron activity (69).

Finally, although amelioration of the cardinal features of parkinsonism by pallidal surgery is certainly consistent with this model, another clinical result observed after pallidal surgery—marked amelioration of drug-induced dyskinesias—is an unexpected result that challenges some of the key features of this model. To understand how this clinical result challenges the model, it is necessary to explore how this model has been used to explain some hyperkinetic movement disorders.

PATHOPHYSIOLOGY OF CHOREOATHETOSIS/HEMIBALLISM

The point of departure for explaining the pathophysiology of chorea and hemiballism is the well known clinical and experimental observation that destruction of the STN produces hemiballism. Further clinical and experimental observations indicate that choreoathetosis and ballism are part of the same spectrum of hyperkinetic movement disorders. Some patients with STN infarcts present with choreoathetosis rather than true hemiballism. The natural history of hemiballism in humans appears to be gradual moderation of the intensity of movements; and as ballism subsides, patients may develop more typically choreoathetoid movements. In some patients with Huntington's disease, as chorea worsens with disease progression the involuntary movements come to resemble ballism rather than classic choreoathetosis.

The consequences of STN destruction are interesting and inferred to produce physiological effects opposite to those thought to occur in parkinsonism (Fig. 3-3). With loss of STN neuron excitation of the GPi and SNr neurons, basal ganglia output to the thalamus decreases. This situation is speculated to result in enhanced thalamocortical activation. Similar phenomena are thought to occur in hyperkinetic disorders resulting from striatal pathology such as Huntington's disease. There is evidence that in the early stages of Huntington's disease there is selective loss of striatal neurons projecting to the GPi with consequent disinhibiton of GPi neurons projecting to the STN (3,62,63). The resulting excessive inhibition of STN neurons produces a physiological analogue of STN destruction with diminished excitation of the GPi and SNr and resulting enhancement of thalamocortical projection neuron activity (Fig. 3-4).

PEAK DOSE DYSKINESIAS

Efforts have been made to explain the treatment-related dyskinesias, particularly peak dose dyskinesias, which occur commonly in PD patients in the context of this model by invoking drug-induced abnormalities in basal ganglia output to the thalamus (15). The basis on which these attempts to explain dyskinesias is based is the clinical observation that the movements of peak dose dyskinesias bear a remarkable resemblance to the choreoathetosis/ballism observed with Huntington's disease. As with the choreoathetosis of Huntington's disease or hemiballism following STN destruction, peak dose dyskinesias are suggested to result from diminished basal ganglia output to the thalamus.

Two animal models of peak dose dyskinesias have been utilized in an effort to explore this hy-

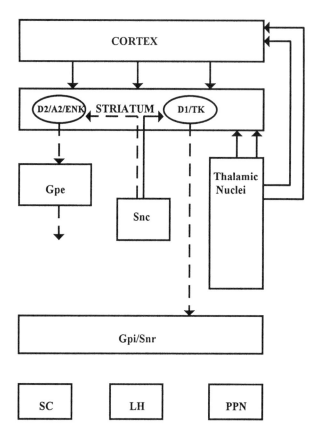

FIG. 3-3. Hemiballism. The consequences of STN destruction are loss of excitation of GPi/SNr with consequent decreased inhibitory basal ganglia output to the thalamus and increased thalamocortical excitation. See Fig. 3-1 for explanation of abbreviations.

pothesis. Treatment of unilaterally 6-OHDA-lesioned rats with L-dopa or dopamine agonists using chronic intermittent schedules (parenteral administration—intramuscular, intraperitoneal, subcutaneous—several times per day) of drug administration results in a heightened rotational response to agonist administration. This "priming" effect has been suggested to be an analogue of peak dose dyskinesias. Similarly, chronic intermittent administration of L-dopa or dopamine agonists to MPTP-lesioned primates results in the rapid development of peak dose dyskinesias analogous to those seen in PD patients. In contrast to chronic intermittent administration, chronic continuous administration of agonists appears to blunt the emergence of priming and peak dose dyskinesias in unilaterally 6-OHDA-lesioned rats and MPTP-lesioned primates, respectively (11,22,30). The difference in outcomes between chronic intermittent and chronic continuous ad-

ministration schedules gives credence to the idea that treatment with L-dopa, at least as practiced at present, contributes to the development of dyskinesias. Regimens aimed at reproducing chronic continuous administration in humans might be useful for forestalling or moderating the emergence of dyskinesias, though reproducing the chronic continuous administration paradigms used in animals is difficult.

Some data indicate that priming in unilaterally 6-OHDA-lesioned rats and peak dose dyskinesias in MPTP-lesioned primates is accompanied by alterations in the activity of striatal output pathways different from those seen in untreated animals. For example, Gnanalingham et al. reported that unilaterally 6-OHDA-lesioned rats treated with a chronic intermittent regimen of L-dopa have normalization of GABA-A receptor expression in the entopeduncular nucleus and SNr (30). Similarly, 6-OHDA-induced lesions

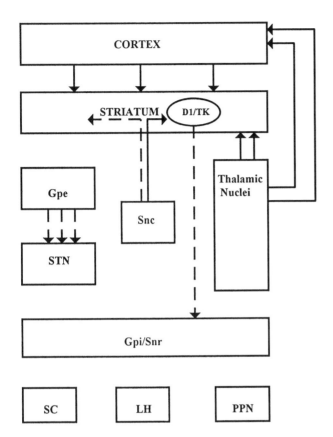

FIG. 3-4. Early stage Huntington's disease. Preferential loss of striato-GPe projection neurons leads to disinhibition of GPe neurons projecting to the STN. The resulting excessive inhibition of STN function results in diminished GPi/SNr output and thalamo-cortical excitation in a manner analogous to STN destruction. See Fig. 3-1 for explanation of abbreviations.

result in ipsilateral sensitivity of SNr neurons to iontophoresed GABA, an alteration reversed by chronic intermittent L-dopa treatment (79). These results suggest that chronic intermittent L-dopa or dopamine agonist therapy results in relative normalization of striato-GPi/SNr projection neuron activity (Fig. 3-5). When chronic intermittent-treated animals are then challenged with L-dopa or a dopamine agonist, both the striato-GPe and striato-GPi/SNr respond to stimulation of their dopamine receptors, with the striato-GPe neurons decreasing in activity and striato-GPi/SNr neurons increasing in activity. The effect of the decrease in striato-GPe activity is to disinhibit the GPe and suppression of STN activity. The increased striato-GPi/SNr activity causes increased inhibition of GPi/SNr neurons; and, coupled with the reduced drive from the STN, basal ganglia output to the thalamus and other targets decreases. In subjects who never re-

ceived chronic intermittent L-dopa or agonist treatment, the result is relative normalization of basal ganglia output to the thalamus; in the chronic intermittent-treated subjects, the restoration of striato-GPi/SNr activity by treatment results in diminished GPi/SNr output as striato-GPi/SNr projection neuron activity is driven above levels seen normally in unlesioned subjects (Fig. 3-6). Other studies, looking at neurochemical or metabolic markers of striatal projection neuron activity are consistent with this proposal (23,24,51,52). It has also been suggested that priming results in increased sensitivity of striato-GPe neurons to agonist effects; if true, this would further enhance the effects of L-dopa or dopamine agonists on basal ganglia output (61).

The major challenge to this model of peak dose dyskinesias has emerged from the recent experience with pallidotomy. The beneficial ef-

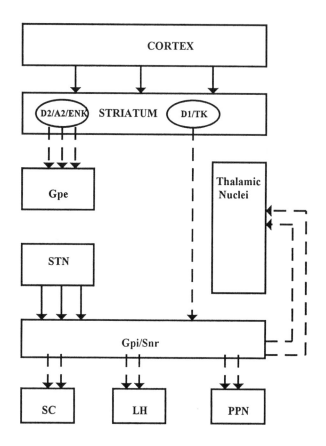

FIG. 3-5. Effects of chronic intermittent L-dopa or dopamine agonist treatment. There is relative normalization of striato-GPi/SNr output but little effect on striato-GPe output. The STN continues to be hyperactive with excessive basal ganglia inhibition of thalamocortical activity. See Fig. 3-1 for explanation of abbreviations.

fects of pallidotomy are inferred to derive from a reduction in basal ganglia output to the thalamus. If dyskinesias result from diminished basal ganglia output to the thalamus, pallidotomy, which reduces basal ganglia output to the thalamus even further, would be expected to exacerbate dyskinesias. This result is the opposite of what has been observed following pallidotomy (6,42,46). It is now well documented that perhaps the most striking improvement after pallidotomy is a marked reduction in dyskinesias. In addition, a relevant animal experiment has been performed by Blanchet et al. (10). This group produced axon-sparing GPe lesions in MPTP-lesioned primates and then attempted to induce peak dose dyskinesias. According to the model, the GPe lesions should blunt peak dose dyskinesias; but in fact, dyskinesias were exacerbated after GPe lesions. These observations indicate that the model does not explain peak dose dyskinesias and in fact contains some serious flaw(s).

DYSKINESIAS: A ROLE FOR THE THALAMUS?

The marked decrease in dyskinesias after pallidotomy suggests that the posteroventral pallidum is in some sense a generator of dyskinesias. How might the increased pallidal output thought to be characteristic of parkinsonism produce dyskinesias? One clue comes from a study performed by Page et al. (53). Lesions of the VA/VL thalamus diminished peak dose dyskinesias in MPTP-treated nonhuman primates. This result suggests that the thalamus might also be considered a generator of dyskinesias. At first glance, this observation and the experience with pallidotomy appears to be contradictory: Pallidotomy should remove an inhibitory influence on the thalamus and result in an increase in thalamic neuron activity, and thalamotomy should do the opposite. In fact, the situation is likely to be much more complex. Thalamocortical projection neurons

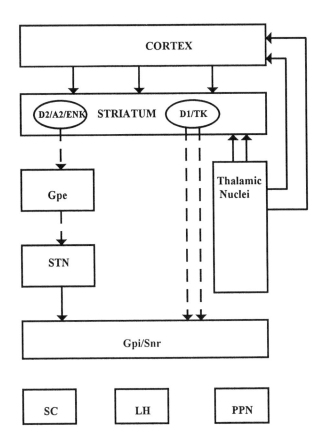

FIG. 3-6. Effects of L-dopa or dopamine agonist stimulation in a chronic intermittent treated subject. The striato-GPe output drops, resulting in less STN excitatory output to the GPi/SNr whereas striato-GPi/SNr output increases above normal levels, resulting in excessive inhibition of GPi/SNr neurons and disinhibition of thalamocortical projection neuron activity, a final pathway analogous to choreoathethosis in Huntington's disease or hemiballism. See Fig. 3-1 for explanation of abbreviations.

are unlikely to be passive transducers of basal ganglia output. Thalamocortical projection neurons have complex and, to some extent, nonlinear properties (69). These neurons have been shown to exist in tonic firing and burst firing modes. The transition from one state to another is regulated by complex interactions between membrane properties and afferent input. Both states are likely to convey information to the cortex but with rather different signal properties. Our naive assumption is that increased GABAergic input, from pallidal neurons for example, should produce decreased thalamocortical neuron activity. Electrophysiological evidence indicates that stimulation of GPi/SNr neurons does reduce thalamocortical projection neuron activity, but it may not be the crucial phenomenon (77). An interesting body of data demonstrates that hyperpolarization of thalamocortical projection neurons by GABA receptors, specifically the GABA-B receptor, regulates the transition from tonic to burst firing (69). Post-

synaptic GABA-B receptors mediate a hyperpolarization that drives the resting membrane potential of thalamocortical neurons into the appropriate range for activation of a low threshold calcium current (the T current), which drives bursting activity.

Most GPi/SNr terminals synapse on thalamocortical projection neurons, but these terminals also innervate inhibitory GABAergic interneurons (41). Projections from the GPe and ventral pallidum reach the inhibitory and GABAergic neurons of the reticular nucleus of the thalamus. The influence of basal ganglia output on GABAergic interneurons is not known, but there are several possible scenarios, including feed-forward inhibition. Similarly, the effects of basal ganglia output on reticular nucleus function is not known, though the change in GAD mRNA expression within reticular neurons in unilaterally 6-OHDA lesioned rats suggests a real functional connection and may indicate increased reticular neuron activity. The activity of reticular nucleus neurons is thought to be particularly important for regulating the transition from tonic to bursting activity in thalamocortical projection neurons. It may be that many of the abnormal motor phenomena seen with basal ganglia disorders have their proximate cause in complex derangements of thalamocortical neuron function.

These speculations suggest new lines of inquiry into dyskinesias based on the possible role of the thalamus. Further investigation of the effects of basal ganglia output on thalamic neuron function is needed. Some studies have been performed, and the initial work has yielded results at variance with the simple transducer conception of the thalamus used in the present model of basal ganglia pathophysiology (43,73,78). Still, most of the studies of thalamic physiology have been performed with reference to the role of the thalamus in sensation or regulation of consciousness and not with respect to motor, specifically basal ganglia-related, function. Functional studies of the basal ganglia-related portions of the thalamus may prove rewarding. Some clinical investigations based on the idea of modulating thalamocortical projection neuron function may also be useful. For example, agents that affect the T current, such as ethosuximide, or GABA-B agonists/antagonists, might be tested for effects on dyskinesias.

CONCLUSIONS

The success of pallidotomy in alleviating dyskinesias indicates the presence of a major flaw in the present model of basal ganglia pathophysiology. It is time to reexamine critically the anatomic conceptions behind this model. It is also necessary to place future hypotheses about movement disorder pathophysiology in a physiological, rather than an anatomical, framework, a task rendered difficult by our relative ignorance of basal ganglia function. The failure of this model has provided some useful clues for future work. For example, the behavior of thalamocortical neurons and their effect of neocortical function is not predictable from the present model, and understanding the regulation of thalamocortical neurons by basal ganglia is crucial to furthering our understanding of movement disorders.

Acknowledgements. Supported by the Geriatrics Research, Education and Clinical Center of the Ann Arbor Veterans Administration Medical Center, AG08671, and NS15655.

REFERENCES

1. Afsharpour S. Light microscopic analysis of Golgi-impregnated rate subthalamic neurons. *J Comp Neurol* 1985;236:1–13.
2. Albin RL, Young AB, Penney JB. The functional anatomy of basal ganglia disorders. *Trends Neurosci* 1989;12:366–375.
3. Albin RL, et al. Abnormalities of striatal projection neurons and *n*-methyl-D-aspartate receptors in presymptomatic Huntington's disease. *N Engl J Med* 1990;322: 1293–1298.
4. Alexander GE, DeLong MR, Strick PL. Parallel organization of functional circuits linking basal ganglia and cortex. *Annu Rev Neurosci* 1986;9:357–381.
5. Aziz TZ, Peggs D, Sambrook MA, Crossman AR. Lesion of the subthalamic nucleus for alleviation of 1-methyl-4-phenyl-1,2,3,6-tetrahydropyridine (MPTP)-induced parkinsonism in the primate. *Mov Disord* 1991; 6:288–293.
6. Baron MS, et al. Treatment of advanced Parkinson's disease by posterior GPi pallidotomy: 1 year results of a pilot study. *Ann Neurol* 1996;40:355–366.
7. Bergman H, Wichmann T, Delong MR. Reversal of experimental parkinsonism by lesions of the subthalamic nucleus. *Science* 1990;249:1436–1438.
8. Bergman H, Wichmann T, Karmon B, Delong MR. The primate subthalamic nucleus. II. Neuronal activity in the MPTP model of parkinsonism. *J Neurophysiol* 1994;72: 5-7–520.
9. Berretta S, Parthasarathy HB, Graybiel AM. Local release of GABAergic inhibition in the motor cortex induces immediate–early gene expression in indirect pathway neurons of the striatum. *J Neurosci* 1997;17: 4752–4763.
10. Blanchet PJ, Boucher R, Bedard PJ. Excitotoxic lateral pallidotomy does not relieve L-DOPA-induced dyskinesia in MPTP parkinsonian monkeys. *Brain Res* 1994; 650:32–39.
11. Blanchet PJ, Calon F, Martel JC, et al. Continuous administration decreases and pulsatile administration increases behavioral sensitivity to a novel dopamine D2 agonist (U-91356A) in MPTP-exposed monkeys. *JPET* 1995;272:854–857.
12. Brotchie JM, Crossman AR. D-[³H]Aspartate and [¹⁴C]GABA uptake in the basal ganglia of rats following lesions in the subthalamic region suggest a role for excitatory amino acid but not GABA-mediated transmission in subthalamic nucleus efferents. *Exp Neurol* 1991;113: 171–181.
13. Ceballos-Baumann AO, et al. Restoration of thalamo-cortical activity after posterioventral pallidotomy in Parkinson's disease. *Lancet* 1994;344:814.
14. Chesselet MF, Delfs JM. Basal ganglia and movement disorders: an update. *Trends Neurosci* 1996;19:417–422.
15. Crossman AR. A hypothesis on the pathophysiological mechanisms that underlie levodopa- or dopamine agonist-

induced dyskinesia in Parkinson's disease: implications for future strategies in treatment. *Mov Disord* 1990; 5:100–108.

16. Crossman A R. Primate models of dyskinesia: the experimental approach to the study of basal ganglia-related involuntary movement disorders. *Neuroscience* 1987; 21: 1–40.

17. Davis K D, et al. Globus pallidus stimulation activates the cgl motor system during alleviation of parkinsonian symptoms. *Nat Med* 1997;71:674.

18. Delfs J M, Ciaramitaro VM, Soghomonian JJ, Chesselet MF. Unilateral nigrostriatal lesions induce a bilateral increase in glutamate decarboxylase messenger RNA in the reticular thalamic nucleus. *Neuroscience* 1996; 71:383–395.

19. Delfs J M, Ciaramitaro VM, Parry TJ, Chesselet M F. Subthalamic nucleus lesions: widespread effects on changes in gene expression induced by nigrostriatal dopamine depletion in rats. *J Neurosci* 1995;15:6562–6575.

20. Delong M R. Primate models of movement disorders of basal ganglia origin. *Trends Neurosci* 1990;13:281–285.

21. Dogali M, et al. Stereotactic ventral pallidotomy for Parkinson's disease. *Neurology* 1995;45:753–761.

22. Engber TM, Susel Z, Juncos JL, Chase TN. Continuous and intermittent levodopa differentially affect rotation induced by D1 and D2 dopamine agonists. *Eur J Pharmacol* 1989;168:291–298.

23. Engber TM, Susel Z, Kuo S, Chase TN. Chronic levodopa treatment alters basal and dopamine agonist-stimulated cerebral glucose utilization. *J Neurosci* 1990;10:3889–3895.

24. Engber TM, Susel Z, Kuo S, Gerfen CR, Chase TN. Levodopa replacement therapy alters enzyme activities in striatum and neuropeptide content in striatal output regions of 6-hydroxydopamine lesioned rats. *Brain Res* 1991;552:113–118.

25. Fuller TA, Russchen FT, Price JL. Sources of presumptive glutamergic/aspartergic afferents to the rat ventral striatopallidal region. *J Comp Neurol* 1987;258: 317–338.

26. Garcia-Munoz M, Young SJ, Groves PM. Terminal excitability of the corticostriatal pathway. I. Regulation by dopamine receptor stimulation. *Brain Res* 1991;551: 195–206.

27. Garcia-Munoz M, Young SJ, Groves PM. Terminal excitability of the corticostriatal pathway. II. Regulation by glutamate receptor stimulation. *Brain Res* 1991;551: 207–215.

28. Gerfen CR. The neostriatal mosaic; multiple levels of compartmental organization in the basal ganglia. *Annu Rev Neurosci* 1992;15:285–320.

29. Gerfen CR, et al. D1 and D2 dopamine receptor-regulated gene expression of striatonigral and striatopallidal neurons. *Science* 1990;250:1429–1432.

30. Gnanalingham K K, Robertson RG. Chronic continuous and intermittent L-3,4-dihydroxyphenylalanine lesioned rats—an autoradiographic study using [^{3}H]flunitrazepam. *Neuroscience* 1993;57:673–681.

31. Grafton ST, Waters C, Sutton J, Lew MF, Couldwell W. Pallidotomy increases activity of motor association cortex in Parkinson's disease: a PET study. *Ann Neurol* 1995;37:776–783.

32. Graybiel AM. Neurotransmitters and neuromodulators in the basal ganglia. *Trends Neurosci* 1990;13:244–254.

33. Hassani OK, Mouroux M, Feger J. Increased subthalamic neuronal activity after nigral dopaminergic lesion independent of disinhibition via the globus pallidus. *Neuroscience* 1996;72:105–115.

34. Hazrati LN, Parent A. Projection from the external pallidum to the reticular thalamic nucleus in the squirrel monkey. *Brain Res* 1991;117:877–897.

35. Holsapple J W, Preston J B, Strick PL. The origin of thalamic inputs to the "hand" representation in the primary motor cortex. *J Neurosci* 1991;11:2644–2654.

36. Hoover J E, Strick PL. Multiple output channels in the basal ganglia. *Science* 1993;259:819–821.

37. Johnson A K, Coirini H, Kallstrom L, Weisel FA. Characterization of dopamine receptor binding sites in the subthalamic nucleus. *Neuroreport* 1994;5:1836–1838.

38. Kawaguchi Y, Wilson CJ, Emson PC. Projection subtypes of rat neostriatal matrix cells revealed by intracellular injection of biocytin. *J Neurosci* 1990;10: 3421–3438.

39. Kincaid A K, Albin R L, Newman SW, Penney J B, Young A B. 6-Hydroxydopamine lesions of the nigrostriatal pathway alter the expression of glutamic acid decarboxylase mRNA in rat globus pallidus projection neurons. *Neuroscience* 1992;51:705–718.

40. Kreiss DS, Anderson LA, Walters J R. Apomorphine and dopamine d(1) receptor agonists increase the firing rates of subthalamic nucleus neurons. *Neuroscience* 1996; 72:863–876.

41. Kultas-Ilinsky K, Ilinsky I, Warton S, Smith K R. Fine structure of nigral and pallidal afferents in the thalamus: an EM autoradiographic study in the cat. *J Comp Neurol* 1983;216:390–405.

42. Laitinen LV, Bergenheim AT, Hariz MI. Leksell's posteroventral pallidotomy in the treatment of Parkinson's disease. *J Neurosurg* 1992;76:53–61.

43. Lavin A, Grace A A. Modulation of dorsal thalamic cell activity by the ventral pallidum: its role in the regulation of thalamocortical activity by the basal ganglia. *Synapse* 1994;18:104–127.

44. Limousin P, et al. Effect of parkinsonian signs and symptoms of bilateral subthalamic nucleus stimulation. *Lancet* 1995;345:91–95.

45. Lin A M, Kao LS, Chai CY. Involvement of nitric oxide in dopaminergic transmission in rat striatum: an in vivo electrochemical study. *J Neurochem* 1995;65: 2043–2049.

46. Lozano AM, et al. Effect of GPi pallidotomy on motor function in Parkinson's diease. *Lancet* 1995;346: 1383–1387.

47. Marsden CD, Obeso JA. The functions of the basal ganglia and the paradox of stereotaxic surgery in Parkinson's disease. *Brain* 1994;117:877–897.

48. Matsumura M, Tremblay L, Richard H, Filion M. Activity of pallidal neurons in the monkey during dyskinesia induced by injection of bicuculline in the external pallidum. *Neuroscience* 1995;65:59–70.

49. Miller WC, DeLong M R. Parkinsonian symptomatology: an anatomical and physiological analysis. *Ann NY Acad Sci* 1988;515:287–302.

50. Mitchell IJ, et al. Neural mechanisms underlying parkinsonian symptoms based upon regional uptake of 2-deoxyglucose in monkeys exposed to 1-methyl-4-phenyl-1,2,3,6-tetrahydropyridine. *Neuroscience* 1989; 32:213–226.

51. Mitchell IJ, Boyce S, Sambrook MA, Crossman A R. A 2-deoxyglucose study of the effects of dopamine agonists on the parkinsonian primate brain. *Brain* 1992; 115:809–824.

52. Mitchell IJ, Luquin R, Boyce S, et al. Neural mechanisms by dystonia: evidence from a 2-deoxyglucose uptake study in a primate model of dopamine agonist-induced dystonia. *Mov Disord* 1990;5:49–54.

53. Page R D, Sambrook MA, Crossman AR. Thalamotomy for the alleviation of levodopa-induced dyskinesia: experimental studies in the 1-methyl-4-phenyl-1,2,3,tetrahydropyridine-treated parkinsonian monkey. *Neuroscience* 1900;55:147–165.

54. Pan HS, Penney JB, Young A B. Gamma-aminobutyric acid and benzodiazepine receptor changes induced by unilateral 6-hydroxydopamine lesions of the medial forebrain bundle. *J Neurochem* 1985;45:1396–1404.

55. Parent A, Hazrati L-N. Functional anatomy of the basal ganglia. I. The corticobasal ganglia-thalamo-cortical loop. *Brain Res Rev* 1995;20:91–127.

56. Parent A, Hazrati L-N. Functional anatomy of the basal ganglia. II. The place of the subthalamic nucleus and external pallidum in basal ganglia circuitry. *Brain Res Rev* 1995;20:128–154.

57. Parent A, Charara A, Pinault D. Single striatofugal axons arborizing in both pallidal segments and in the substantia nigra in primates. *Brain Res* 1995;698:280–284.

58. Parry TJ, Eberle-Wang K, Lucki I, Chesselet MF. Dopaminergic stimulation of subthalamic nucleus elicits oral dyskinesia in rats. *Exp Neurol* 1994;128:181–190.

59. Parthasarathy HB, Graybiel AM. Cortically driven immediate-early gene expression reflects modular influence of sensorimotor cortex on identified striatal neurons in the squirrel monkey. *J Neurosci* 1997;17:2477–2491.

60. Playford ED, et al. Impaired mesial frontal and putamen activation in Parkinson's disease: a positron emision tomography study. *Ann Neurol* 1992;32:151–161.

61. Pollack A K, Turgeon SM, Fink JS. Apomorphine priming alters the response of striatal outflow pathways to D2 agonist stimulation in 6-hydroxydopamine-lesioned rats. *Neuroscience* 1997;79:79–93.

62. Reiner A, et al. Differential loss of projection neurons in Huntington disease. *Proc Natl Acad Sci USA* 1988; 85:5733–5737.

63. Richfield EK, Herkenham M. Selective vulnerability in Huntington's disease: preferential loss of cannabinoid receptors in lateral globus pallidus. *Ann Neurol* 1994; 36:577–584.

64. Robertson RG, Clarke CA, Boyce S, Sambrook MA, Crossman AR. The role of striatopallidal neurones utilizing gamma-aminobutyric acid in the pathophysiology of M PTP-induced parkinsonism in the primate: evidence from [³H]flunitrazepam autoradiography. *Brain Res* 1990;531:95–104.

65. Robertson RG, Graham WC, Sambrook MA, Crossman AR. Further investigations into the pathophysiology of M PTP-induced parkinsonism in the primate: an intracerebral microdialysis study of gamma-aminobutyric acid in the lateral segment of the globus pallidus. *Brain Res* 1991;563:278–280.

66. Robledo P, Feger J. Excitatory influence of rat subthalamic nucleus to substantia nigra pars reticulate and the pallidal complex: electrophysiological data. *Brain Res* 1990;S18:366–370.

67. Schiffmann SN, Vanderhaegen JJ. Adenosine A2 receptors regulate the gene expression of striatopallidal and striatonigral neurons. *J Neurosci* 1993;12:3591–3600.

68. Sellal F, Lisovoski F, Hirsch E, Mutschler V, Collard M, Marescaux C. Contralateral disappearance of parkinsonian signs after subthalamic hematoma. *Neurology* 1992; 42:255–256.

69. Sherman SM, Guillery RW. Functional organization of thalamocortical relays. *J Neurosci* 1996;76:1367–1395.

70. Sidibe M, Smith Y. Differential synaptic innervation of striatofugal neurones projecting to the internal or external segments of the globus pallidus by thalamic afferents in the squirrel monkey. *J Comp Neurol* 1996;365: 445–465.

71. Smith A D, Bolam J P. The neural network of the basal ganglia as revealed by the study of synaptic connections of identified neurones. *Trends Neurosci* 1990;13:259–265.

72. Spencer H J. Antagonism of cortical excitation of striatal neurons by glutamic acid diethyl ester: evidence for glutamic acid as an excitatory transmitter in the rat striatum. *Brain Res* 1976;102:91–101.

73. Storey E, Beal M F. Neurochemical substrates of rigidity and chorea in Huntington's disease. *Brain* 1993;116: 1201–1222.

74. Surmeier DJ, Kitai ST. Dopaminergic regulation of striatal efferent pathways. *Curr Opin Neruobiol* 1994; 4:915–919.

75. Tallaksen-Greene SJ, Wiley RG, Albin R L. Localization of striatal excitatory amino acid binding site subtypes to striatonigral neurons. *Brain Res* 1992;594:165–170.

76. Uhl GR, Navia B, Douglas J. Differential expression of preproenkephalin and preprodynorphin mRNAs in striatal neurons: high levels of preproenkephalin expression depend on cerebral cortical afferents. *J Neurosci* 1988; 8:4755–4764.

77. Uno M, Ozama N, Yoshida M. The mode of pallido-thalamic transmission investigated with intracellular recording from cat thalamus. *Exp Brain Res* 1978; 33:493–507.

78. Voloshin MY, et al. Influence of *N*-methyl-4-phenyl-1,2,3,6-tetrahydropyridine-induced injury of dopaminergic nigrostriatal system on movement components of the instrumental reflex and motor thalamic reactions in the cat. *Neuroscience* 1991;45:291–305.

79. Weick BG, Engber TM, Susel Z, Chase TN, Walters JR. Responses of substantia nigra pars reticulate neurons to GABA and SKF 38393 in 6-hydroxydopamine-lesioned rats are differentially affected by continuous and intermittent levodopa administration. *Brain Res* 1990;523: 16–22.

80. Wichmann T, Bergman H, DeLong M R. The primate subthalamic nucleus. III. Changes in motor behavior and neuronal activity in the internal pallidum induced by subthalamic inactivation in the MPTP model of parkinsonism. *J Neurophysiol* 1994;72:621–530.

Pallidal Surgery for the Treatment of Parkinson's Disease and Movement Disorders, edited by
J. K. Krauss, R. G. Grossman, and J. Jankovic.
Lippincott-Raven Publisher, Philadelphia © 1998.

4

Rationales for Pallidal Surgery: What are the Mechanisms?

Allen S. Mandir and *Frederick A. Lenz

*Departments of Neurology and *Neurosurgery, Johns Hopkins Hospital, Baltimore, Maryland 21287, USA*

Posteroventral pallidal surgery ameliorates a variety of motoric symptoms in patients with idiopathic Parkinson's disease (PD). Reported benefits following pallidotomy for the PD patient include improvement of all the cardinal symptoms of this disease: bradykinesia, akinesia, rigidity, tremor, and postural instability (2,26,33,59). Most pallidal surgery to date is performed for parkinsonian patients who do not respond sufficiently to levodopa administration or who suffer from troublesome side effects of pharmacological therapy (e.g., on–off phenomenon). Of the benefits reported from pallidotomy, improvement of levodopa-induced dyskinesias is the most consistent (2,25,32, 33,45,52,55). More recently, pallidotomy has been applied to purely hyperkinetic disorders (e.g., hemiballism and dystonia) with good effect (50,57,65,102,112). How these far-reaching benefits come about is unclear, although with advances in our understanding of basal ganglia physiology and molecular biology the mechanisms of pallidotomy effects should follow.

Currently, the major advances in understanding basal ganglia physiology and pathophysiology stem from nonhuman primate animal models (20). Similarities of neuronal activity in patients with movement disorders to that in animal models helps validate theories of basal ganglia physiology. To review plausible mechanisms of motoric improvements following pallidotomy, it is necessary to refer to these physiological models. The reader may wish to refer to the chapters of this book that discuss these points in greater detail.

BASAL GANGLIA MOTOR CIRCUITRY: PATHOPHYSIOLOGY IN PARKINSONISM

A simplified model of the basal ganglia motor circuit connecting the putamen (the major motoric input structure of the striatum) to the globus pallidus internus segment (GPi, the major motoric output structure) distinguishes *direct* and *indirect* pathways (Fig. 4-1). The *indirect* pathway connects the putamen first to the external segment of globus pallidus (GPe) and then via the subthalamic nucleus (STN) to the GPi. There also exists a reciprocal connection to the GPe from the STN (38,96). In nonhuman primates, the target of GPi efferents in the basal ganglia motor loop are thought to be the ventral lateral pars oralis (VLo), corresponding to the ventralis oralis posterior (Vop) in humans (41).

The GPi neurons utilize GABA to inhibit its thalamic targets (83,116). From these thalamic areas, projections exist to the cortex prominently to the supplementary motor area (SMA) and primary motor cortex (MI). Another projection from GPi targets the pedunculopontine nucleus (PPN), which in turn has excitatory projections to the spinal cord.

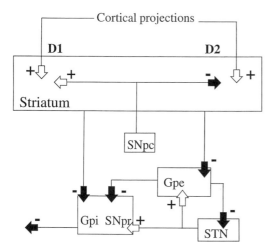

FIG. 4-1. Basal ganglia connections. Cortical projections to the striatum are excitatory, whereas dopaminergic inputs from the substantia nigra, pars compacta (*SNpc*) are excitatory at D1-type receptors and inhibitory at D2-type receptors. The "direct" pathway includes an inhibitory projection from the striatum to the internal segment of the globus pallidus (*Gpi*). The "indirect" pathway includes an inhibitory projection to the external segment of the globus pallidus (*Gpe*), which in turn sends an inhibitory projection to the subthalamic nucleus (*STN*); to complete this pathway, the STN sends an excitatory pathway to the GPi. In addition to these projections of these classic pathways, note the excitatory projection from the STN to the GPe and an inhibitory pathway from the GPe to the GPi. Outflows from the GPi and substantia nigra pars reticulata (*SNpr*) are inhibitory. *Arrowheads* demonstrate direction of connections; *dark arrowheads* represent inhibitory projections and *white arrowheads* the excitatory projections.

Cortical projections to the putamen (glutamergic) activate both the direct and indirect pathways. Dopaminergic projections from substantia nigra pars compacta (SNpc) excite the direct pathway through activation of D1-type receptors and inhibit the indirect pathway (D2 type receptors). Because putaminal neurons have a GABAergic projection to the GPi, activation of the *direct* pathway inhibits GPi activity and disinhibits the thalamus. Similarly, decreased inhibition of the PPN ultimately results in greater excitation of the spinal cord.

Putaminal projections to the GPe via the *indirect* pathway are GABAergic, as are GPe projec-

tions to the STN. STN projections to the GPi (and GPe) are excitatory (glutamergic); and thus cortical excitation of the *indirect* pathway ultimately increases the inhibition of GPi outflow to the thalamus and PPN. Note that the presence of dopamine decreases GPi activity in both the *direct* and *indirect* pathways because of the differential effects on D1 and D2 receptors. With dopaminergic deficiency, such as in parkinsonism, the predicted result is that of increased tonic activity of GPi (35,100).

It is important to remember that output from the GPi projects to brainstem structures and completes an anatomical loop back to the cortex via thalamic relays. Furthermore, somatotopic segments of the GPi may ultimately project to different motor and premotor cortices (20,22).

PALLIDAL SURGERY
FOR PARKINSON'S DISEASE

Extracellular recordings of human GPi have not been carried out in normal subjects, but in parkinsonian patients they demonstrate increased GPi activity compared to that of the GPe (6,113). That GPi activity is increased following dopaminergic deficiency in these patients is supported by positron-emission tomography (PET) findings and regional cerebral blood flow (rCBF) studies (28). In addition, GPi extracellular recordings in parkinsonian patients demonstrate firing patterns similar to those in the nonhuman primate model of *N*-methyl-4-phenyl-1,2,3,6-tetrahydropyridine (MPTP)-induced parkinsonism (6,113). Note that there is some argument whether GPe activity is increased in PD compared to that in control subjects. Some physiological PET studies in primate models have failed to show a significant decrement of GPe activity in parkinsonian patients compared to that in controls (87,93). Molecular analysis examining levels of messenger RNA (mRNA) for co-localized neurotransmitters may also argue against such a change in activity (109). However, these findings may still be compatible with neuronal recordings in nonhuman primates and the model of basal ganglia physiology. These former methods of PET and mRNA quantification lack temporal resolution and thus could be consistent with a change in neuronal firing pattern of overall decreased baseline firing with increased bursting type of activity. Indeed, this type of pattern is reported in parkinsonian basal ganglia and may indicate the importance of patterned activity within the corticobasal ganglia-thalamic loop for producing parkinsonian pathophysiology (5,36).

Using the schema above and these data, one may begin to formulate a rationale why pallidal surgery alleviates many of the motor manifestations of PD. Using the guidelines of the basal ganglia physiological model, we may distinguish motor function related to changes in the motoric output nuclei of the basal ganglia, the GPi, and the SNpr. The following disorders are hypothesized to result from increased inhibitory output of the GPi (hypokinetic disorders) or from decreased basal ganglia output (hyperkinetic disorders).

DISORDERS RESULTING FROM INCREASED BASAL GANGLIA OUTPUT ACTIVITY

Akinesia/Bradykinesia

Bradykinesia (slowed movement) and akinesia (defective initiation of movement) are cardinal symptoms of PD. Overall, the movements that require self-initiation are more affected than those initiated following a stimulus (115). The voluntary nature of these movements requires the ultimate expression of dysfunction at the cortical level (114). The primary motor cortex is most directly involved in producing skilled voluntary movements and receives prominent projections from the supplementary motor area (SMA). The SMA, in turn, is thought to function in the preparation and execution of voluntary movements. The GPi influences the primary motor cortex (MI) in part via thalamocortical relay directed from the VLo to the MI as well as through the VLo first to the SMA and then to the MI (40,42,54,58,92,101). Bradykinetic parkinsonian movements lack the classic triphasic burst pattern used to produce ballistic movements (37). This pattern is further disrupted during self-initiated movements compared to stimulus-initiated movements (115). Extracellular record-

ings in MPTP-induced parkinsonian monkey MI and SMA directly reflect this disorganization (114). Interestingly, common characteristics of parkinsonian recordings throughout the basal ganglia and thalamus are increased receptive field responses compared to normal states (6,111).

In cortical areas as well, there is loss of directional specificity of neuronal firing preceding and during movements (114). Specifically, a reduction of directional specificity of GPi neurons that fire in response to limb perturbations has been reported in MPTP-treated monkeys (19,71). The alterations of SMA neuronal activity in the parkinsonian state are also reflected in clinical studies by abnormal cortical "readiness" potentials (*bereitschaftspotential*), abnormal cerebral blood flow studies, and PET imaging (24,51,85,94,95). Disruption of normal preparatory responses in the SMA may be sufficient to produce akinesia and may explain the increased difficulties during self-initiated movements seen in PD.

Abnormal activity in projections to the MI from the GPi via the thalamus directly and the SMA indirectly could explain these signs of parkinsonism. Akinesia and bradykinesia are alleviated after pallidotomy (59). PET studies show normalization of cortical metabolism during voluntary movements of PD subjects undergoing pallidotomy (28). It appears that removal of the increased inhibitory drive of the GPi assists in allowing return of some organization of electromyographic (EMG) activity. Conversely, in parkinsonism thalamotomy has been suggested to increase bradykinesia or have no effect on movement times (81,105). The alleviation of akinesia and bradykinesia following subthalamotomy further supports the notion that it is the increased tonic output of the GPi in parkinsonism that is responsible for these clinical signs (4).

Tremor

The 3- to 6-Hz parkinsonian rest tremor is produced by alternating contraction of opposing muscle groups. Voluntary activation of the muscles diminishes the resting tremor at least initially. In parkinsonism, extracellular recordings throughout the thalamus and basal ganglia demonstrate oscillatory firing patterns not seen in the normal state (77). Thalamic neurons in particular have been implicated in the generation of resting tremor. As such, thalamic recordings in PD patients reveal oscillatory activity that is significantly correlated with tremor (63). Thalamotomy may produce immediate and long-lasting relief of tremor (53,80).

In parkinsonism, increased inhibitory activity from the GPi to the Vop may serve to hyperpolarize thalamic neurons. *In vitro* studies demonstrate two distinct modes of thalamic firing: the"transfer" mode and the "oscillatory" mode (49,70). The transfer mode occurs when thalamic neurons are held in a subthreshold depolarized state. In this state, depolarizing inputs into thalamic cells result in a steady firing rate of action potentials. In theory, when in the transfer mode thalamic neurons receiving oscillating inhibitory inputs from GPi should oscillate. Activity consistent with this mechanism is seen during recordings of the thalamus of PD patients (117).

When *in vitro* thalamic cells are placed in hyperpolarized states they exhibit properties of the oscillatory mode (49,70). In this state, high-frequency bursts of action potentials result, mediated by calcium spikes (slow time- and voltage-dependent calcium potentials) (48,49). A relative refractory period follows activation of the calcium channels. Thus bursts of action potentials may be seen in the oscillatory mode. In PD patients, neuronal bursting patterns of GPi may be seen at a rate of 12 to 15 Hz (34,111). One theory holds that this firing pattern may result in 4- to 6-Hz firing rates of thalamic neurons via thalamic filtering of the calcium spike oscillator. Moreover, in parkinsonian monkeys, neurons in the GPi (77) may be seen in phase with the bursts detected in human parkinsonian thalamus (117). An alternating hyperpolarizing input from the GPi thus would result in thalamic firing at tremor frequency.

This theory is supported clinically, as pallidotomy can ameliorate tremor in PD patients (59,103). In fact, tremor diminishment may correlate with the percentage of oscillatory GPi neurons in the field of the pallidotomy lesion (105).

Stereotactic thalamotomy targeting the Vim in parkinsonian patients also abolishes tremor, although this thalamic area is the cerebellar and pallidal relay. Alternative theories have suggested that tremor results from altered peripheral inputs involved in long loop reflex arcs. This theory is more compatible with Vim thalamotomy results, as sensory inputs traversing the long loop reflex arc are thought to include the Vim on the way to the motor cortex. In MPTP-treated parkinsonian monkeys, neurons in the GPi demonstrate altered responsiveness to peripheral sensory inputs. In turn, the VLo in MPTP-treated parkinsonism monkeys shows more frequent, less specific responses to peripheral somatosensory inputs (111). The gain of long latency reflexes in parkinsonian patients is increased (107,108). Computer simulations suggest that long loop reflexes with increased gain have the potential to oscillate at the frequency of parkinsonian tremor (100). In PD patients, peripheral input producing reflex activity and sectioning of dorsal roots both can alter the phase of the tremor (86,88,89,98,107).

A full explanation of tremor etiology in PD may require the combination of oscillatory activity inherent to the basal ganglia and contributions from sensory input. Disruptions of this loop, particularly in terms of diminished altered pallidal outputs to the thalamus may address the effectiveness of tremor relief from pallidotomy.

Rigidity

Increased joint resistance to passive movement independent of speed and position characterizes parkinsonian rigidity. Theories exist that this parkinsonian sign results from increased tonic activity of cells in the GPi projecting to the thalamus. Supportive of this claim is the alleviation of rigidity of PD patients who undergo pallidotomy (59).

It has been proposed that parkinsonian rigidity results from supraspinal mechanisms, as no fundamental change in mechanical muscle properties or short latency reflexes are observed in PD patients (90). Furthermore, microneuronal recordings of fusimotor activity in PD suggest that Ia discharges are not increased with rigidity (10). Explanation of a cortically mediated mechanism of rigidity in PD has been suggested by alterations of long loop reflexes. As described above, the long-latency reflex in parkinsonian patients has an increased, relatively fixed gain (90), which would occur through the connection from the SMA to the motor cortex (1). The EMG response to stretch is thus increased, leading to rigidity or increased resistance to joint movement. Furthermore, the resting EMG activity in PD is elevated, implying tonic motoneuron activity, perhaps cortically mediated.

An alternative supraspinal mechanism of parkinsonian rigidity was proposed by Delwaide et al. (23). They suggested that Ib interneurons, which normally exert an inhibitory influence on alpha motoneurons, are less active in parkinsonian patients. They proposed that this change in Ib activity results from changes in basal ganglia output in PD and implicates a pathway from the basal ganglia projecting to the pontine nucleus gigantocellularis and reticulospinal projection pathways in the dorsal longitudinal fasciculus. Rigidity, as expected by these models, would be reduced by disrupting altered GPi outflow by stereotactic lesions. The effect of pallidotomy in reducing rigidity is supportive of both cortically mediated and reticulospinally mediated theories of long-latency reflex pathways.

DISORDERS RESULTING FROM DECREASED BASAL GANGLIA OUTPUT ACTIVITY

Levodopa-induced Dyskinesias

That pallidotomy can alleviate hypokinetic and hyperkinetic movement dysfunction simultaneously seems paradoxical. However, we encounter this type of paradox commonly when L-dopa or dopamine agonists are applied to alleviate both negative and positive movement disorders of parkinsonism. Moreover, selective D1 antagonists may lessen levodopa-induced dyskinesias (LIDs) without worsening the negative parkinsonian symptoms. Thus although lending great insight into basal ganglia function, current physiological models must be extended to explain the variety of motor behavior observed during basal ganglia dysfunction.

The LIDs commonly seen in PD patients following years of treatment with L-dopa are still poorly understood. There is agreement that they are in part attributable to a deficiency in dopamine buffering capacity that occurs in PD (31,97). Patients with more severe parkinsonism exhibit greater LID, giving credence to this hypothesis. Among the MPTP-induced parkinsonian primates given dopaminergic agonists, only those with severe parkinsonism developed dyskinesias (36). Likewise, more severe LIDs tend to be displayed on the more parkinsonian side of patients, and PET studies have inversely correlated ^{18}F-fluorodopa retention with severity of fluctuations of PD patients on L-dopa (61). In addition, in animal models of parkinsonism, presynaptic and postsynaptic changes occur within the dopaminergic system to produce LIDs (17,18, 74,75). Normal subjects, with normal dopamine buffering capacity and physiological synaptic organization, do not demonstrate LIDs (79). Dyskinesias observed in nonhuman primates do not occur immediately but only after weeks of dopamine agonist administration (36).

There are differing opinions whether the *direct or indirect* pathways are more involved in producing LIDs (3,67). Levels of co-localized neurotransmitters unique to D1 and D2 neurons following nigral lesions and L-dopa treatment have been reported, suggesting that one or the other pathway is predominant in producing LIDs (110). Other studies have examined the effects of selective D1 or D2 agonists on producing LIDs (14). Still requiring clarification, at least to some degree, D1 and D2 receptor pathways may contribute to LIDs (30). In MPTP-induced parkinsonian primates, levodopa and dopamine agonists were able to produce dyskinesias similar to LIDs in PD patients (36). The firing rate of GPi in MPTP-induced parkinsonian animals is increased compared to that in the normal state; but during apomorphine-induced dyskinesias, GPi activity demonstrated firing rates even lower than those in the normal state (36). Primate parkinsonian model studies of 2-deoxyglucose uptake demonstrated parallel results, suggesting lower than normal GPi activity during periods of drug-induced dyskinesia (73).

Applying the basal ganglia physiological model, we may examine the theoretical contributions of direct and indirect pathways to LID. With fluctuation of dopamine, from decreased buffering capacity and receptor supersensitivity, LIDs may result from overactivation of D1 receptors, which would lead to hypoactivity of the GPi by direct inhibition (Fig. 4-1). The cyclical fluctuations of the dopaminergic response could quickly change the firing rates from hyperactivity to hypoactivity of the GPi, relating to "off" and "on" states, respectively. The indirect (D2) pathway would then predict cyclical periods of increased excitation of the GPe, as dopamine has an inhibitory effect on the GABAergic projections of the putamen that serve to inhibit the GPe. In turn, increased firing of the GPe should hyperpolarize and thus inhibit STN neurons, leading ultimately again to hypoactivity in the GPi. Cortical glutaminergic projections to the striatum also may contribute to on–off fluctuations and dyskinesias. N-Methyl-D-aspartate (NMDA) antagonists oppose production of dyskinesia without worsening the negative parkinsonian symptoms in PD and in MPTP-induced parkinsonian monkeys (8,82). Presumably it is the heightened sensitivity of glutaminergic receptor in the striatum that contributes to expression of LIDs (56).

It is tempting to believe the inverse corollary to increased GPi activity producing parkinsonian symptoms as discussed above: that decreased GPi activity produces hyperkinesis. However, experimental lesions of the GPi (decreasing GPi activity) did not produce dyskinesia (21). Abnormal hyperkinetic movements are reported with partial lesions of the GPi rather than more complete lesions (43,44,47,72). Furthermore, the benefits of pallidotomy in reducing LIDs may not be explained by decreased activity of the GPi alone, as one would predict heightened levels of dyskinesias with decreased GPi inhibitory output. Thus it is likely that decreased activity in the GPi is necessary but insufficient to cause LIDs. Other studies suggest a plausible explanation for mechanisms of dyskinesia following pallidotomy as discussed below.

According to the model, increased activity of GPe in the indirect pathway is correctly predicted during dyskinesia. In MPTP-induced parkinsonian primates, hyperactivity of GPe seemed highly correlated to the production of LIDs, which in turn was correlated to hypoactivity of the GPi. Lesion-

ing the GPe accordingly should decrease dyskinesia, yet GPe destruction is shown to worsen LIDs (7). In addition, Filion et al. (36) consistently found neurons in the GPe that decreased activity and in the GPi that demonstrated increased activity during dyskinesias. They suggested that it is not decreased GPi alone that produces dyskinesias but perhaps the coexistence of populations within the GPi that show hyper- and hypoactivity. Moreover, because segments of the GPi may ultimately project to differing end-targets, selective lesions may impart differing results. In nonhuman animal models, the excitatory agent bicuculline injected into the GPe was shown to produce dyskinesias but with resultant populations of hyperactive and hypoactive neurons in the GPe and GPi. Together with the discussion above, these findings suggest that the patterned output from the GPi is equally instrumental in producing dyskinesia as hypoactivity. Accordingly, Levy et al. (66) suggested that the GPe not only causes hyperactivity of the STN but fine-tunes STN patterning of firing. In fact, rat models demonstrate increased rates of firing and more bursting type of neuronal patterns in the STN following GPe lesions (39,91). Destruction of the GPi by pallidotomy may then disconnect these abnormal firing patterns on the thalamus, producing relief from dyskinesia.

The circuit structure of the basal ganglia-thalamo-cortical motor loop suggests that lesioning anywhere in this circuit may produce remote effects. In fact, it should not be surprising that despite being an "output" relay GPi lesions can influence responses in "upstream" structures of the basal ganglia. In fact, pallidal lesions in the rat can significantly reduce the inhibitory response seen in the STN following cortical stimulation (91). Thus both physical isolation and modification of other loop structures could help correct effects caused by an abnormally patterned output in the GPi.

Hemiballism

The prototypical lesion for producing hemiballism is contralateral destruction of the STN. According to the basal ganglia physiological model, resultant activity in the GPi should be decreased. This point is supported in human and nonhuman primates by extracellular recordings (102,112). As discussed for LIDS, hypoactivity of the GPi alone does not explain the resulting movement disorder. It is the patterning of GPi output that contributes to this disorder. In fact, the GPi activity recorded was described as tonic activity interrupted by prolonged periods of silence. This spontaneous activity differed from that in PD patients and normal individuals. Pallidotomy successfully alleviated hemiballismus in these patients, perhaps by disrupting the transmission of these abnormally patterned outputs from the GPi to the thalamus. In fact, thalamotomy and chronic thalamic stimulation successfully controlled cases of persistent hemiballism, suggesting a mechanism of improvement that involves removal of abnormally patterned activity on motor cortices via the thalamus that results from the GPi (15,57,108). In addition, those areas of thalamus relaying cerebellar projections (Vim) help diminish the symptoms of dyskinesia. As with dystonia, discussed below, a contribution of somatosensory derangement may play a role in the production of hemiballismus. Unlike that seen with LIDs, the activity of the GPe is diminished in hemiballism (103,112). This finding may be supported by the basal ganglia model (Fig. 4-1). The reciprocal innervation between the STN and the GPe may successfully predict decreased activity in the GPe following lesions of the STN. The GPe activity in LIDs and hemiballism thus superficially differs, which may additionally support the importance of the abnormal patterned activity of the GPi in the production of dyskinesias. Hemiballism differs from LIDs in part by the amplitude of movement, and it is tempting to speculate that perhaps a relatively decreased GPe in hemiballism may contribute to these differences perhaps by projections through the GPi. More traditionally, it is thought that it is the destruction of excitatory glutaminergic projections to the GPi from the STN that produces this profound movement.

Dystonia

Dystonia is characterized by excessive activity in reflexive and voluntary movements (69). Attempting voluntary movement usually exacerbates dystonia, increasing the spread of involved musculature. Conversely, sleep or rest may di-minish the level of dystonic signs. The etiology of this movement disorder is still unknown.

That pallidotomy alone may alleviate some forms of dystonia suggests that it is a central phenomenon. In fact, other evidence suggests that dystonia is a central, rather than a peripheral, mechanism. Studies of nerve conduction, evoked potentials, and EMG have not revealed peripheral abnormalities in idiopathic torsion dystonia. Furthermore, voluntary movements of muscles involved in task-specific dystonia may be undertaken without difficulty. For example, those with chewing dystonia may have no symptoms of speech disorder or of similar mouth movements; patients who have focal lower limb dystonias while walking forward may walk backward with ease. Lesions of the putamen, caudate, and thalamus that usually spare the globus pallidus are sufficient to cause secondary dystonia (11,27, 68,76,84). This finding lends credence to the suggestion that dystonia results from basal ganglia dysfunction.

Contributions from peripheral afferents to the production of dystonia, however, are also likely. There are abnormalities of peripheral reciprocal inhibition in dystonic patients (69), which may reflect presynaptic changes of Ia afferents (69). These findings may result from descending pathways or perhaps from changes in muscle spindle afferents. Following peripheral botulinum toxin treatments for writer's cramp, some cortical areas (including the supplementary area) return to a more normal activation state, although underactivity in the primary motor cortex remains (9,16). Sensory training has been employed in an attempt to alleviate dystonia (62), and upstream changes following peripheral treatment may relate to reorganization of somatosensory cortical maps seen with some forms of dystonia.

In an animal model of dystonia similar to that of writer's cramp, monkeys demonstrated a focal dystonia following repetitive distal forelimb gripping tasks (12), associated with reorganization of the somatosensory cortical map of this limb. Furthermore, microstimulation in these corresponding cortical areas produces increased contraction of associated muscles (78). In patients with writer's cramp, transcranial magnetic stimulation produces a larger area of muscle contraction than control (46). Thalamic recordings in the Vim of dystonic patients reveal a reorganization of sensorimotor maps (64). This area of the thalamus is involved with cerebellar—thalamic relays and relates to the results of single-photon emission computed tomography (SPECT) studies showing rCBF changes in deep cerebellar nuclei (60). The proportion of cells in the GPi responding to sensory stimulation was higher in a patient undergoing pallidotomy for focal dystonia than that observed in hemiballism patients, supporting the idea of somatosensory reorganization during dystonia (65).

Overactivation of agonist and co-contraction of agonist and antagonist muscles is characteristic of dystonia. The first EMG burst in the classic triphasic agonist-antagonist-agonist EMG pattern of ballistic movement is affected (37), as are abnormalities in antagonist firing and timing of reciprocal inhibition (69). There is greater activity in secondary agonists during reflexive and voluntary movements in dystonic patients. Moreover the duration of the long-latency stretch reflex in patients with dystonia is prolonged.

Basal ganglia outflow is thought to be diminished (less inhibitory) in dystonia. Indirect evidence is seen in those peak dose dystonias, as seen with PD. Furthermore, PET studies demonstrate dissociation between activity in the lentiform nuclei and the thalamus consistent with increased activity in the *direct* pathway (29). Other studies have reported decreased D2 receptors in dystonic patients, suggesting reduced activity in the *indirect* pathway. Overactivation of the *direct* pathway and underactivation of the *indirect* pathway would lead to decreased GPi activity. This would fit with other hyperkinetic disorders; and dystonia is often thought of as ultimate overactivity. However, some patients with PD develop dystonias at the end of their L-dopa dose, and primates receiving MPTP may demonstrate dystonia prior to L-dopa treatment. For these cases and with dystonia with diurnal variation, L-dopa treatment may palliate dystonic symptoms. Interestingly, recordings in Vop of dystonic patients undergoing thalamotomy for treatment of pain show decreased firing (64). This finding is more in agreement with the schema of hypokinetic disorders. Perhaps, as with other symptoms relieved by pallidal surgery,

it is by minimizing disrupting output from the basal ganglia that pallidal surgery demonstrates its effectiveness in the treatment of dystonia.

CONCLUSION

Pallidotomy is paradoxical in that it is used to treat both hyperkinetic and hypokinetic movement disorders. Despite advances in our understanding of the physiological and molecular mechanisms, clearly our knowledge of the true mechanisms of the diseases and treatments are deficient. There seems to be a deeper complexity of basal ganglia interactions with motor and sensory systems not explainable by current models. This is emphasized by the influences of structures quite distant within the traditional cortical-basal ganglia—thalamic loop as well as structures outside this schema. It is likely that higher order properties of neuronal firing also contribute to motor programming and execution, which probably includes the firing pattern in addition to the rate. Moreover, synaptic plasticity within the cortical-basal ganglia—thalamic loop is likely involved in pathophysiological and restorative mechanisms of the movement disorders. The dynamics of somatosensory system maps are strongly implicated in dystonia; and plasticity in glutaminergic projections (13) may contribute to LIDs and parkinsonian symptoms.

REFERENCES

1. Aizawa H, Tanji J. Corticocortical and thalamocortical responses of neurons in the monkey primary motor cortex and their relation to a trained motor task. *J Neurophysiol* 1994;71:550–560.
2. Baron MS, Vitek JL, Bakay RA, et al. Treatment of advanced Parkinson's disease by posterior GPi pallidotomy: 1-year results of a pilot study. *Ann Neurol* 1996;40:355–666.
3. Bennett JPJ, Landow ER, Schuh LA. Suppression of dyskinesias in advanced Parkinson's disease. II. Increasing daily clozapine doses suppress dyskinesias and improve parkinsonism symptoms. *Neurology* 1993; 43:1551–1555.
4. Bergman H, Wichmann T, DeLong MR. Reversal of experimental parkinsonism by lesions of the subthalamic nucleus. *Science* 1990;249:1436–1438.
5. Bergman H, Wichmann T, Karmon B, DeLong MR. The primate subthalamic nucleus. II. Neuronal activity in the MPTP model of parkinsonism. *J Neurophysiol* 1994;72:507–520.
6. Beric A, Sterio D, Dogali M, Fazzini E, Eidelberg D, Kolodny E. Characteristics of pallidal neuronal dis-

charges in Parkinson's disease patients. *Adv Neurol* 1996;69:123–188.

7. Blanchet PJ, Boucher R, Bedard PJ. Excitotoxic lateral pallidotomy does not relieve L-dopa-induced dyskinesia in MPTP parkinsonian monkeys. *Brain Res* 1994;650:32–39.

8. Blanchet PJ, Metman LV, Mouradian MM, Chase TN. Acute pharmacologic blockade of dyskinesias in Parkinson's disease. *Mov Disord* 1996;11:580–581.

9. Brooks DJ. PET studies on the early and differential diagnosis of Parkinson's disease. *Neurology* 1993; 43:S6–S16.

10. Burke D, HagLarth KE, Wallin G. Reflex mechanisms in parkinsonian rigidity. *Scand J Rehabil Med* 1977; 9:15–23.

11. Burton K, Farrell K, Li D, Calne DB. Lesions of the putamen and dystonia: CT and magnetic resonance imaging. *Neurology* 1984;34:962–965.

12. Byl NN, Merzenich MM, Jenkins WM. A primate genesis model of focal dystonia and repetitive strain injury. I. Learning-induced dedifferentiation of the representation of the hand in the primary somatosensory cortex in adult monkeys. *Neurology* 1996;47:508–520.

13. Calabresi P, Pisani A, Mervuri NB, Bernardi G. The corticostriatal projection: from synaptic plasticity to dysfunctions of the basal gangla. *TINS* 1996;19:19–24.

14. Calon F, Goulet M, Blanchet PJ, et al. Levodopa or D2 agonist induced dyskinesia in MPTP monkeys: correlation with changes in dopamine and GABAA receptors in the striatopallidal complex. *Brain Res* 1995; 680:43–52.

15. Cardoso F, Jankovic J, Grossman RG, Hamilton W. Outcome after stereotactic thalamotomy for dystonia and hemiballismus. *Neurosurgery* 1995;36:501–508.

16. Ceballos-Baumann AO, Sheean G, Passingham RE, Marsden CD, Brooks DJ. Botulinum toxin does not reverse the cortical dysfunction associated with writer's cramp: a PET study. *Brain* 1997;120:571–582.

17. Chase TN, Baronti F, Fabbrini G, Heuser IJ, Juncos JL, Mouradian MM. Rationale for continuous dopaminomimetic therapy of Parkinson's disease. *Neurology* 1989;39[suppl 2]:7–10.

18. Chase TN, Engber TM, Mouradian MM. Contribution of dopaminergic and glutamatergic mechanisms to the pathogenesis of motor response complications in Parkinson's disease. *Adv Neurol* 1996;69:497–501.

19. DeLong MR. Primate models of movement disorders of basal ganglia origin. *TINS* 1990;13:281–285.

20. DeLong MR. Primate models of movement disorders of basal ganglia origin. *Trends Neurosci* 1990; 13:281–285.

21. DeLong MR, Coyle JT. Globus pallidus lesions in the monkey produced by kainic acid: histologic and behavioral effects. *Appl Neurophysiol* 1979;42:95–97.

22. DeLong MR, Georgopoulos AP, CrutcherMD, Mitchell SJ, Richardson RT, Alexander GE. Functional organization of the basal ganglia: contributions of single-cell recording studies. *Ciba Found Symp* 1984;107:64–82.

23. Delwaide PJ, Pepin JL, Maertens DN. Short-latency autogenic inhibition in patients with parkinsonian rigidity. *Ann Neurol* 1991;30:83–89.

24. Dick JP, Rothwell JC, Day BL, et al. The Bereitschafts potential is abnormal in Parkinson's disease. *Brain* 1989;112:233–244.

25. Dogali M, Fazzini E, Kolodny E, et al. Stereotactic ventral pallidotomy for Parkinson's disease. *Neurology* 1995;45:753–611.

26. Dogali M, Sterio D, Fazzini E, Kolodny E, Eidelberg D, Beric A. Effects of posteroventral pallidotomy on Parkinson's disease. *Adv Neurol* 1996;69:585–590.

27. Dooling EC, Adams RD. The pathological anatomy of posthemiplegic athetosis. *Brain* 1975;98:29–48.

28. Eidelberg D, Moeller JR, Ishikawa T, et al. Regional metabolic correlates of surgical outcome following unilateral pallidotomy for Parkinson's disease. *Ann Neurol* 1996;39:450–459.

29. Eidelberg D, Moeller JR, Ishikawa T, et al. The metabolic topography of idiopathic torsion dystonia. *Brain* 1995;118:1473–1484.

30. Engber TM, Boldry RC, Kuo S, Chase TN. Dopaminergic modulation of striatal neuropeptides: differential effects of D1 and D2 receptor stimulation on somatostatin, neuropeptide Y, neurotensin, dynorphin and enkephalin. *Brain Res* 1992;581:261–288.

31. Fabbrini G, Mouradian MM, Juncos JL, Schlegel J, Mohr E, Chase TN. Motor fluctuations in Parkinson's disease: central pathophysiological mechanisms. Part I. *Ann Neurol* 1988;24:366–371.

32. Favre J, Taha JM, Nguyen TT, Gildenberg PL, Burchiel KJ. Pallidotomy: a survey of current practice in North America. *Neurosurgery* 1996;39:883–890; discussion 890–892.

33. Fazzini E, Dogali M, Sterio D, Eidelberg D, Beric A. Stereotactic pallidotomy for Parkinson's disease: a long-term follow-up of unilateral pallidotomy. *Neurology* 1997;48:1273–1277.

34. Filion M, Tremblay L. Abnormal spontaneous activity of globus pallidus neurons in monkeys with MPTP-induced parkinsonism. *Brain Res* 1991;547:142–151.

35. Filion M, Tremblay L, Bedard PJ. Abnormal influences of passive limb movement on the activity of globus pallidus neurons in parkinsonian monkeys. *Brain Res* 1988;444:165–176.

36. Filion M, Tremblay L, Bedard PJ. Effects of dopamine agonists on the spontaneous activity of globus pallidus neurons in monkeys with MPTP-induced parkinsonism. *Brain Res* 1991;547:152–161.

37. Hallett M, Marsden CD. Ballistic flexion movements of the human thumb. *J Physiol (Lond)* 1979; 294:33–50.

38. Hazrati LN, Parent A. Striatal and subthalamic afferents to the primate pallidum: interactions between two opposite chemospecific neuronal systems. *Prog Brain Res* 1993;99:89–104.

39. Hassani OK, Mouroux M, Feger J. Increased subthalamic neuronal activity after nigral dopaminergic lesion independent of disinhibition via the globus pallidus. *Neuroscience* 1996;72:105–115.

40. Hedreen J, Martini LJ, Koliatsos VE, Hamada I, Alexander GE, DeLong MR. Organization of primate basal ganglia "motor circuit." 4. Ventrolateral thalamus links internal pallidum (GPi) and supplementary motor area (SMA). *Soc Neurosci Abstr* 1988;14:721 (abst).

41. Hirai T, Jones KG. A new parcellation of the human thalamus on the basis of histochemical staining. *Brain Res Rev* 1989;14:1–34.

42. Holsapple JW, Preston JB, Strick PL. The origin of thalamic input to the "hand" representation in the primary motor cortex. *J Neurosci* 1991;11:2644–2654.

43. Horak FB, Anderson ME. Influence of globus pallidus on arm movements in monkeys. I. Effects of kainic acid-induced lesions. *J Neurophysiol* 1984; 52:290–304.

44. Hore J, Vilis T. Arm movement performance during reversible basal ganglia lesions in the monkey. *Exp Brain Res* 1980;39:217–228.

45. Iacono RP, Shima F, Lonser RR, Kuniyoshi S, Maeda G, Yamada S. The results, indications, and physiology of posteroventral pallidotomy for patients with Parkinson's disease [see comments]. *Neurosurgery* 1995; 36:1118–1125, discussion 1125–1127.

46. Ikoma K, Samii A, Mercuri B, Wassermann EM, Hallett M. Abnormal cortical motor excitability in dystonia. *Neurology* 1996;46:1371–1376.

47. Inase M, Buford JA, Anderson ME. Changes in the control of arm position, movement, and thalamic discharge during local inactivation in the globus pallidus of the monkey. *J Neurophysiol* 1996;75:1087–1104.

48. Jahnsen H, Llinas R. Electrophysiological properties of guinea pig thalamic neurones: an in vitro study. *J Physiol (Lond)* 1984;349:205–226.

49. Jahnsen H, Llinas R. Ionic basis for the electroresponsiveness and oscillatory properties of guinea pig thalamic neurones in vitro. *J Physiol (Lond)* 1984; 349:247–349.

50. Jankovic J, Ondo WO, Lai E, Grossman RG. Pallidotomy for dystonia. *Ann Neurol* 1997;42:446–447.

51. Jasper HH, Bertrand G. Thalamic units involved in somatic sensation and voluntary and involuntary movements in man. In: Purpura DP, Yahr MD, eds. *The thalamus.* New York: Columbia University Press, 1966:365–390.

52. Johansson F, Malm J, Nordh E, Hariz M. Usefulness of pallidotomy in advanced Parkinson's disease. *J Neurol Neurosurg Psychiatry* 1997;62:125–132.

53. Kelly P, Gillingham FJ. Long-term results of stereotactic surgery and L-dopa therapy in patients with Parkinson's disease: a ten year follow-up study. *J Neurosurg* 1980;53:332–337.

54. Kim R, Nakano K, Jayaraman A, Carpenter MB. Projections of the globus pallidus and adjacent structures: an autoradiographic study in the monkey. *J Comp Neurol* 1976;169:263–289.

55. Kishore A, Turnbull IM, Snow BJ, et al. Efficacy, stability and predictors of outcome of pallidotomy for Parkinson's disease: six-month follow-up with additional 1-year observations. *Brain* 1997;120: 729–737.

56. Kotter R. Postsynaptic integration of glutamatergic and dopaminergic signals in the striatum. *Prog Neurobiol* 1994;44:163–196.

57. Krauss JK, Mundinger F. Functional stereotactic surgery for hemiballism. *J Neurosurg* 1996;85:278–286.

58. Kuo JS, Carpenter MB. Organization of pallidothalamic projections in rhesus monkey. *J Comp Neurol* 1973;151:201–236.

59. Laitinen LV, Bergenheim AT, Hariz MI. Ventroposterolateral pallidotomy can abolish all parkinsonian symptoms. *Stereotact Funct Neurosurg* 1992; 58:14–21.

60. LeDoux MS, Rutledge SL, Mountz JM, Darji JT. SPECT abnormalities in generalized dystonia. *Pediatr Neurol* 1995;13:5–10.

61. Leenders KL, Palmer AJ, Quinn N, et al. Brain dopamine metabolism in patients with Parkinson's disease measured with positron emission tomography. *J Neurol Neurosurg Psychiatry* 1986;49:853–860.

62. Leis AA, Dimitrijevic MR, Delapasse JS, Sharkey PC. Modification of cervical dystonia by selective sensory stimulation. *J Neurol Sci* 1992;110:79–89.

63. Lenz FA, Dostrovsky JO, Tasker RR, Yamashiro K, Kwan HC, Murphy JT. Single unit analysis of the human ventral thalamic nuclear group: correlation of thalamic "tremor cells" with the 3–6 Hz component of parkinsonian tremor. *J Neurosci* 1988;8:754–764.

64. Lenz FA, Seike M, Jaeger CJ, et al. Single unit analysis of thalamus in patients with dystonia. *Mov Disord* 1992;7:371 (abst).

65. Lenz FA, Suarez JI, Verhagen Metman SG, et al. *Ann Neurol* 1997 (*submitted*).

66. Levy R, Hazrati LN, Herrero MT, et al. Re-evaluation of the functional anatomy of the basal ganglia in normal and parkinsonian states. *Neuroscience* 1997; 76:335–343.

67. Marconi R, LefeLvre-Caparros D, Bonnet AM, Vidailhet M, Dubois B, Agid Y. Levodopa-induced dyskinesias in Parkinson's disease: phenomenology and pathophysiology. *Mov Disord* 1994;9:2–12.

68. Marsden CD, Obeso JA, Zarranz JJ, Lang AK. The anatomical basis of symptomatic hemidystonia. *Brain* 1985;108:463–483.

69. Marsden CD, Rothwell JC. The physiology of idiopathic dystonia. *Can J Neurol Sci* 1987;14[suppl]: 521–577.

70. McCormick DA, Feeser HR. Functional implications of burst firing and single spike activity in lateral geniculate relay neurons. *Neuroscience* 1990;39:103–113.

71. Miller WC, DeLong MR. Parkinsonian symptomatology: an anatomical and physiological analysis. *Ann NY Acad Sci* 1988;515:287–302.

72. Mink JW, Thach WT. Basal ganglia motor control. III. Pallidal ablation: normal reaction time, muscle cocontraction, and slow movement. *J Neurophysiol* 1991; 65:330–351.

73. Mitchell IJ, Boyce S, Sambrook MA, Crossman AR. A 2-deoxyglucose study of the effects of dopamine agonists on the parkinsonian primate brain. *Brain* 1992; 115:809–824.

74. Mouradian MM, Heuser IJ, Baronti F, Chase TN. Modification of central dopaminergic mechanisms by continuous levodopa therapy for advanced Parkinson's disease. *Ann Neurol* 1990;27:18–23.

75. Mouradian MM, Heuser IJ, Baronti F, Fabbrini G, Juncos J, Chase TN. Pathogenesis of dyskinesias in Parkinson's disease. *Ann Neurol* 1989;25:523–526.

76. Narbona J, Obeso JA, Tunon T, Martinez-Lage JM, Marsden CD. Hemi-dystonia secondary to localised basal ganglia tumour. *J Neurol Neurosurg Psychiatry* 1984;47:704–709.

77. Nini A, Feingold A, Slovin H, Bergman H. Neurons in the globus pallidus do not show correlated activity in the normal monkey, but phase-locked oscillations appear in the MPTP model of parkinsonism. *J Neurophysiol* 1995;74:1800–1805.

78. Nudo RJ, Milliken GW, Jenkins WM, Merzenich MM. Use dependent alterations of movement representations in primary motor cortex of adult squirrel monkeys. *J Neurosci* 1996;16:785–807.

79. Nutt JG. On-off phenomenon: relation to levodopa pharmacokinetics and pharmacodynamics. *Ann Neurol* 1987;22:535–540.

80. Ohye C, Hirai T, Miyazaki M, Shibazaki T, Nakajima H. Vim thalamotomy for the treatment of various kinds of tremor. *Appl Neurophysiol* 1982;45:275–280.

81. Oyesika N, Mandir AS, Bakay RA, Freeman A, Watts RL. Stereotactic thalamotomy for Parkinson's disease: quantitative assessment of tremor and bradykinesia before and after surgery. Presented at the Congress of Neurological Surgeons, 1991 (abst).

82. Papa SM, Chase TN. Levodopa-induced dyskinesias improved by a glutamate antagonist in parkinsonian monkeys [see comments]. *Ann Neurol* 1996; 39:574–578.

83. Penney JB, Young AB. GABA as the pallidothalamic neurotransmitter: implications for basal ganglia function. *Brain Res* 1981;207:195–199.

84. Pettigrew LC, Jankovic J. Hemidystonia: a report of 22 patients and a review of the literature. *J Neurol* 1985; 48:650–657.

85. Playford ED, Jenkins IH, Passingham RE, Nutt J, Frackowiak RS, Brooks DJ. Impaired mesial frontal and putamen activation in Parkinson's disease: a positron emission tomography study. *Ann Neurol* 1992;32:151–161.

86. Pollack LJ, Davis L. Muscle tone in parkinsonian states. *Arch Neurol Psychiatry* 1930;23:303–319.

87. Porrino LJ, Burns RS, Crane AM, Palombo E, Kopin IJ, Sokoloff L. Local cerebral metabolic effects of L-dopa therapy in 1 methyl-4-phenyl-1,2,3,6- tetrahydropyridine induced parkinsonism in monkeys. *Proc Natl Acad Sci USA* 1987;84:5995–5999.

88. Rack PM, Ross HF. The role of reflexes in the resting tremor of Parkinson's disease. *Brain* 1986;109:115–141.

89. Renou G, Rondot P, Bathien N. Influence of peripheral stimulation on the silent period between bursts of parkinsonian tremor. In: Desmedt JE, ed. *New developments electromyography and clinical neurophysiology.* Basel: Karger, 1973:635–640.

90. Rothwell JC, Obeso JA, Troub MM, Marsden CD. The behaviour of long-lotenage stretch reflex in patients with Parkinson's disease. *J Neurol Neurosurg Psychiatry* 1983;46:35–44.

91. Ryan LJ, Clark KB. Alteration of neuronal responses in the subthalamic nucleus) following globus pallidus and neostriatal lesions in rats. *Brain Res Bull* 1992; 29:319–327.

92. Schnider SM, Kwong RH, Kwan HC, Lenz FA. Detection of feedback in the central nervous system of parkinsonian patients. *Biol Cybern* 1989;60:203–212.

93. Schwartzman RJ, Alexander GM, Ferraro TN, Grothusen JR, Stahl SM. Cerebral metabolism of parkinsonian primates 21 days after MPTP. *Exp Neurol* 1988;102:307–313.

94. Shibasaki H, Shima F, Kuroiwa Y. Clinical studies of the movement related cortical potential and the relationship between the dentatorubrothalamic pathway and readiness potential. *J Neurol* 1978;219:15–25.

95. Simpson JA, Khuraibet AJ. Readiness potential of cortical area 6 preceding self paced movement in Parkinson's disease. *J Neurol Neurosurg Psychiatry* 1987; 50:1184–1191.

96. Smith Y, Parent A. Neurons of the subthalamic nucleus in primates display glutamate but not GABA immunoreactivity. *Brain Res* 1988;453:353–356.

97. Spencer SE, Wooten GF, Altered pharmaco kinetics of L-dopa metabolism in rat striatum deprived of dopaminergia innervation. *Neurology* 1984;34: 1105–1188.

98. Stein R B, Lee RG. Tremor and clonus. In: Brooks UB, ed. *Handbook of Physiology.* Sect. I: *Nervous system.* Vol II: *Motor control part II.* Bethesda: American Physiological Society, 1981:325–343.

99. Stein R B, Oguztoreli MN. Tremor and other oscillations in neuromuscular systems. *Biol Cybern* 1976; 22:147–157.

100. Sterio D, Beric A, Dogali M, Fazzini E, Alfaro G, Devinsky O. Neurophysiological properties of pallidal neurons in Parkinson's disease. Ann Neurol 1994; 35:586–591.

101. Strick PL. Anatomical analysis of ventrolateral thalamic input to primate motor cortex. *J Neurophysiol* 1976;39:1020–1031.

102. Suarez JI, Verhagen-Metman L, Reich SG, Dougherty PM, Hallett M, Lenz FA. Pallidotomy for hemiballismus: efficacy and characteristics of neuronal activity. *Ann Neurol* 1997 (*in press*).

103. Svennilson E, Torvik A, Lowe R, Leksell L. Treatment of parkinsonism by stereotactic thermolesions in the pallidal region. *Acta Psychiatr Neurol Scand* 1960; 35:358–377.

104. Taha JM, Favre J, Baumann TK, Burchiel KJ. Tremor control after pallidotomy in patients with Parkinson's disease: correlation with microrecording findings. *J Neurosurg* 1997;86:642–647.

105. Tasker R R, Siqueira J, Hawrylyshyn PA, Organ LW. What happened to VIM thalamotomy for Parkinson's disease? *Appl Neurophysiol* 1983;46:68–83.

106. Tatton WG, Bedingham W, Verrier MC, Blair RD. Characteristic alterations in repsonses to imposed wrist displacements in parkinsonian rigidity and dystonia musculorum deformans. *J Can Sci Neurol* 1984; 11:281–287.

107. Teravainen H, Evarts E, Calne D. Effects of kinesthetic inputs on parkinsonian tremor. *Adv Neurol* 1979; 24:161–173.

108. Tsubokawa T, Katayama Y, Yamamoto T. Control of persistent hemiballismus by chronic thalamic stimulation: report of two cases. *J Neurosurg* 1995; 82: 501–505.

109. Vila M, Herrero MT, Levy R, et al. Consequences of nigrostriatal denervation on the gamma-aminobutyric acidic neurons of substantia nigra pars reticulate and superior colliculus in parkinsonian syndromes. *Neurology* 1996;46:802–809.

110. Vila M, Levy R, Herrero MT, et al. Metabolic activity of the basal ganglia in parkinsonian syndromes in human and nonhuman primates: a cytochrome oxidase histochemistry study. *Neuroscience* 1996; 71:903–912.

111. Vitek JL, Ashe J, DeLong MR, Alexander GE. Altered somatosensory response properties of neurons in the "motor" thalamus of MPTP treated parkinsonian monkeys. *Soc Neurosci Abstr* 1990;16:425 (abst).

112. Vitek JL, Evatt M, Zhang J, et al. Pallidotomy as a treatment for medically intractable dystonia. *Ann Neurol* 1997;42:409–442.

113. Vitek JL, Kaneoke Y, Turner R, Baron M, Bakay R, DeLong MR. Neuronal activity in the internal (GPi) and external (GPe) segments of the globus pallidus (GP) of parkinsonian patients is similar to that in the MPTP-treated primate model of parkinsonism. *Soc Neurosci Abstr* 1993;19:1584 (abst).

114. Watts RL, Mandir AS. The role of motor cortex in the pathophysiology of voluntary movement deficits associated with parkinsonism. *Neurol Clin* 1992; 10:451–469.

115. Watts RL, Mandir AS, Montgomery EB. Neuronal, kinematic and electromyographic characterization of self- and stimulus-initiated motor tasks in normal and MPTP parkinsonian nonhuman primates. *Soc Neurosci Abst* 1990;16:115 (abst).

116. Young AB, Penney JB. Neurochemical anatomy of movement disorders. *Neurol Clin* 1984;2:417–433.

117. Zirh TA, Lenz FA, Reich SG, Dougherty PM. Patterns of bursting occurring in thalamic cells during parkinsonian tremor. Neuroscience (*in press*).

Pallidal Surgery for the Treatment of Parkinson's Disease and Movement Disorders, edited by J. K. Krauss, R. G. Grossman, and J. Jankovic. Lippincott-Raven Publishers, Philadelphia © 1998.

5

Parkinson's Disease

William G. Ondo and Joseph Jankovic

Department of Neurology, Baylor College of Medicine, Houston, Texas 77030, USA

The disease that would eventually bear his name was first described by James Parkinson in 1817 (302), when he described six people with slowness of movement (bradykinesia), slow shuffling gaits with postural instability, and tremor. Rigidity, the remaining cardinal feature of Parkinson's disease (PD), was not included in his initial description because Parkinson did not examine most of the people he described; rather, he observed them from a distance in various cafes and other public gathering areas.

EPIDEMIOLOGY

Although numerous epidemiological studies of PD have failed in their goal to identify the cause of PD, they have resulted in a wealth of detailed demographic data. The reported incidence of PD has ranged from 4.5/100,000 to 21/100,000 cases per year (12,134,141,325,340). Although the true incidence is the best determinant of disease frequency, several factors make this parameter difficult to determine for PD. First, early PD is often not recognized or is misdiagnosed. Conversely, some cases diagnosed as PD evolve into other parkinsonian conditions. Second, there may be a long preclinical period prior to symptom onset; and third, PD is a disease of later life. Therefore the incidence becomes a function of the age demographics for any population.

The estimated prevalence of PD ranges from 18/100,000 to 328/100,000 cases per year in the general population (23,48,70,244,249,266,272, 281,361,372,395). The prevalence in the geriatric population (age > 65 years) is usually cited at more than 1%, making PD one of the most common neurological diseases of the elderly.

Although not a consistent finding, PD appears to be slightly more common in men. The condition is found worldwide, but it is reported more commonly in European whites than in Asians and least commonly in Africans, even when examining mixed ancestry populations in the United States (184,330,351). Prevalence studies suffer from a variety of ascertainment biases; therefore these epidemiological data represent only best estimates.

Parkinson's disease is clearly diagnosed more often now than earlier in the century. The population incidence, however, has probably not increased significantly (61). Therefore the increasing frequency may be due to improved diagnostic skills, older population demographics, or both. Likewise, data on PD-associated mortality are difficult to interpret, as few patients die directly from their PD. The preponderance of data suggests that PD moderately shortens the life-span. Louis et al. reported that PD patients had a mortality risk of 2.7 compared to nondemented age-matched elderly controls (229). Mortality from PD decreased after the introduction of levodopa (408), but more recently seems to have remained relatively constant (68). In fact, absolute PD-associated mortality has increased recently, but it may be due to the older age of the PD population and improvements in the treatment of other conditions, a mortality "ceiling" effect (23).

The various modes of onset and clinical subtypes of PD carry different prognoses. Patients who present with prominent tremor seem to experience less morbidity, slower disease progression, and a longer life-span than those who present with postural instability and gait disorder (PIGD) (326). A large number of PIGD patients, however, do not meet the pathological criteria for PD, so this may represent a separate disease process. Other predictors of mortality include an older age at disease onset, dementia, and autonomic dysfunction (87).

Symptom onset is typically between the ages of 50 and 60. Most investigators suspect that early-onset PD (age < 40 years) represents one end of the normal distribution spectrum of age at onset. There are, however, several distinguishing clinical characteristics between young-onset and older-onset PD. Young-onset PD more commonly presents with appendicular dystonia. The initial response to levodopa is more robust but quickly results in levodopa-induced motor complications, especially dyskinesias (126,169, 195). This presents a particular treatment dilemma, as these patients often demand more aggressive pharmacological treatment to maintain work proficiency.

CLINICAL FEATURES

The diagnosis of PD is based on clinical symptoms and neurological examination. Onset is typically unilateral, but the contralateral side usually becomes involved within 6 months. Rest tremor is the presenting complaint in about 70% of patients at the time of initial diagnosis, although most of these patients have concurrent rigidity and hypokinesia that may be subtle. Rest tremor occurs in a position that does not require volitional muscle contraction. It may be first noticed during the passive arm swing of walking. The tremor typically begins in the thumb as a pill-rolling motion before spreading to include other fingers and the wrist. Eventually the entire arm, leg, and perioral muscles can be involved. The tremor occurs at a uniform frequency throughout the body, usually at 4 to 5 Hz. Head tremor (oscillating at the neck) and voice tremors rarely occur with PD, and their presence suggests essential tremor (ET). Many PD patients also demonstrate postural tremor.

This may be clinically and electrophysiologically similar to either ET or enhanced physiological tremor (PT), and it may respond to ET treatments such as β-blockers and primidone (147,189,199,382). Because of its low amplitude, the postural tremor of PD usually causes little functional disability. Some patients, however, also demonstrate a large-amplitude postural tremor that typically begins shortly after a new static position is achieved—hence the term reemergent tremor—and crescendos in amplitude for several more seconds. This reemergent postural tremor has the same frequency as the rest tremor and, similar to rest tremor, responds to levodopa; it is considered a postural form of rest tremor. The exact relation between rest tremor and the various types of postural tremor associated with PD, however, remains unclear.

The rigidity of PD is usually termed "cogwheel" because upon passive movement the limbs demonstrate rhythmic resistance at a frequency of about 6 to 10 Hz. Therefore the rigidity is probably not a passive manifestation of the 4 to 5-Hz rest tremor, as was long assumed. Unlike spasticity, the rigidity of PD is seen equally during flexion and extension, is not velocity-dependent, and is not associated with any pathological reflexes. In other cases, patients demonstrate a more constant "lead pipe" rigidity. Axial rigidity is also present and may account for much of the subjective neck and back pain that accompanies PD. Volitional muscle contraction of the contralateral limb may be required to unmask subtle rigidity.

Bradykinesia and hypokinesia are the most common and characteristic findings in PD. They are best demonstrated by rapid distal movements such as finger and foot tapping. Patients may begin these tasks at a normal speed but typically decrease both velocity and amplitude until they "reset" the task at a higher frequency and larger amplitude. This is distinct from pyramidal motor disorders, where motor speed is uniformly slower and the amplitude does not decrease. Functionally, bradykinesia often manifests as small writing (micrographia) or difficulty with buttoning. The absence of facial expression seen with PD (hypomimia) is due to both bradykinesia and rigidity in the muscles of facial expression. Drooling is attributed to slowed swallowing, rather than increased saliva production (15).

Gait abnormalities often manifest initially with asymmetrically diminished arm swing. The steps then become shorter and begin to take on a shuffling characteristic. Patients may look as though they are constantly falling forward and trying to reestablish their center of gravity (festination). They may later develop leg "freezing" or "motor blocks," which most commonly occurs while initiating the first step (start hesitation) and while turning. Freezing may be overcome by a variety of visual cues and self-imposed physical maneuvers that require the patient to lift the foot consciously and propel it forward. Common "tricks" to overcome freezing include stepping over real or imagined objects and marching rhythmically in cadence.

Stooped posture is another common feature of PD. Patients who have prolonged unilateral involvement may also develop scoliosis and unilateral paraspinal hypertrophy on the contralateral side. Other orthopedic complications include ulnar deviation of the digits and flexion of the metacarpophalangeal joints (striatal hand).

A variety of autonomic symptoms and signs often accompany PD. Many patients develop autonomic symptoms, including constipation, erectile dysfunction, urinary urgency and nocturia, and symptomatic orthostasis. Constipation is reported by most PD patients. Although it is often ascribed to medication use, de novo patients consistently demonstrate slowed gastrointestinal transport time, and pathological degeneration of the myenteric plexus (180). Urinary urgency and nocturia are also frequent complaints. Cystographic studies demonstrate detrusor hyperreflexia in 90% of PD patients (20,33). Other common cystographic findings of PD include desynchronized external sphincter activity during detrusor contractions, an inability to relax the external sphincter at the onset of voiding, and impaired detrusor contractility. Orthostatic hypotension occurs in most PD patients and may be complicated by medical treatment (116). Sexual dysfunction results from both diminished libido and pure autonomic dysfunction (308). It should be noted that excessive autonomic symptoms suggest a diagnosis other than that of idiopathic PD (see Multiple System Atrophy, below).

Depression occurs in many PD patients (129). Initially it may resemble bradyphrenia (slowed thought processing), but careful questioning demonstrates symptoms typical of idiopathic depression: fluctuating mood and changes in appetite and sleep. Depression should be specifically queried, as it responds to antidepressant medications. Sleep disturbances are common with PD. Patients have difficulty both achieving and maintaining sleep. The etiology of this problem is multifactorial and includes nocturia, depression, medication "wearing off," and akinesia. Rapid eye movement (REM) behavioral disorder has been shown to be a risk factor for the subsequent development of PD (349).

Although bradyphrenia and facial hypomimia often combine to give a demented appearance, cognitive function is only mildly affected until late in the course of PD. Patients may demonstrate mild deficits in executive function, attention set shifting difficulties, and visuospatial relations (216). Language is almost always preserved, although patients may experience a form of anomia called "tip-of-the-tongue" phenomenon (243). This pattern of dementia is often referred to as subcortical. The presence of marked dementia is suggestive of other parkinsonian diseases (see Dementia with Lewy Bodies, below).

Patients with PD frequently report nonspecific visual complaints. A specific pattern of diminished contrast sensitivity that is not elicited by normal visual acuity testing is common (31,73, 142,143,159,322) and may respond to dopaminergic treatment (158,242,254). The pathophysiological substrate resulting in the condition is unknown but may involve dopaminergic neurons in the retina. Oculomotor function is relatively preserved in PD patients except for limitation of upward gaze, which may be an age-related phenomenon. Spontaneous eye blink frequency is reduced, and patients may demonstrate a Meyerson's (glabellar) sign in which eye blinking elicited from tapping between the eyes does not extinguish with repeated tapping.

Olfactory function is typically impaired with PD, even in the early stages (81,218,367). Although patients seldom subjectively complain of anosmia, both smell discrimination and sensitivity are dramatically reduced compared to those of controls. The severity of anosmia does not correlate with the duration, severity, subtype, or treatment of PD (80,81). The anterior olfactory nucleus in PD patients shows significant cell loss and Lewy bodies (309). Interestingly, olfaction is relatively spared in other parkinsonian diseases and may even be used as a diagnostic tool for PD (81,405).

Weight loss is almost always present in PD. Patients generally lose 5 to 10 kg, often early in the course of the disease. The etiology of this weight loss is unclear. A variety of theories, including increased caloric expenditure secondary to increased rigidity or levodopa-induced dyskinesia and diminished caloric intake secondary to diminished appetite or dysphagia (or both), have been proposed, but none has been consistently substantiated (1,183,215,237,386). Other possibilities include hypothalamic dysfunction, diminished olfactory acuity, or the effects of elevated central nervous system (CNS) tumor necrosis factor-alpha (TNFα) (170,262), which is associated with weight loss in other conditions, such as acquired immuno deficiency syndrome (AIDS). Interestingly, patients gain weight shortly after pallidotomy (200,287). This weight gain correlates only with improved "off" motor scores and therefore is probably not due to reduced dyskinesia or improved bulbar function (287).

Finally, many PD patients develop chronic seborrhea, often on their forehead. The pathogenesis of this dermatological finding is unknown.

PARKINSON'S DISEASE
RATING SCALES

A variety of quantified timed tests for dexterity and speed, measures of rigidity, accelerometry testing, computerized posturography, and a variety of cognitive test batteries are employed to test the severity of the PD (167,400). Clinical scales, however, most reliably demonstrate disability associated with PD (47,93,205,354,401,414). The most widely used scale is the Unified Parkinson's Disease Rating Scale (UPDRS) (Fig. 5-1) (see also Chapter 8). The latest version is divided into six sections. The first section briefly evalu-

ates mental status, the second reports on subjective activities of daily living, the third is a motor examination, the fourth concerns treatment complications, the fifth is the Hoehn and Yahr scale, and the sixth is the Schwab and England activities of daily living scale.

ATYPICAL PARKINSONISM

Idiopathic PD is the most common form of parkinsonism. Several conditions share some clinical similarities with PD but have different pathologies, prognosis, treatment responses, and probably etiologies (Table 5-1). No definitive diagnostic tests are available, so a careful history and neurological examination are required to differentiate these conditions. The correct diagnosis is particularly important when surgery is considered because the atypical parkinsonian disorders do not respond to pallidotomy.

Progressive Supranuclear Palsy

Progressive supranuclear palsy (PSP) (Steele-Richardson-Olszewski syndrome) constitutes up to 6% of all parkinsonian cases and has an overall estimated prevalence of 1/100,000 to 2/100,000 (118). Onset of symptoms is typically during the seventh decade, somewhat later than for PD (118,168). The range of age at onset is narrower than for PD. Patients younger than 55 or older than 75 at onset are rare. The condition may be more common in men. Death from disease complications (aspiration pneumonia, sequelae of immobility, or falls) usually occurs within 6 to 10 years after symptom onset (224).

At least 60% of patients with PSP present with gait disturbances and unexplained falls (168,222,223). Gait in PSP differs from that of PD in that: (a) arms are not flexed and arm swing is relatively preserved; (b) patients attempt to walk quickly with apparent disregard for falls, rather than slowly and cautiously; and (c) patients typically turn quickly by pivoting on their heels rather than taking numerous small steps (en block turns), resulting in frequent backward falls that often result in serious injury. Patients are typically wheelchair-bound within 5 years from symptom onset.

Unified Parkinson's Disease Rating Scale

I. Mentation, Behavior and Mood

1. Intellectual Impairment
0 = None.
1 = Mild. Consistent forgetfulness with partial recollection of events and no other difficulties.
2 = Moderate memory loss, with disorientation and moderate difficulty handling complex problems. Mild but definite impairment of function at home with need of occasional prompting.
3 = Severe memory loss with disorientation for time and often to place. Severe impairment in handling problems.
4 = Severe memory loss with orientation preserved to person only. Unable to make judgements or solve problems. Requires much help with personal care. Cannot be left alone at all.

2. Thought Disorder *(Due to dementia or drug intoxication.)*
0 = None.
1 = Vivid dreaming.
2 = "Benign" hallucinations with insight retained.
3 = Occasional to frequent hallucinations or delusions; without insight; could interfere with daily activities.
4 = Persistent hallucinations, delusions, or florid psychosis. Not able to care for self.

3. Depression
0 = Not present.
1 = Periods of sadness or guilt greater than normal, never sustained for days or weeks.
2 = Sustained depression (1 week or more).
3 = Sustained depression with vegetative symptoms (insomnia, anorexia, weight loss, loss of interest).
4 = Sustained depression with vegetative symptoms and suicidal thoughts or intent.

4. Motivation/Initiative
0 = Normal.
1 = Less assertive than usual; more passive.
2 = Loss of initiative or disinterest in elective (non-routine) activities.
3 = Loss of initiative or disinterest in day to day (routine) activities.
4 = Withdrawn, complete loss of motivation.

II. Activities of Daily Living *(For both "on" and "off.")*

5. Speech
0 = Normal.
1 = Mildly affected. No difficulty being understood.
2 = Moderately affected. Sometimes asked to repeat statements.
3 = Severely affected. Frequently asked to repeat statements.
4 = Unintelligible most of the time.

6. Salivation
0 = Normal.
1 = Slight but definite excess of saliva in mouth; may have nighttime drooling.
2 = Moderately excessive saliva; may have minimal drooling.
3 = Marked excess of saliva with some drooling.
4 = Marked drooling, requires constant tissue or handkerchief.

7. Swallowing
0 = Normal.
1 = Rare choking.
2 = Occasional choking.
3 = Requires soft food.
4 = Requires NG tube or gastrostomy feeding.

8. Handwriting
0 = Normal.
1 = Slightly slow or small.
2 = Moderately slow or small; all words are legible.
3 = Severely affected; not all words are legible.
4 = The majority of words are not legible.

9. Cutting food and handling utensils
0 = Normal.
1 = Somewhat slow and clumsy, but no help needed.
2 = Can cut most foods, although clumsy and slow; some help needed.
3 = Food must be cut by someone, but can still feed slowly.
4 = Needs to be fed.

10. Dressing
0 = Normal.
1 = Somewhat slow, but no help needed.
2 = Occasional assistance with buttoning, getting arms in sleeves.
3 = Considerable help required, but can do some things alone.
4 = Helpless.

11. Hygiene
0 = Normal.
1 = Somewhat slow, but no help needed.
2 = Needs help to shower or bathe; or very slow in hygienic care.
3 = Requires assistance for washing, brushing teeth, combing hair, going to bathroom.
4 = Foley catheter or other mechanical aids.

12. Turning in bed and adjusting bed clothes
0 = Normal.
1 = Somewhat slow and clumsy, but no help needed.
2 = Can turn alone or adjust sheets, but with great difficulty.
3 = Can initiate, but not turn or adjust sheets alone.
4 = Helpless.

13. Falling *(Unrelated to freezing.)*
0 = None.
1 = Rare falling.
2 = Occasionally falls, less than once per day.
3 = Falls an average of once daily.
4 = Falls more than once daily.

14. Freezing when walking
0 = None.
1 = Rare freezing when walking; may have start-hesitation.
2 = Occasional freezing when walking.
3 = Frequent freezing. Occasionally falls from freezing.
4 = Frequent falls from freezing.

15. Walking
0 = Normal.
1 = Mild difficulty. May not swing arms or may tend to drag leg.
2 = Moderate difficulty, but requires little or no assistance.
3 = Severe disturbance of walking, requiring assistance.
4 = Cannot walk at all, even with assistance.

16. Tremor *(Symptomatic complaint of tremor in any part of body.)*
0 = Absent.
1 = Slight and infrequently present.
2 = Moderate; bothersome to patient.
3 = Severe; interferes with many activities.
4 = Marked; interferes with most activities.

17. Sensory complaints related to parkinsonism
0 = None.
1 = Occasionally has numbness, tingling, or mild aching.
2 = Frequently has numbness, tingling, or aching; not distressing.
3 = Frequent painful sensations.
4 = Excruciating pain.

III. Motor Examination

18. Speech
0 = Normal.
1 = Slight loss of expression, diction and/or volume.
2 = Monotone, slurred but understandable; moderately impaired.
3 = Marked impairment, difficult to understand.
4 = Unintelligible.

19. Facial Expression
0 = Normal.
1 = Minimal hypomimia, could be normal "Poker Face".
2 = Slight but definitely abnormal diminution of facial expression
3 = Moderate hypomimia; lips parted some of the time.
4 = Masked or fixed facies with severe or complete loss of facial expression; lips parted 1/4 inch or more.

20. Tremor at rest
0 = Absent.
1 = Slight and infrequently present.
2 = Mild in amplitude and persistent. Or moderate in amplitude, but only intermittently present.
3 = Moderate in amplitude and present most of the time.
4 = Marked in amplitude and present most of the time.

21. Action or Postural Tremor of hands
0 = Absent.
1 = Slight; present with action.
2 = Moderate in amplitude, present with action.
3 = Moderate in amplitude with posture holding as well as action.
4 = Marked in amplitude; interferes with feeding.

22. Rigidity *(Judged on passive movement of major joints with patient relaxed in sitting position; ignore cogwheeling.)*
0 = Absent.
1 = Slight or detectable only when activated by mirror or other movements.
2 = Mild to moderate.
3 = Marked, but full range of motion easily achieved.
4 = Severe, range of motion achieved with difficulty.

23. Finger Taps *(Patient taps thumb with index finger in rapid succession with widest amplitude possible, each hand separately.)*
0 = Normal.
1 = Mild slowing and/or reduction in amplitude.
2 = Moderately impaired. Definite and early fatiguing. May have occasional arrests in movement.
3 = Severely impaired. Frequent hesitation in initiating movements or arrests in ongoing movement.

FIG. 5-1. Modified Unified Parkinson's disease rating scale.

4 = Can barely perform the task.

24. **Hand Movements** *[Patient opens and closes hands In rapid succession with widest amplitude possible, each hand separately.]*
0 = Normal.
1 = Mild slowing and/or reduction in amplitude.
2 = Moderately impaired. Definite and early fatiguing. May have occasional arrests in movement.
3 = Severely impaired. Frequent hesitation in initiating movements or arrests in ongoing movement.
4 = Can barely perform the task.

25. **Rapid Alternating Movements of Hands** *[Pronation-supination movements of hands, vertically or horizontally, with as large an amplitude as possible, each hand separately.]*
0 = Normal.
1 = Mild slowing and/or reduction in amplitude.
2 = Moderately impaired. Definite and early fatiguing. May have occasional arrests in movement.
3 = Severely impaired. Frequent hesitation in initiating movements br arrests in ongoing movement.
4 = Can barely perform the task.

26. **Leg Agility** *[Patient taps heel on ground in rapid succession, picking up entire leg. Amplitude should be about 3 Inches.]*
0 = Normal.
1 = Mild slowing and/or reduction in amplitude.
2 = Moderately impaired. Definite and early fatiguing. May have occasional arrests in movement.
3 = Severely impaired. Frequent hesitation in initiating movements or arrests inongoing movement.
4 = Can barely perform the task.

27. **Arising from chair** *[Patient attempts to arise from a straight-back wood or metal chair with arms folded across chest.]*
0 = Normal.
1 = Slow; or may need more than one attempt.
2 = Pushes self up from arms of seat.
3 = Tends to fall back and may have to try more than one time, but can get up without help.
4 = Unable to arise without help.

28. **Posture**
0 = Normal erect.
1 = Not quite erect, slightly stooped posture; could be normal for older person.
2 = Moderately stooped posture, definitely abnormal; can be slightly leaning to one side.
3 = Severely stooped posture with kyphosis; can be moderately leaning to one side.
4 = Marked flexion with extreme abnormality of posture.

29. **Gait**
0 = Normal.
1 = Walks slowly, may shuffle with short steps, but no festination (hastening steps) or propulsion.
2 = Walks with difficulty, but requires little or no assistance; may have some festination, short steps, or propulsion.
3 = Severe disturbance of gait, requiring assistance.
4 = Cannot walk at all, even with assistance.

30. **Postural Stability** *[Response to sudden, strong posterior displacement produced by pull on shoulders while patient erect with eyes open and feet slightly apart. Patient is prepared, and can have had some practice runs.]*
0 = Normal.
1 = Retropulsion, but recovers unaided.
2 = Absence of postural response; would fall if not caught by examiner.
3 = Very unstable, tends to lose balance spontaneously.
4 = Unable to stand without assistance.

31. **Body Bradykinesia and Hypokinesia** *[Combining slowness, hesitancy, decreased armswing, small amplitude, and poverty of movement in general.]*
0 = None.
1 = Minimal slowness, giving movement a deliberate character; could be normal for some persons. Possibly reduced amplitude.
2 = Mild degree of slowness and poverty of movement which is definitely abnormal. Alternatively, some reduced amplitude.
3 = Moderate slowness, poverty or small amplitude of movement.
4 = Marked slowness, poverty or small amplitude of movement.

IV. Complications of Therapy *[In the past week.]*

A. DYSKINESIAS

32. **Duration: What proportion of the waking day are dyskineslas present?** *[Historical information.]*
0 = None
1 = 1–25% of day.
2 = 26–50% of day.
3 = 51–75% of day.
4 = 76–100% of day.

33. **Disability: How disabling are the dyskineslas?** *[Historical Information; may be modified by office examination.]*
0 = Not disabling.
1 = Mildly disabling.
2 = Moderately disabling.
3 = Severely disabling.
4 = Completely disabled.

34. **Painful Dyskinesias: How painful are the dyskinesias?**
0 = No painful dyskinesias.
1 = Slight.
2 = Moderate.
3 = Severe.
4 = Marked.

35. **Presence of Early Morning Dystonia** *[Historical information.]*
0 = No
1 = Yes

B. CLINICAL FLUCTUATIONS

36. **Are any "off" periods predictable as to timing after a dose of medication?**
0 = No
1 = Yes

37. **Are any "off" periods unpredictable as to timing after a dose of medication?**
0 = No
1 = Yes

38. **Do any of the "off" periods come on suddenly, e.g., over a few seconds?**
0 = No
1 = Yes

39. **What proportion of the waking day is the patient "off" on average?**
0 = None
1 = 1–25% of day.
2 = 26–50% of day.
3 = 51–75% of day.
4 = 76–100% of day.

FIG. 5-1. (*Continued*)

The PSP patients typically exhibit severe bulbar symptoms (178). Their speech is dysarthric and associated with impaired guttural sounds, voice spasticity, and reduced ability to modulate volume. This contrasts to the voice of PD patients, which is typically hypophonic (reduced volume). Dysphagia becomes severe and contributes significantly to morbidity and mortality.

Tremor is uncommon in PSP patients but may occur early in the course of their illness. Along with bradykinesia, rigidity, and a moderate early levodopa response, such a tremor often results in the misdiagnosis of PD. The most reliable factors that differentiate PSP from PD include a history of falls early in the disease, oculomotor abnormalities, and a poor levodopa response (222,223). Computerized posturography may also aid the diagnosis (288). PSP patients have significantly worse limits of stability and significantly lower percentages of maximum stability in conditions that limit visual and proprioception when compared to patients with PD.

TABLE 5-1. *Clinical comparison of parkinsonian conditions*

Characteristic	Parkinson's disease	Progressive supranuclear palsy	Multiple system atrophy	Dementia with Lewy bodies	Cortico-basal degeneration	Vascular Parkinsonism	Drug-induced Parkinson's
Unilateral onset	++	—	—	—	+++	—	—
Rest tremor	+++	+	+	++	+	+	++
Action tremor	+	+	+	+	++	+	++
Rigidity	+++	++	++	++	+++	+	++
Bradykinesia	+++	+	++	++	++	+	+++
Gait problems	+	+++	++	+	+++	+++	+
Oculomotor dysfunction	+	+++	++	+	++	++	—
Blepharospasm	—	+++	+	+	++	+	—
Cognitive decline	+	+++	+	+++	++	++	+
Autonomic dysfunction	+	+	+++	++	+	++	—
Dystonia	+	++	+	—	++	—	—
Contractures	—	—	+	—	+++	—	—
Bulbar symptoms	+	+++	++	+	++	++	+
Apraxia	—	—	—	—	+++	—	—

The facial appearance of those with PSP is characteristic and involves an astonished expression with deep facial folds. Dystonia may occur in the limbs or neck. Classically, patients demonstrate axial extension and retrocollis, but this sign is often absent. About 30% of patients develop "apraxia of eyelid opening" (120). The specific phenomenology and pathophysiology of this condition are debated but involve varying degrees of dystonic muscle contraction followed by an inability to open the lids volitionally.

Despite the condition's name, supranuclear vertical gaze palsy is neither sensitive nor specific for PSP (102). Down-gaze palsy overcome by the oculocephalic (dolls' eyes) maneuver is more specific than up-gaze palsy. Almost all patients with PSP have slowed vertical saccadic eye movements, often early in the disease course. Square wave jerks (spontaneous 5- to 10-degree saccades) are another common but nonspecific feature.

Neuropsychiatric evaluation of PSP demonstrates deficits in executive function with relative sparing of language and memory (90,130,225). These deficits may become severe during the later stages. Personality changes are common, and patients frequently become withdrawn and seemingly unconcerned about their condition. Pseudobulbar affect with emotional lability and other frontal lobe features are common.

The etiology of PSP is unknown. Although a few familial cases have been reported (38), most do not demonstrate any genetic component. No clear environmental risk factors have emerged other than a possible higher risk in rural areas and in people with lower levels of education (118,125).

Radiological findings are neither sensitive nor specific. In more advanced cases there is atrophy of the midbrain tectum and colliculi, with subsequent enlargement of the third ventricle (413). ^{18}F-Fluorodopa positron emission tomography (PET) in PSP patients demonstrates less uptake in the caudate than in PD patients (41), but PET has not gained wide acceptance as a diagnostic test because of its unclear specificity and high cost.

Despite several similar clinical characteristics, pathological changes seen with PSP are different from those seen with PD. PSP brains show neurofibrillary fibers and neuropil threads throughout the basal ganglia and brainstem (144). They are present within the cell body and contain abnormally phosphorylated tau protein (416). Neuron loss in the substantia nigra occurs uniformly throughout the structure rather than just in the lateral pars compacta, as is seen with PD. There is also significant loss of striatal neurons and postsynaptic dopaminergic receptors, which may account for the poor response to levodopa treatment. Numerous other neurotransmitters, including the GABAergic, cholinergic, and adrenergic systems, are also involved.

Treatment of PSP is largely unsatisfactory. About 35% of patients have moderate improvement with dopaminergic drugs, but this benefit usually wanes (277). Tricyclic antidepressants subjectively improve some patients, probably as a result of their antidepressant properties and improvement in pseudobulbar affect. Idazoxan, a presynaptic α_2 blocker, demonstrated some efficacy but is not widely available (108). Botulinum toxic injections often alleviate blepharospasm and other focal dystonias.

Multiple System Atrophy

Multiple system atrophy (MSA) is currently the preferred nosology for three conditions: Shy-Drager syndrome (SDS), striatonigral degeneration (SND), and olivopontocerebellar atrophy (OPCA). Although the acquisition of good epidemiological data has been hampered by inconsistent diagnostic criteria, one meta-analysis reported a mean age at onset of 54.2 ± 9.0 years (range 31–78 years) and a mean survival of 6.2 years after disease onset (19). MSA may present clinically as one of the classic subtypes or have overlapping features (404). Although they are discussed as one entity, SDS tends to have the most severe autonomic dysfunction, OPCA has the most prominent ataxia, and SND most resembles PD, although tremor is uncommon and bulbar symptoms are more severe.

Autonomic dysfunction eventually occurs in almost all cases of MSA. Bladder and sexual functions are typically most impaired at onset. Beck et al. reported that all 62 patients clinically diagnosed with MSA had electromyographic anal and urethral sphincter abnormalities (17). Erectile dysfunction may precede other features by several years and approaches 100% as the disease progresses. Orthostatic hypotension is common and may be described vaguely as "weakness," "light-headedness," "dizziness," or "worsening parkinsonism." Actual syncope is surprisingly uncommon given the dramatic falls in standing blood pressure. Inspiratory stridor while awake and asleep are common in MSA, especially the SND variant (164,271). Sleep apnea has also

been postulated to account for the high rate of nocturnal sudden death in this population.

The differentiation of PD from mild MSA based solely on autonomic symptoms can be difficult. Autonomic symptoms may be present in PD, especially constipation, but PD patients seldom present with these symptoms, which are usually mild unless exacerbated by medications.

The extrapyramidal features of MSA mimic those of PD, except that onset is usually bilateral, a lower percentage of patients have rest tremor, and improvement with dopaminergic therapy is inconsistent and less robust (13,129). Cerebellar features in MSA include gait ataxia, scanning speech, nystagmus, and to a lesser degree appendicular ataxia. Pyramidal signs such as extensor reflexes and spasticity may be present but are often masked by rigidity. Cognitive function is not severely impaired, but moderate executive dysfunction, pseudobulbar affect, personality changes, and depression may be present (316,338).

Magnetic resonance imaging (MRI) is a useful aid for MSA diagnosis. The SND and SDS variants may show increased putamen hypodensity on T2 images that correlates with iron deposition (201,345). A linear hyperdensity may also be seen along the lateral border of the putamen. OPCA often demonstrates cerebellar and pontine atrophy. PET studies are varied but tend to show reduced activity in the putamen and cerebellum (310).

Neuropathology demonstrates cell loss and gliosis diffusely throughout the subcortical gray matter. A relatively specific glial cytoplasmic inclusion (GCI) is now accepted as the pathological hallmark of MSA (264). These inclusions stain for ubiquitin, have a tubular structure, and are most abundant in the cortex and supraspinal autonomic system (295).

The parkinsonian features of MSA often respond to dopaminergic medications but not as well as in PD. Adverse effects, especially orthostatic hypotension, limit their use to a greater degree in MSA patients. Interestingly, patients with the SND variant often have levodopa-induced oromandibular dyskinesias without clinical benefit from the drug. Continuous biphasic positive airway pressure may benefit patients with central sleep apnea and nocturnal stridor. Tracheostomy is required in some cases.

Dementia with Lewy Bodies

Dementia with Lewy bodies (DLB) is gaining recognition as a distinct and underdiagnosed form of dementia accompanied by parkinsonian traits. Depending on inclusion criteria, it may be the second most common form of dementia behind Alzheimer's disease (AD) (182,194). Clinically, the disease may present with parkinsonism or cognitive dysfunction (227,228). The motor examination generally mimics that of PD except that a smaller percentage of DLB patients have rest tremor (55% versus 85%), more patients have myoclonus (18% versus 0%), and the age of onset may be older (68 versus 62 years) (227). The two conditions, however, cannot be reliably differentiated by the motor examination alone. Cognitive deficits are largely "cortical": memory loss, dyspraxia, and dysphasia (186). In contrast to AD, DLB has a higher rate of well formed visual hallucinations and psychosis and a more fluctuating course (16). Autonomic symptoms are also more common in DLB than in PD or AD.

Pathologically, DLB demonstrates Lewy bodies spread throughout the cerebral cortex and subcortical gray matter (105). In many cases they are accompanied by neurofibrillary tangles and senile plaques identical to those seen with AD. There is, in fact, considerable debate on whether this disorder represents a variant of AD or PD or is a distinct pathological entity.

The motor components of DLB generally respond well to dopaminergic therapy. Treatment, however, is frequently complicated by an exacerbation of hallucinations and symptomatic orthostasis.

Corticobasal Degeneration

Corticobasal degeneration (CBD) is a neurodegenerative disease of insidious onset that usually occurs during the seventh decade (221). Epidemiological data are scarce, but the disease probably affects both genders equally. Cases appear sporadically, and no risk factors have been identified. Symptoms typically present unilaterally as hand or leg clumsiness or numbness (334). The symptoms develop into a significant motor and sensory apraxia, often accompanied by action myoclonus, joint contractures, dystonic posturing, and bradykinesia. Eventually, patients are left with a useless limb, which they may dissociate from the rest of their body (alien limb). Typically, the contralateral side becomes affected about 3 years after initial presentation. Dysphagia and speech apraxia are also common. Gait and balance become impaired to the point that patients are wheelchair-bound within 3 to 5 years. A variety of abnormal eye movements, including supranuclear palsies, impaired smooth pursuit, and slowed saccades, may appear.

Cognitive compromise occurs in many cases but is variable. Some patients initially present with aphasia, but memory is relatively preserved (241). Death from bulbar dysfunction or the sequelae of immobility ensues within 5 to 10 years from onset. The condition resembles PD only during its early stages when patients have rigidity, loss of dexterity, and a mixed tremor that evolves into myoclonus. Later the disease is often confused with PSP or even cerebral vascular disease because of its marked asymmetry.

The MRI scans often show asymmetrical frontoparietal atrophy contralateral to the affected side (345). Electroencephalography may show asymmetrical slowing late in the disease, and somatosensory evoked potentials may exhibit diminished thalamocortical potentials. ^{18}F-Labeled 2-deoxyglucose PET shows significantly reduced glucose metabolism in the cortex contralateral to the affected side. (273).

Pathological examination demonstrates swollen "achromatic" cells in cortical layers 3 and 5 (223). There is associated neuron loss and gliosis in the frontal and parietal lobes, substantia nigra, and subthalamic nucleus.

Patients usually do not respond to levodopa, even in the early stages. The myoclonus and rigidity may be alleviated by clonazepam or baclofen. Dystonic posturing and pain usually diminish with botulinum toxin injections. Speech, occupational therapy, and physical therapy help some patients, but the overall treatment response is unsatisfactory.

Vascular Parkinsonism

Vascular parkinsonism remains the most difficult parkinsonian condition to define accurately. The nosology has evolved over time, resulting in a variety of conditions that clinically overlap: lower body parkinsonism, Binswanger's disease, atypical normal-pressure hydrocephalus, and arteriosclerotic parkinsonism. Critchley contrasted vascular parkinsonism to PD as having more dementia and emotional incontinence, more bladder incontinence, more bulbar signs, possible pyramidal signs, a shuffling gait with frequent freezing but no festination, retained arm swing, and the absence of tremor (67). Subsequent descriptions have emphasized the relative prominence of leg symptoms over arm symptoms, a moderately broad-based gait, possible cerebellar signs, and an association with hypertension (99,384). The onset of VP is usually symmetrical. Age at onset tends to be older than that of PD, and the course is more acute with a possible stepwise progression. Vascular parkinsonism may also clinically resemble PSP (82,409).

Pathological examination and MRI may show discrete basal ganglia lacunar infarcts, but more commonly demonstrate periventricular diffuse deep white matter (DWM) changes (leukoariosis). The significance of leukoariosis is debated but seems to correlate with slowed gait, worse balance, and slowed cognitive processing time in elderly patients (378).

Patients with vascular parkinsonism may demonstrate a moderate response to levodopa, but chronic treatment is usually unsatisfactory. Control of cardiovascular risk factors and gait training may improve some cases.

Drug-Induced Parkinsonism

The frequency of drug-induced parkinsonism (DIP) varies considerably according to the inclusion criteria and observer vigilance but probably averages between 10% and 20% of all patients taking dopamine blocking medications. Many nonpsychiatric medications, such as chlorpromazine (Compazine), promethazine (Phenergan), metoclopramide (Reglan), the antidepressant amoxapine (Ascenden), and the calcium channel blockers cinnarizine and flunarizine, may cause DIP. Recognition of this common problem is poor among both psychiatric and medical professionals (403). In 90% of cases, DIP begins within 3 months of medication initiation or dose augmentation (238). No irrefutable risk factors have emerged, although some suggest that older age, female gender, and a family history of tremor or PD predispose toward the development of DIP (193,263). Low urinary free dopamine levels correlated with the subsequent development of DIP in one study (68). DIP may also be associated with tardive dyskinesia.

Clinically, the condition may closely mimic PD. The onset, however, is characteristically bilateral and more acute (187). Bradykinesia is typically the most prominent feature. Rigidity is common but tends not to be of the cogwheel type. The tremor has both postural and rest components and is typically 5 to 7 Hz—somewhat faster than the tremor of PD.

The pathogenesis may simply involve blockade of the dopamine receptors, but the clinical symptoms do not correlate with drug dosing or serum levels. Some patients with DIP have subclinical PD that is unmasked by dopaminergic blockade (327).

Treatment involves discontinuation of the offending agent or switching to an "atypical" antipsychotic with fewer extrapyramidal side effects, such as clozapine. Improvement after drug withdrawal may take up to several months. If it is not practical to discontinue the offending agent, the addition of anticholinergic medications or amantadine, which has dopaminergic, glutaminergic, and anticholinergic properties, should be considered. Dopamine agonists and even levodopa can also be used, but these agents may exacerbate the underlying psychosis or other problem that initially required dopamine blocking medications.

Toxin-Induced Parkinsonism

Several toxins can result in parkinsonism. Manganese toxicity results in parkinsonism associated with personality changes and dementia, dystonia, postural tremor, and a peculiar "cock-like" gait (44,251). Pathological abnormalities are seen predominantly in the globus pallidus internus (GPi) and the subthalamic nucleus (STN) (415). Levodopa benefits some patients (250).

Carbon monoxide (CO) poisoning, as seen with smoke inhalation, results in a characteristic scenario of initial recovery, followed in several days by the development of persistent parkinsonism (112,225). Typically, patients also have significant frontal lobe dysfunction that may result in varying degrees of akinetic mutism (210). MRI typically demonstrates bilateral GPi lesions. Prognosis varies from a nearly full recovery to death. Levodopa and anticholinergics benefit some patients.

Other toxins that can result in parkinsonism include cyanide (341,389), carbon disulfide (311), and methanol (247). The drug 1-methyl-4-phenyl-1,2,3,6-tetrahydropyridine (MPTP) also results in a condition similar to that of idiopathic PD (see Parkinson's Disease, Etiology, below).

PATHOLOGY OF PARKINSON'S DISEASE

Despite extensive characterization, no specific pathological criteria have been established to diagnose PD. Most neuropathologists require the histological presence of Lewy bodies (LB) (110). These 5- to 25-μm eosinophilic cytoplasmic inclusion bodies can be found diffusely in neurons throughout the subcortical gray matter in PD (109,217). Classically, they have three concentric layers: a core (variably present), a body, and a halo. A more homogeneous, less eosinophilic version of the LB is also found in the cortex. Histochemical staining of the LB reveals proteins, fatty acids, sphingomyelin, polysaccharides, and α-synuclein (365). The outer layer also contains high levels of phosphorylated neurofilament (100). The biochemical processes that result in LB formation are unresolved.

Unfortunately, the presence of LBs is not specific for PD. They can be found in a variety of neurodegenerative diseases including DLB, MSA, PSP, Hallervorden-Spatz disease, and ataxia-telangiectasia (109). They can also be found in a small percentage of clinically normal controls, where they are an age-dependent phenomenon. It is unclear whether these cases represent subclinical PD. A less sensitive but more specific pathological marker, called a pale body, is found in the substantia nigra (SN) and locus ceruleus of patients with PD (111,296). They resemble a round, granular vacuole and are often found near an LB; they consist of short, branched filaments and usually stain for ubiquitin.

Cell loss, gliosis, and loss of dendritic length occurs most prominently in the lateral ventral tier of the pars compacta in the SN (95). Cell loss in PD, however, can occur throughout the subcortical gray matter. The most affected SN cells are the A9 dopaminergic neurons that project to striatal spiny neurons. Anatomical and physiological evidence suggests that 50% to 80% cell loss is required prior to any clinical manifestation (21,62,95,153). Therefore the pathological process that results in PD probably starts at least 4 to 5 years before the onset of symptoms.

It should be noted that natural aging results in significant cell loss in the SN, marked reduction of striatal dopamine, and reduced levels of enzymes that catalyze dopamine synthesis (50,68). In contrast to PD, however, this cell loss occurs diffusely throughout the SN and, in fact, is least prominent in the ventrolateral tier (95).

PATHOPHYSIOLOGY OF PARKINSON'S DISEASE

Five parallel cortico-striato-thalamic circuits run through the basal ganglia (69). Three of these circuits subserve cognitive and personality function, one subserves ocular motion, and one subserves motor function. Although all five are modulated by dopaminergic input from the substantia nigra (SN), it is perturbation of the motor circuit that has been most studied and is most responsible for the symptoms of PD.

The striatum (caudate and putamen) receives glutamatergic input from all areas of the cortex (Fig. 5-2). This is then modified by dopaminergic input from the pars compacta of the SN. From the striatum, the basal ganglia diverges into two pathways that converge on the globus pallidus internus (GPi): the direct pathway and the indirect pathway. The effects of SN dopaminergic input to the indirect and direct pathways are different and depend on the receptor type (107). D1 receptors predominate in the direct pathway, whereas D2 receptors predominate in the indirect pathway. Therefore with diminished dopaminergic input from the SN, as is seen with PD, there is decreased direct striatal output, which subserves the GPi, but increased indirect striatal output, which subserves the globus pallidus externa (GPe) (Fig. 5-3).

Other dopaminergic receptor types have been identified, but their role in PD is not well established. D5 receptors (D1B) are located throughout the cortex, thalamus, and striatum. D3 (D2B) receptors probably serve as autoreceptors in the SN and are abundant in limbic connections; D4 (D2C) receptors are poorly localized but seem to play a role in behavior.

Physiological models of the direct and indirect basal ganglia pathways have been refined (74, 407). In the direct pathway, after receiving dopaminergic input from the SN, the striatum directly inhibits the GPi via γ-aminobutyric acid (GABA) and substance P. The indirect pathway is

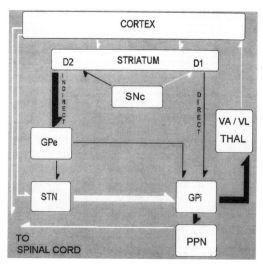

FIG. 5-3. Changes seen in the basal ganglia in Parkinson's disease: *thin arrows* represent reduced activity, *wide arrows* represent increased activity. See Fig.1 for abbreviations.

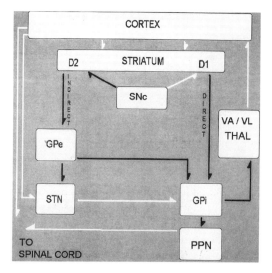

FIG. 5-2. Normal basal ganglia circuitry: *black arrows* are inhibitory, *white arrows* are excitatory. The SNc uses dopamine as the primary neurotransmitter. All other nuclei use GABA (*black arrows*) or glutamate (*white arrows*) as their primary neurotransmitters. *SNc,* substantia nigra pars compacta; *GPe,* globus pallidus externa; *GPi,* globus pallidus internus; *STN,* subthalamic nucleus; *PPN,* pedunculopontine nucleus; *VA/VL Thal,* ventral anterior and ventral lateral thalamus.

less well understood (58). After receiving dopaminergic input, the striatum inhibits the GPe via GABA. The GPe then inhibits the subthalamic nucleus (STN) and the GPi to a lesser extent via GABA. The STN then stimulates the GPi via glutamate. The GPi (the main basal ganglia outflow of both pathways) then inhibits the ventral lateral thalamus, which subsequently stimulates the supplementary motor area (SMA). In agreement with that model, PET and single-photon emission computed tomography (SPECT) studies in PD patients demonstrate reduced activity of the cortical SMA (317,331) that is reversed by both dopaminergic treatment and GPi lesioning (131,171,331).

In PD, therefore, the net effect of diminished SN dopaminergic output via both direct and indirect pathways is increased GPi activity and reduced ventral lateral (VL) thalamic activity. In the direct circuit, inhibitory input to the GPi from the striatum is reduced. In the indirect pathway, excitatory input to the GPi from the STN is increased.

This model is somewhat simplistic and has been challenged. Some doubt the existence of any "indirect" pathway and posit a direct connection from the GPe to the thalamus (145,297). There are clearly several subcircuits, autoreceptors, and alternate pathways (SN–thalamic and basal ganglia–brainstem connections), that further complicate the physiology (176,207), and the relative effects of tonic versus phasic basal ganglia activity are still poorly understood. The greatest criticism of the model, however, is its inability to account for all the clinical manifestations of surgical PD treatment. First, ventral anterior (VA)/VL thalamic lesions do not result in parkinsonian signs, as would be predicted. Second, GPe lesions do not ablate levodopa-induced dyskinesia; and, most importantly, the model does not explain the simultaneous reduction in contralateral dyskinesia and alleviation of bradykinesia that is seen after GPi lesioning (90). This last phenomenon may be the result of segregated function within the GPi (157). Furthermore, dyskinesia may be only indirectly caused by dopaminergic influences and directly caused by relative overactivity of glutamatergic output from the STN (293).

The pathophysiology of PD tremor is somewhat unique. Although even isolated "benign" rest tremor shows reduced SN function (36), unlike the other cardinal features of PD, especially bradykinesia, tremor severity does not correlate with ^{18}F-dopa PET studies (291,393). There are also minor pathological differences between tremor-dominant cases of PD and patients who exhibit tremor as a minor feature (150). There is evidence that the tremor of PD is pathophysiologically integrated into the same olivocerebellar-thalamic pathways that have been implicated in the pathogenesis of ET. Thalamic stimulation that improves PD tremor decreases cerebellar hemisphere activity but has no demonstrable effect on the basal ganglia (72).

Despite the progress achieved, it is apparent that a definitive understanding of basal ganglia physiology remains elusive. Further characterization of this physiology and the perturbations that result from PD will greatly facilitate future surgical and pharmacological treatment.

CELL DEATH IN PARKINSON'S DISEASE

A better understanding of the processes that cause neuronal death should result in more effective treatment and possibly a cure for PD. Although the initiating event remains unknown, several lines of evidence support the concept that oxidative stress and endogenous toxin production may perpetuate cell death.

In essence, oxidative stress is the mechanism by which superoxide and hydroxyl radicals are converted to water (Fig. 5-4). O_2^- is first converted to hydrogen peroxide (H_2O_2). Both enzymatic monoamine oxidase (MAO) and nonenzymatic oxidation of dopamine and levodopa result in equal molar production of H_2O_2 (172,286), which probably serves as the relevant entry point for oxidative stress reactions in PD. H_2O_2 is then catalyzed via transition metals (iron) into a hydroxyl radical (39). This highly reactive compound oxidizes lipid membranes, resulting in lipid peroxidation and water production. The lipid radicals trigger a series of events that lead to cellular demise. The main enzymatic protection from oxidative stress reactions is afforded by glutathione peroxidase, superoxide dismutase, and catalase. Ascorbate, β-carotene, and α-tocopherol also inhibit this process.

The evidence for increased oxidative stress in PD is multifactorial. First, several intermediates of the lipid peroxidation pathway are increased in PD (77,286). Second, the SN of PD patients shows histological evidence of oxidative damage to lipid membranes (286). Third, there are significantly diminished levels of reduced glutathione in PD and in patients who had Lewy bodies at autopsy but did not yet demonstrate symptoms or signs of PD (286). This finding is not seen in MSA despite similar medication usage. These findings can be interpreted two ways: (a) There is a primary deficiency in the glutathione peroxidase enzymatic pathway that may directly diminish the brain's ability to defend against oxidative stress and, in turn, primarily cause PD; or (b) reduced glutathione levels are diminished because the defensive mechanism (redox reaction) is "exhausted" from constant oxidation caused by an increase in H_2O_2, a secondary phenomenon. The fact that similar glutathione levels are seen in incidental Lewy body disease, prior to any symptoms of PD, suggests that it is an early phenomenon. Fourth, iron levels are significantly increased in

$$O^{\cdot}_2 \quad + \quad 2H+ \ggg \quad H_2O_2 \quad + \quad {}^3O_2$$

superoxide   hydrogen   triplet
radical   peroxide   oxygen

$$H_2O_2 \quad + \quad Fe^{2+} \ggg \quad {}^{\cdot}OH \quad + \quad OH\text{-} \ + \ Fe^{3+}$$

                                         hydroxyl   hydroxide
                                         radical   ion

$${}^{\cdot}OH \quad + \quad RH \ggg \quad R^{\cdot} \quad + \quad H2O$$

                             lipid   lipid   water
                                          radical

FIG. 5-4. Oxidative stress pathways. The Fenton reaction catalyzes step II. Dopamine turnover enters this cycle by producing H_2O_2.

the SN of PD patients despite normal ferritin levels (65,77,363). The reason for this excess accumulation is unknown, although the iron could catalyze hydroxy radical formation via the Fenton reaction (39).

If oxidative stress is primarily etiological, it appears to be a localized condition, perhaps initiated by the H_2O_2 produced in monoamine oxidation. It should be noted that PD is not associated with conditions that trigger generalized oxidative stress, such as vitamin E deficiency, radiation exposure, or iron overload; nor have anti-oxidant drugs shown any irrefutable clinical benefit (305).

The second major avenue of research regarding cellular demise in PD involves mitochondrial dysfunction. Shapira et al. reported a 30% reduction in NADH-CoQ1 reductase activity (complex I) in the SN of patients with PD, but not in those with MSA (347,348). The functional loss is patchy and occurs unevenly among cells. Reasons for the anatomic selectivity of complex I dysfunction are unknown. Data on complex I activity in other organs in PD patients are mixed. Some research has found that complex I activity is reduced in platelets (196,298,417) and in skeletal muscle (26,49,274), whereas other studies have been unable to reproduce these results (5,78,232).

Mitochondrial DNA encodes for part of complex I, and evaluation of this DNA has revealed numerous different point mutations and one dele-

tion in patients with PD (160,290). Mitochondrial point mutations, however, are not uncommon in normal controls. The absence of any consistent mutations and of any maternal inheritance pattern suggest that they represent spontaneous mutations rather than inherited abnormalities. They therefore probably account for only a small percentage of PD.

ETIOLOGY OF PARKINSON'S DISEASE

Despite an improving physiological understanding of the PD brain, the underlying pathogenesis of PD is unknown. Basic questions such as whether PD is a specific disease or a syndrome, and the relative influence of genetic and environmental factors are still debated. Current thinking supports the concept that some endogenous or exogenous toxins perpetuate cell death through oxidative stress in genetically predisposed individuals. The genetic predisposition may involve increased production or decreased elimination of the toxin or a general deficiency in defenses against subsequent cellular demise. Likely, there are multiple genetic and environmental factors.

The case for environmental toxin culpability in PD is most strongly supported by consistent epidemiological data that demonstrate higher rates of PD in rural areas (123,151,190, 373–375). Several related risk factors include herbicide and pesticide exposure (123,148,155, 201,220,359,419), agrarian profession (14,151,376), and the use of well water (46,173,190). Other possible risk factors include industrial chemical exposure (8,373) and minor head trauma (368).

Exposure to the neurotoxin MPTP produces a condition that closely resembles PD and now serves as an invaluable research tool that has facilitated better understanding of idiopathic PD. MPTP first came to clinical attention in 1982 when a number of intravenous drug users in California acutely developed parkinsonism (204). MPTP was subsequently identified as an impurity during the illicit production of a heroin substitute. The condition resembles PD in almost every way except that tremor is less prominent and the course is much more acute. Patients are levodopa responsive but develop dyskinesias and acute motor fluctuations within weeks of initiating therapy (13). Pathological examination demonstrates highly selective cell loss in the SN.

The pathophysiology of MPTP toxicity is now well understood. In the CNS, MPTP is oxidized via MAO-B to the 1-methyl-4-phenylpyridinium ion (MPP$^+$) (60). The compound is actively internalized through dopamine transporters (58), which explains its predilection for the SN. In fact, experimental models of MPTP toxicity can be prevented by pretreating with MAO-B or dopamine reuptake inhibitors (146,248,329,344). Once inside the cell, MPP$^+$ is actively taken into the mitochondria as a function of the negative mitochondrial electron gradient. Inside the mitochondria MPP$^+$ inhibits complex I of the oxidative phosphorylation chain (276,328), resulting in decreased adenosine triphosphate (ATP) production, which in turn may lead to cell death (258).

The MPTP may also perturb the tricarboxylic acid (TCA) cycle by inhibiting α-ketoglutarate dehydrogenase, which is often considered to be the rate-limiting step. This would further impair cell energy production. In fact, reduced α-ketoglutarate levels have been reported in the SN of patients with PD, but this finding has not been confirmed (257).

Smoking and Parkinson's Disease

Numerous epidemiological studies have reported an inverse relation between smoking behavior and PD (24,133,175,185,191,245,265,360,402). Even identical twin pairs discordant for PD demonstrate this tendency (24). The relative risk for nonsmoking ranges between 0.2 to 0.8 (median 0.5). The causal relation underlying this consistent inverse correlation, however, remains controversial.

Several metabolites of tobacco smoke can increase dopamine release (186). Elevated dopamine levels can explain the mild alleviation of PD symptoms reported shortly after smoking (163) but are unlikely to account for reduced rates of PD. Other smoking metabolites can reduce dopamine turnover, which could reduce oxidative stress (6,10,113). Moreover, MAO-B activity appears to be reduced in smokers (45, 101,252,418).

Several epidemiological studies argue against any biochemical protective effect from smoking. First, symptom onset in PD patients who smoke tends to be at a younger age (368). If smoking were protective, they should present at a relatively older age. Second, there is no correlation between smoking and the severity, or progression, of PD (118). Third, much of the difference in smoking rates is accounted for by PD patients who smoked when young but subsequently stopped (185,360).

The opposing argument suggests that PD patients have less urge to smoke. A PD personality type of aversion to risk-taking and conformity to societal mores has emerged and can be demonstrated from childhood (307,360). In accordance with this observation, PD patients have lower rates of alcohol consumption but normal coffee/caffeine consumption (174). It is also well established that common pleasure-seeking behavior is dopaminergically mediated, and that dopaminergic blockade reduces the urge to smoke (306).

Infectious Processes and Parkinson's Disease

Subsequent to the worldwide influenza outbreak of 1917–1926, up to 80% of survivors developed a parkinsonian condition called von Economo's encephalitis (85,89,152). It differed from idiopathic PD in that it affected all ages, was accompanied by more hyperkinetic movements, was not progressive, and pathologically demonstrated neurofibrillary tangles in the SN (149). Other viruses, such as those causing Western equine encephalitis (270,353), coxsackie B encephalitis (394), and Japanese B encephalitis (128), have also resulted in nonprogressive parkinsonian conditions. Antibodies to herpes simplex virus have been found in brains of PD patients (239,240), but these antibody titers are common in the general population, and no virus particles or herpes DNA have been reported (356,406). Theories of intrauterine viral infections have not been supported (88). Overall, it is unlikely that a virus or an infectious process plays a significant role in the pathogenesis of idiopathic PD.

Neuroimmunology

Although a generalized immune process does not appear likely, increasing evidence suggests that specific aspects of autoimmune reactions are active in patients with PD (197). Antibodies against dopaminergic neurons are found in 78% of PD patients versus 3% of controls (52). Serum and cerebrospinal fluid (CSF) from PD patients also retard dopaminergic cell growth in cell culture (141). Pathological changes in the PD brain show HLA-DR-positive activated microglia, complement proteins in Lewy bodies, and elevated β_2-microglobulin (246,259,260).

A variety of non-antigen-specific markers of an immunological response, including interleukin-1β (IL-1β), IL-6, transforming growth factor-α (TGFα), transforming growth factor-1β (TGF1β), and epidermal growth factor (EGF), are elevated in PD (197,259,260). Elevated levels of TNFα have been demonstrated in the striatum and CSF fluid of PD patients (209,262). This may lead to increased nitric oxide (NO) production and cytotoxicity. In all cases it is unclear whether these immunological changes are etiological, secondary, or an epiphenomenon associated with cell death. Therapeutic investigations based on these findings are ongoing (226,366).

Genetics

Although idiopathic PD has generally been considered to be a sporadic disease, advances in human genetics have rekindled interest in possible contributing genetic factors. Identical twin studies of PD patients initially reported low concordance for PD (85,396). Subsequent reevaluation, however, has shown that a higher number of "unaffected" twins have since developed symptoms of PD (119,178). Furthermore, many of the asymptomatic siblings do have ^{18}F-fluorodopa PET scans consistent with PD (40).

Epidemiological studies have consistently shown a higher than expected rate of PD in first-degree relatives of affected persons (4,32,75, 208,233,235,358,390). The odds ratio usually ranges from 2.0 to 3.0. These cases are clinically indistinct from PD and are consistent with an autosomal dominant inheritance with incomplete penetrance. To date, there is no compelling evidence that supports mitochondrial inheritance.

Several large families have been reported (25,121,124,364,398). In most cases these families have some atypical features, including young onset, lack of tremor, and poor levodopa response. In one large family with a clinical syndrome identical to PD, except for a younger age of onset and more rapid progression, the abnormality mapped to chromosome 4q21-q74 (122,319). A specific gene mutation was subsequently shown to code for the protein α-synuclein, a presynaptic nerve terminal protein with an unknown function (320). It is found in Lewy bodies in patients with idiopathic PD (365). Although analysis of a large number of other familial cases has not shown a link to this area (357), evaluation of the first PD genetic marker should advance our understanding of PD.

DYSKINESIA

Drug-induced dyskinesias eventually complicate the course of most PD patients treated with levodopa. Most PD patients develop dyskinesias within 5 years after the introduction of levodopa (28,279,318). One-third of all patients enrolled in the DATATOP trial developed dyskinesias within 2 years of levodopa therapy (305). For reasons that are still unclear, patients who develop PD at a younger age are more prone to develop early and more severe dyskinesias (126,169,195).

Phenomenologically, dyskinesias usually consist of appendicular or neck choreiform and stereotypical movements. Dystonia and myoclonus may also occur but are less common. Dyskinesias usually start in the foot on the most affected side, although these symptoms often go unrecognized by the patient (234). Although they can be painful and functionally incapacitating, most patients prefer dyskinesias to being "off" (no benefit from dopaminergic therapy), and typically it is the caregiver who is more concerned by their presence.

In most patients the appearance of dyskinesias correlates with the highest levels of serum and CSF levodopa: "peak dose dyskinesia." This condition is referred to as the improvement–dyskinesia–improvement (I-D-I) pattern. About 10% of patients, however, develop a pattern consisting of dyskinesia (as serum levels rise), followed by clinical improvement (at the highest serum levels), followed by dyskinesia (as levels fall) (269). This dyskinesia–improvement–dyskinesia (D-I-D) pattern is particularly difficult to manage.

The pathology of dyskinesia is not clearly understood. The general notion that a reduction in dopaminergic striatal input results in postsynaptic hypersensitivity is supported by the absence of dyskinesias in diseases that reduce postsynaptic receptor function (i.e., PSP). Apomorphine, which acts directly at the postsynaptic receptor, results in a steeper response curve in patients who have clinical fluctuations, suggesting postsynaptic culpability (389).

The overall severity of the underlying PD may be the major risk factor for developing dyskinesia (154). As the disease progresses, the loss of dopaminergic dendrites in the striatum may lead to a reduction in dopaminergic buffering capacity, which could result in the all-or-none response that characterizes motor fluctuations. PET studies do indeed show a significant reduction in striatal ^{18}F-fluorodopa in advanced and fluctuating, but not stable, PD patients (211).

Apomorphine response curves are much steeper in patients with more advanced disease, but these data are complicated by the fact that all of these patients have taken levodopa (64).

Levodopa administration clearly affects the onset and severity of dyskinesia. Mouradian et al. showed that even 1 week of continuous intravenous levodopa reduced the threshold for the subsequent development of dyskinesia (267). The total levodopa dose (42,378) and duration of treatment (154,339) correlate with the development of dyskinesias in several studies. The mode of levodopa administration may also be important. Animal studies demonstrate that intermittent dopaminergic infusions result in more dopaminergic sensitization than continuous infusion (181). Less well controlled human studies have also reported fewer dyskinesias and fluctuations with continuous infusions than with pulsatile administration (56,57,268,352). Clinical trials comparing dyskinesia development in patients taking slow-release levodopa (relatively more stable levels) and regular levodopa have been mixed. Some have shown that long-acting preparations delay the development of dyskinesias (337), whereas others have failed to show any significant clinical difference (29,83).

Evidence suggests that glutamate and relatively overactive NMDA channels may result in dyskinesias. NMDA blockade reduces apomorphine and levodopa induced dyskinesias in animal models of PD (28,293). Furthermore, it is well established that pallidal surgery reduces contralateral dyskinesias. This is not adequately explained by traditional views of basal ganglia physiology and, in fact, may be the result of perturbed glutaminergic tracts. This and other evidence suggests that dyskinesias result from relative overactivity of the D2-mediated indirect pathway in contrast to the D1-mediated direct pathway. (179). D1-specific agonists tend to reduce dyskinesia in animal models of PD, but no such drug has been tested in humans (362).

TREATMENT

The pharmacological treatment options for PD are rapidly increasing (169a). Numerous existing medications, including amantadine, anticholinergics, dopamine agonists, and various preparations of levodopa, significantly diminish morbidity. Several newer agents, including additional dopamine agonists, catechol-*O*-methyl transferase (COMT) antagonists, and neuroprotective and neurotrophic factors, are undergoing testing in humans and may be available in the near future.

Clinical trials have yet to determine whether any agent slows the progression of disease through neuroprotection. If one believes in the neuroprotective effects of MAO-B inhibitors or dopamine agonists, treatment with these agents should begin immediately upon diagnosis. Otherwise, treatment should begin when it is thought that there is some functional limitation. This is sometimes difficult to determine and must be individualized. For example, a working individual may be symptom-free other than micrographia, which may cause significant functional problems, whereas another individual may have much more obvious symptoms yet not require treatment.

Treatment strategies also must consider long-term ramifications. Today the average patient survives 25 years after initial presentation of PD symptoms. Overly aggressive initial treatment, especially with levodopa preparations, may prematurely lead to a variety of problems (e.g., dyskinesias, reduced duration of effect, and the on–off phenomenon) that could be delayed by more conservative therapy. Therefore the treatment strategy must be individualized to the needs of the patient. As a general rule, if an early or medium stage PD patient has no clinical evidence of PD, they are probably overmedicated for that stage of their disease.

Monoamine Oxidase-B Inhibitors

Selegeline (Eldepryl, Deprenyl) is an irreversible inhibitor of MAO-B that prevents the enzymatic breakdown of dopamine into dihydroxyphenylacetic acid (DOPAC). Therefore selegeline not only increases synaptic dopamine levels but should also reduce production of hydrogen peroxide, which may be the initial step implicated in oxidative stress-mediated cell death. Evidence also suggests that selegeline may reduce apoptosis by triggering cellular protein synthesis independently from its MAO-B properties (139, 379–381).

Retrospective data showed an increased life expectancy in PD patients who took selegeline (27,383). Subsequently, the DATATOP study reported that selegeline (10 mg/day) delayed the clinical need for levodopa, and that patients on selegeline and levodopa required lower levodopa doses (305). Although the study was designed based on the hypothesis that selegeline provides neuroprotection, the results demonstrated an unexpected clinical improvement, making the study design unable to determine any true neuroprotective effect. Subsequent data interpretation, however, has not supported true neuroprotection (282,285). One retrospective study, in fact, suggested higher overall mortality rate among patients taking selegeline (10 mg/day) (212,303), although this report has not been widely accepted (283). No increase in mortality was found, however, in patients treated with Deprenyl during the first five years of the DATATOP study (305a).

Nevertheless, selegeline, at 5 to 10 mg per day, clearly results in symptomatic improvement of PD with few adverse effects. Reports of adverse drug reactions between selegeline and tricyclic antidepressants and between selegeline and serotonin-specific reuptake inhibitors (SSRI) (314) are not justified in the opinion of most movement disorder specialists (333).

Selegeline is hepatically metabolized to L-amphetamine and L-methamphetamine. Although both metabolites further augment dopamine synaptic concentrations, they are potential pro-oxidants that may offset any potential antioxidant properties of selegeline. They may also account for much of the medication's antidepressant and stimulating effects. Newer sublingual and transdermal preparations of selegeline that bypass hepatic metabolism are currently being investigated. Preliminary data suggest that these compounds significantly increase serum selegeline levels while reducing metabolite levels. Other MAO-B inhibitors, such as lazabolide and rasagaline, are being investigated (236,304).

Anticholinergic Agents

Anticholinergic medications such as trihexy-phenidyl (Artane) and benztropine (Cogentin) were once the mainstay of PD treatment but have been replaced by dopaminergic medications. These medications may particularly benefit those with refractory tremor and can be used in that scenario. Otherwise, their moderate efficacy seldom outweighs their significant adverse effect profile (constipation, dry mouth, hypotension, blurred vision, sedation, and cognitive slowing).

Amantadine

Amantadine (Symmetrel) is an aliphatic primary amine antiviral agent that has been used to treat PD since the early 1970s (7,71). Amantadine probably improves PD patients by several mechanisms. It increases dopamine release from presynaptic terminals and has anticholinergic properties (135,371,392). Amantadine was also found to possess NMDA antagonist properties via blockade of open ion channels, resulting in diminished glutaminergic activity (231). NMDA antagonism presents two potential benefits in PD patients. Overexcitation of this system is thought to potentiate cell death in several neurodegenerative conditions including PD. Clinical support for the possible neuroprotective properties of amantadine was demonstrated when it was reported to be an independent predictor for survival in PD patients (387). Glutamate antagonism may also directly benefit patients with dyskinesia associated with levodopa use by reducing glutamatergic outflow from the subthalamic nucleus (293).

Early clinical studies clearly demonstrated its efficacy and good tolerability as monotherapy for early PD. Although no formal practice guidelines exist, amantadine is most commonly employed for early, mild PD prior to initiating other treatments (42,301,355). Other studies have shown additional benefit from amantadine when it is added to other medications (43,94, 300,385,393).

Though generally considered a less potent agent than dopamine agonists, amantadine clearly provides symptomatic benefit and augments the efficacy of other medications. There also appears to be a subset of patients in whom rest tremor is significantly reduced. Amantadine has been used to treat fatigue associated with other neurological conditions. The typical dose is 200 to 400 mg per day in two or three divided doses. The medicine is well tolerated but may cause mild nausea and anticholinergic side effects. Other peculiar adverse effects are the development of leg edema and livedo reticularis, a lattice-like, mottling discoloration of the skin, seen especially around the shin. This problem is purely cosmetic and usually resolves after drug discontinuation.

Dopamine Agonists

Currently available dopamine agonists in the United States include bromocriptine (Parlodel), pergolide (Permax), pramipexole (Mirapex), ropinirole (Requip), and cabergolide (Dostinex) (Table 5-2). The latter, a long-acting agonist, is not marketed for PD. Apomorphine and lisuride are also used in countries outside the United States. Although there are numerous pharmacokinetic differences, all the medications are designed to stimulate postsynaptic dopamine type 2 (D2) receptors (9,79,412). D1 receptor stimulation may also alleviate symptoms, but it is less well established (97,136). The relative affinities for D2 receptors, other dopaminergic sites, and other neurotransmitters vary among the drugs.

Although the ratio of clinical improvement to adverse effects is less than that for levodopa, these medications offer several theoretical and practical advantages. There is a growing body of evidence that dopamine agonists prevent dopaminergic cell death in vitro and in MPTP and 6-hydroxydopamine (6-OHDA) models of PD (11,134,203). They seem to retard normal age-related loss of dopaminergic cells (52,95) and reduce dopamine turnover (76,315,420). Dopamine agonists have also demonstrated neuroprotection in non-PD models of oxidative stress (165,278) and protect against experimental ischemia (138). This may be due to their ability to reduce dopamine turnover, thereby reducing H_2O_2 production; or it may be due to a direct effect as free radical scavengers (106,278). Clinically, therapy with dopamine agonists almost

TABLE 5-2. *Properties of dopamine agonists*

Agonist	Route	Daily-dose dosing	$t_{1/2}$ (hour)	D1	D2	D3	$\alpha2$	Distinctive adverse events
Apomorphine	SC, SL, IV	Variable	0.5–1.5	+++	+++	0	?	Stomatitis (SL)
Bromocriptine	PO	7.5-40.0 mg t.i.d. / o.i.d.	3–8	+	+++	+	+	Hair loss, erythro-myagia, retro-peritoneal fibrosis
Pergolide	PO	0.5–6.0 mg t.i.d. mg	27	+++	+++	+	++	Similar to bromo-criptine, hypotension
Pramipexole	PO	0.25–4.5 mg t.i.d.	8–12	0	+++	+++	+	?
Ropinirole	PO	0.75–24 mg t.i.d.	6	0	+++	+++	0	?
Cabergoline	PO	0.25–4.0 mg q.d. / q.o.d.	60–100	+	+++	0	+	?

never results in dyskinesia or the on–off phe-nomenon. When used as monotherapy, they delay the need for levodopa and can subse-quently reduce the necessary dose of levodopa. Treatment with dopamine agonists may also prevent the subsequent development of levo-dopa-induced dyskinesias (336). One retrospec-tive study of pergolide-treated patients, how-ever, failed to demonstrate improved survival (346).

All dopamine agonists have demonstrated ef-ficacy in placebo-controlled trials as monother-apy or add-on therapy for patients receiving levodopa (2,3,36,37,115,156,208,219,256,264, 284,298,312,321,330,335,399). Comparing these trials is difficult, and they have not demonstrated the superiority of any single agent. Several clin-ical comparisons between dopamine agonists have been performed. Two crossover studies re-ported that pergolide was generally superior, in terms of efficacy and adverse event profile, to bromocriptine as add-on therapy (30,313). An-other study showed that pergolide increased the duration of benefit from levodopa more than bromocriptine (34). One long-term parallel de-sign study reported that cabergoline resulted in more "on" time than did bromocriptine when used as add-on therapy, but other measures were equal (162). Ropinirole has also demonstrated more "on" time than bromocriptine (192). Pramipexole tended to show more "on" time and improved UPDRS II scores when compared to bromocriptine in fluctuating patients, but it did not reach statistical significance (137).

Adverse events complicate the use of dopa-mine agonist in 40% to 60% of patients. Nausea, orthostatic hypotension, sedation/confusion, and hallucinations occur most frequently. Erythro-melalgia (St. Anthony's fire) can complicate the use of ergotamine derivatives (pergolide, bromo-criptine, cabergolide) and necessitate dose reduc-tion or elimination.

Levodopa Preparations

For more than 25 years levodopa preparations, levodopa/carbidopa (Sinemet) and levodopa/ benserazide (Madopar), have been the most po-tent pharmacological agents against PD. The ex-cellent clinical response and relatively good ad-verse event profile is superior to that of any other medication option; however, experts still debate the potential long-term effects from chronic levodopa use. There is considerable lab-oratory evidence and some indirect clinical evi-dence that levodopa use may accelerate cell death, expedite tolerance, and result in clinical fluctuations (280). Conversely, levodopa clearly alleviates symptoms, reduces mortality among patients with PD, and according to the patho-logical evidence has not produced neuronal damage in autopsied patients who did not have PD (323,408).

As a rule, levodopa should be titrated to the lowest dose that provides adequate occupational and social functioning. There is usually no rea-son to give levodopa prior to sleep unless the pa-tient needs to awaken frequently and walk during the night. The exact timing of doses thus requires a careful history to determine these individual needs.

Sustained-release levodopa is available as Sinemet CR and Madopar HR, which gradually release levodopa in the stomach. Compared to regular levodopa, the duration of therapeutic plasma levels is doubled (8 versus 4 hours), the peak plasma levels require more time after ingestion (120 versus 40 minutes), and the total bioavailability is about 20% less (54,292,370). Clinically, this translates into a longer latency and more gradual onset, followed by a longer duration of action and gradual wearing off. The amount of improvement is somewhat less consistent than with regular Sinemet, but the longer duration allows a more convenient dosing schedule. Dosing is variable and must be carefully individualized. A typical initial dose is 300 mg of levodopa per day in three divided doses.

The most common initial adverse effects are nausea and hypotension. Higher doses may lead to sedation, confusion, and visual hallucinations. Difficulties with dyskinesia and the on–off phenomenon typically begin after 2 to 5 years of use.

New and Experimental Medications

A variety of novel agents designed to treat PD are currently being developed and tested. Two COMT antagonists, tolcopone (Tasmar) and entacopone, have been shown to increase "on" time, and reduce and improve "off" time by a variety of measures (198,324,342,397). Both drugs also increase dopaminergic adverse events such as dyskinesias. They clearly benefit patients with a severe wearing-off phenomenon, but their role in other scenarios is undefined.

Several antiglutamatergic medications, including remacemide, riluzide, and nematine, are being investigated for both symptomatic and neuroprotective properties. A new class of immunotrophins, including GM1 ganglioside, thalidomide, and GPi-1046, have shown promise as potential neuroprotective agents (226,350,366). Glial cell line-derived neurotrophic factor (GDNF) has regenerated experimentally damaged do-

paminergic cells and is undergoing testing in humans (206).

Surgical pallidotomy significantly alleviates most aspects of PD and is now considered to be an accepted treatment in patients with moderately advanced PD complicated by levodopa-induced dyskinesias (202). Deep brain simulators placed in the thalamus greatly improve contralateral tremor in patients with PD or essential tremor (188). Placement of these devices into the STN and GPi are currently being investigated as alternatives to surgical lesioning. Surgical techniques are beyond the scope of this text but are the focus of the remaining chapters.

Specific Treatment Issues: Nausea, Orthostatic Hypotension, Hallucinations, Dyskinesia

Nausea may occur in patients with PD as a consequence of gastrointestinal dysmotility or as one of the most frequent complications of dopaminergic medications. These medications produce nausea by stimulating the area postrema, which is not protected by the blood–brain barrier. Nausea can often be eliminated simply by taking the medicine with or shortly after meals. High-protein foods should be avoided, as large neutral amino acids interfere with the absorption of levodopa. Nausea usually resolves over time, making ingestion on an empty stomach once again possible. If this measure is not adequate, dopaminergic-induced nausea may resolve by augmenting the dose of carbidopa, which prevents dopamine accumulation in the area postrema. Excessive levels of carbidopa, more than 300 mg per day, however, may penetrate the brain and result in diminished CNS dopamine availability. Carbidopa is available in the form of Lodosyn (25 mg pills). In severe cases patients may require domperidone (Motilium, 10–60 mg per day in TID dosing) a dopamine blocking agent that does not penetrate the CNS. This drug is not currently available in the United States. Standard dopamine blocking antiemetic medications such as promethazine (Phenergan) or prochlorperazine (Compazine) are generally contraindicated in PD patients, but hydroxyzine (Visteral), odansetron (Zofran), or benzodiazepines may be employed with some success.

Orthostatic hypotension and other autonomic symptoms are common with PD. When autonomic symptoms are particularly prominent, a diagnosis of MSA may be considered. Currently, there is no clear evidence that chronic hypotension is deleterious; therefore the goal of treatment is to eliminate symptomatic orthostasis. A careful history must be taken to determine if there is a consistent temporal relation between levodopa ingestion and symptomatic orthostasis, suggesting levodopa culpability.

Initial treatment of orthostatic hypotension usually involves increasing the intravascular volume. Supplemental salt (NaCl) may adequately elevate blood pressure. Fluorocortisone (Florinef) at doses of 0.1 to 0.3 mg per day may also elevate blood pressure, often in conjunction with salt. This regimen requires caution in the setting of any cardiovascular compromise.

Midodrine, an α_2-adrenergic antagonist, is well tolerated by PD patients and is more effective than other sympathomimetics (166,230). Patients report good subjective improvement from the medication, although demonstrable objective data have been less impressive. The dosing ranges from 7.5 to 40 mg per day in three or four divided doses. Adverse effects include supine hypertension, flushing, and tingling scalp sensations.

Several physical measures may also alleviate symptomatic orthostasis. Compression stockings may be of some benefit, but compression must be applied up to the torso to be consistently helpful. All patients with symptomatic hypotension should sleep with the bed in reverse Trendelenburg position (simply elevating the head with pillows is not adequate). This measure reduces the CNS effects of supine hypertension and recalibrates internal homeostatic blood pressure control at the carotid sinus.

Several simple maneuvers may be employed by the patient just prior to standing to increase blood pressure transiently. Adducting the legs together at the hips against some fixed pressure (usually the patient's hands), bouncing up and down on the toes while standing, elevating one leg from the ground, or simply leaning forward at the waist may alleviate symptoms.

Hallucinations are a common side effect of levodopa, especially in the elderly. They are also associated with dementia, visual loss, and poor sleep (97,214,275,343). When they occur independently of levodopa therapy and cognitive deficits are present, a diagnosis of DLB should be considered. Hallucinations caused by dopaminergic drugs occur more commonly at night and generally are not frightening to the patient. They are almost always visual, rather than auditory, and typically involve children or animals. They are of concern to family members and frequently result in institutionalization (117). Hallucinations in those with PD resolve with discontinuation of levodopa, but this is often not possible. Reduction of nighttime levodopa, dopamine agonists, and anticholinergic agents may also diminish hallucinations.

Clozapine, an atypical D4 blocker, is highly effective for eliminating levodopa-associated hallucinations without compromising motor function (55,103,410). In fact, both tremor and dyskinesias may disappear (104). Generally, only 12.5 to 100 mg given at night (a small dose when compared to its use for schizophrenia) is required to eliminate hallucinations. The medicine's most common adverse effects include sedation, confusion, and sialorrhea. A potentially fatal granulocytopenia occurs in approximately 1% of cases, usually within the first year of use. Therefore weekly complete blood counts are required. Small doses of olanzapine, risperidone, ondansetron, remoxipride, and mianserin may also alleviate dopaminergic hallucinations and are much more convenient to use (161,253,411,421).

Dyskinesias complicate the course of most patients subsequent to chronic levodopa therapy. Simple reduction of dopaminergic medications benefits those with peak dose dyskinesia, but this may be difficult without worsening motor symptoms. As a rule, dosing must be changed so the patient takes a smaller individual dose more frequently. Extended-release levodopa preparations make these adjustment responses less predictable and usually must be discontinued. Some practitioners attempt to reduce levodopa preparations while augmenting the use of dopamine agonist, but this regimen is often difficult for the patient to tolerate.

Amantadine may reduce dyskinesias, presumably through glutamatergic mechanisms, and improve the "off" time. Clozapine effectively reduces dyskinesia without worsening motor function, but it is cumbersome to use (18). Other "atypical" antipsychosis medications may also alleviate dyskinesia, but their effect on motor function is inconsistent. Low doses of propranolol have also been reported to diminish choreic dyskinesia (51). The mechanism for this action though unclear, may involve altered dopamine release or may simply be a result of an anxiolytic effect. Fluoxetine may also diminish dyskinesias, but its effect on motor function is unpredictable (84). Neither peak dose dystonia nor wearing-off dystonia respond well to medications. Botulinum toxin injections, however, can significantly improve dystonia and muscle spasm pain (291). Pallidal surgery dramatically reduces dyskinesia contralateral to the lesion site and should strongly be considered in cases of disabling dyskinesia.

REFERENCES

1. Abbott RA, Cox M, Markus H, et al. Diet, body size and micronutrient status in Parkinson's disease. *Eur J Clin Nutr* 1992;46:879–884.
2. Adler CH, Sethi KD, Hauser RA, et al. Ropinirole for the treatment of early Parkinson's disease. *Neurology* 1997;49:393–399.
3. Ahlskog JE, Muenter MD, Maraganore DM, et al. Fluctuating Parkinson's disease: treatment with the long acting dopamine agonist cabergoline. *Arch Neurol* 1994;51:1236–1241.
4. Alonso ME, Otero E, D'Regules R, et al. Parkinson's disease: a genetic study. *Can J Neurol Sci* 1986;13:248–251.
5. Anderson JJ, Ferrari R, Davis TL, et al. No evidence for altered muscle mitochondrial function in Parkinson's disease. *J Neurol Neurosurg Psychiatry* 1993;56:477–480.
6. Anderson K, Fuxe R, Agnati LF. Effects of single injections of nicotine on the ascending dopamine pathways in the rat. *Acta Physiol Scand* 1981;112:345–347.
7. Aoki F, Sitar D. Clinical pharmacokinetics of amantadine hydrochlorate. *Clin Pharmacokinet* 1988;14:35–51.
8. Aquilonius SM, Hartvig P. A Swedish county with unexpectedly high utilization of anti-parkinsonian drugs. *Acta Neurol Scand* 1986;74:379–382.
9. Arai N, Isaji M, Miyata H, et al. Differential effects of three dopamine receptor agonists in MPTP-treated monkeys. *J Neural Trans* 1995;10:55–62.
10. Arqueros L, Naquira D, Zunino E. Nicotine-induced release of catecholamines from rat hippocampus and striatum. *Biochem Pharmacol* 1978;27:2667–2674.
11. Asanuma M, Ogawa N, Nishibayashi S, et al. Protective effects of pergolide on dopamine levels in the 6-hydroxydopamine—lesioned mouse brain. *Arch Int Pharmacodyn Ther* 1995;329:221–230.
12. Ashok PF, Radhakrishan K, Sridharan R, et al. Parkinsonism in Benghazi, East Libya. *Clin Neurol Neurosurg* 1986;88:109–113.
13. Ballard PA, Tetrud JW, Langston JW. Permanent human parkinsonism due to 1-methyl-phenyl-1,2,3,6-tetrahydropyridine (MPTP): seven cases. *Neurology* 1985;35:949–956.
14. Barbeau A, Roy M. Uneven prevalence of Parkinson's disease in the province of Quebec. *Can J Neurol Sci* 1985;12:169.
15. Bateson MC, Gibberd FB, Wilson RSE. Salivary symptoms in Parkinson's disease. *Arch Neurol* 1973;29: 274–275.
16. Beck BJ. Neuropsychiatric manifestations of diffuse Lewy body disease. *J Geriatr Psychiatry Neurol* 1995;8:189–196.
17. Beck RO, Betts CD, Fowler CJ. Genitourinary dysfunction in multiple systems atrophy: clinical features and treatment in 62 cases. *J Urol* 1994;151:1331–1341.
18. Bennet J, Landow E, Dietrich S, et al. Suppression of dyskinesias in advanced Parkinson's disease: moderate daily clozapine doses provide long-term dyskinesia reduction. *Mov Disord* 1994;9:409–414.
19. Ben-Shlomo Y, Wenning GK, Tison F, et al. Survival of patients with pathologically proven multiple system atrophy: a meta-analysis. *Neurology* 1997;48:384–393.
20. Berger Y, Blaivas J, DeLaRocha ER, et al. Urodynamic findings in Parkinson's disease. *J Urol* 1987;138: 836–838.
21. Bernheimer H, Birkmayer W, Hornykiewicz O, et al. Brain dopamine and the syndromes of Parkinson and Huntington: clinical, morphological, and neurochemical correlations. *J Neurol Sci* 1973;20:415–455.
22. Bharucha NE, Bharucha EP, Bharucha AK, et al. Prevalence of Parkinson's disease in the Parsi community of Bombay, India. *Arch Neurol* 1988;45:1321–1323.
23. Bharucha NE, Chandra V, Schoenberg BS. Mortality data for the US for deaths due to and related to twenty neurologic diseases. *Neuroepidemiology* 1984; 3:149–168.
24. Bharucha NE, Stokes L, Schoenberg BS, et al. A case-control study of twin pairs discordant for Parkinson's disease: a search for environmental risk factors. *Neurology* 1986;36:284–288.
25. Bhatia KP, Daniel SE, Marsden CD. Familial parkinsonism with depression: a clinicopathological study. *Ann Neurol* 1993;34:842–847.
26. Bindoff LA, Birch-Machin M, Cartlidge NEF, et al. Respiratory chain abnormalities in skeletal muscle from patients with Parkinson's disease. *J Neurol Sci* 1991;104:203–208.
27. Birkmayer W, Knell J, Rjederer P, et al. Increased life expectancy resulting from addition of L-deprenize to Modopar® treatment in Parkinson's disease: a long term study. *J Neurol Transm* 1985;64:113–127.
28. Blanchet PJ, Allard P, Gregoire L, et al. Risk factors for peak dose dyskinesia in 100 levodopa treated parkinsonian patients. *Can J Neurol Sci* 1996;23:189–193.
29. Block G, Liss C, Reines S, et al. Comparison of immediate release and controlled release carbidopa/levodopa in Parkinson's disease. *Eur Neurol* 1997;37:23–27.

30. Boas J, Worm-Petersen J, Dupont E, et al. The levodopa sparing capacity of pergolide compared with that of bromocriptine in an open label, cross-over study. *Eur J Neurol* 1996;3:44–49.

31. Bodis-Wollner I, Tagliati M. The visual system in Parkinson's disease. *Adv Neurol* 1993;60:390–394.

32. Bonifati V, Fabrizio E, Vanacore N, et al. Familial Parkinson's disease: a clinical genetic analysis. *Can J Neurol Sci* 1995;22:272–279.

33. Bonnet AM, Pichon J, Vidailhet M, et al. Urinary disturbances in striatonigral degeneration and Parkinson's disease: clinical and urodynamic aspects. *Mov Disord* 1997;12:509–513.

34. Bonnet AM, Serre I, Marconi R, et al. A "combined" levodopa test as a useful method for evaluating the efficacy of dopamine agonists: application to pergolide and bromocriptine. *Mov Disord* 1995;10:668–671.

35. Bravi D, Nohria V, Megas LF. Dopamine agonists in the clinical management of Parkinson's disease: symptomatic or neuroprotective effect. *Eur J Neurol* 1996;3:13–18.

36. Brooks D, Playford ED, Ibanez V, et al. Isolated tremor and disruption of the nigrostriatal dopaminergic system: an ^{18}F-dopa PET study. *Neurology* 1992; 42:1554–1560.

37. Brooks DJ, Torjanski N, Burn DJ. Ropinirole in the symptomatic treatment of Parkinson's disease. *J Neural Trans Suppl* 1995;45:231–238.

38. Brown J, Lantos P, Stratton M, et al. Familial progressive supranuclear palsy. *J Neurol Neurosurg Psychiatry* 1993;56:473–476.

39. Burkitt ML, Bilbert BC. Model studies of the iron catalyzed Haber-Weiss cycle and the ascorbate driven Fenton reaction. *Free Radic Res Commun* 1990; 10:265–280.

40. Burn DJ, Mark MH, Playford ED, et al. Parkinson's disease in twins studied with ^{18}F-dopa and positron emission tomography. *Neurology* 1992;42:1894–1900.

41. Burn DJ, Sawle GV, Brooks DJ. Differential diagnosis of Parkinson's disease: multiple system atrophy, and Steele-Richardson-Olszewski syndrome: discriminating analysis of striatal ^{18}F-dopa PET data. *J Neurol Neurosurg Psychiatry* 1994;57:278–284.

42. Butzer JF, Silver D, Sahs AL. Amantadine in Parkinson's disease. *Neurology* 1975;25:603–606.

43. Callaghan N, Mcilroy M, O'Conner M. An extended clinical trial to compare levodopa and amantadine used as single drugs with both drugs used in combination in Parkinson's disease. *Ir J Med Sci* 1974;143:79–85.

44. Calne DB, Chu NS, Huang CC, et al. Manganism and idiopathic parkinsonism: similarities and differences. *Neurology* 1994;44:1583–1586.

45. Calne DB, Langston JW. Aetiology of Parkinson's disease. *Lancet* 1983;2:1457–1459.

46. Campanella G, Filla A, De Michele G, et al. Etiology of Parkinson's disease: results of two case-control studies. *Mov Disord* 1990;5[suppl 1]:31.

47. Canter CJ, de la Torre R, Mier M. A method of evaluating disability in patients with Parkinson's disease. *J Nerv Mental Dis* 1961;133:43–47.

48. Caradoc-Davies TH, Weatherall M, Dixon GS, et al. Is the prevalence of Parkinson's disease in New Zealand really changing? *Acta Neurol Scand* 1992;86:40–44.

49. Cardellach F, Marti MJ, Fernandez-Solri J, et al. Mitochondrial respiratory chain activity in skeletal muscle from patients with Parkinson's disease. *Neurology* 1993;43:2258–2262.

50. Carlson A, Winblad B. Influence of age and time interval between death and autopsy on dopamine and 3-methoxytyramine levels in human basal ganglia. *J Neural Transm* 1976;38:271–276.

51. Carpentier A, Bonnet A, Vidailhet M, et al. Improvement of levodopa-induced dyskinesia by propranolol in Parkinson's disease. *Neurology* 1996;46:1548–1551.

52. Carvey PM, Lin DH, Faselis CJ, et al. Loss of striatal DA innervation increases striatal trophic activity directed at DA neurons in culture. *Exp Neurol* 1996; 140:184–197.

53. Carvey PM, Pieri S, Ling ZD. Attenuation of levodopa-induced toxicity in mesencephalic cultures by pramipexole. *J Neurol Trans* 1997;104:209–228.

54. Cedarbaum JM, Kutt H, McDowell FH. A pharmacokinetic and pharmacodynamic comparison of Sinemet CR (50/200) and standard Sinemet (25/100). *Neurology* 1989;39(Suppl 2):38–44.

55. Chacko RC, Hurley DA, Harper RG, et al. Clozapine for acute and maintenance treatment of psychosis in Parkinson's disease. *J Neuropsychiatry Clin Neurosci* 1995;7:471–475.

56. Chase TN, Baronti F, Fabbrini G, et al. Rationale for continuous dopamimetic therapy of Parkinson's disease. *Neurology* 1989;39[suppl 2]:7–10.

57. Chase TN, Engber TM, Mouradian MM. Palliative and prophylactic benefits of continuously administered dopamimetics in Parkinson's disease. *Neurology* 1994; 44(Suppl 6):515–518.

58. Chesselet MF, Delfs JM. Basal ganglia and movement disorders: an update. *Trends Neurosci* 1996;19:417–422.

59. Chiba K, Trevor A, Castagnoli N. Active uptake of MPP[+], metabolite of MPTP, by brain synaptosomes. *Biochem Biophys Res Commun* 1985;128:1228–1232.

60. Chiba K, Trevor Al, Castagnoli N. Metabolism of the neurotoxic tertiary amine, MPTP, by brain monoamine oxidase. *Biochem Biophys Res Commun* 1984; 120: 574–578.

61. Clarke CE. Mortality from Parkinson's disease in England and Wales 1921–89. *J Neurol Neurosurg Psychiatry* 1993;56:690–693.

62. Cohen G. The pathobiology of Parkinson's disease: biochemical aspects of dopamine neuron senescence. *J Neural Trans Suppl* 1983;19:89–103.

63. Colosimo C, Albanese A, Hughes AJ, et al. Some specific clinical features differentiate multiple system atrophy (striatonigral variety) from Parkinson's disease. *Arch Neurol* 1995;52:294–298.

64. Colosimo C, Merello M, Hughes AJ, et al. Motor response to acute dopaminergic challenge with apomorphine and levodopa in Parkinson's disease: implications for the pathogenesis of the on-off phenomenon. *J Neurol Neurosurg Psychiatry* 1996;60:634–637.

65. Conner JR, Snyder BS, Arosio P, et al. A quantitative analysis of isoferritins in select regions of aged, parkinsonian, and Alzheimer's diseased brains. *J Neurochem* 1995;65:717–724.

66. Cote W, Kremzner LT. Biochemical changes in normal aging in human brain. *Adv Neurol* 1983;38:19–30.

67. Critchley M. Arteriosclerotic parkinsonism. *Brain* 1929;2:23–83.

68. Crowley TJ, Rutledge CO, Hoehn MM, et al. Low urinary dopamine and prediction of phenothiazine induced

parkinsonism: a preliminary report. *Am J Psychiatry* 1971;118:509–518.

69. Cummings J. Frontal-subcortical circuits and human behavior. *Arch Neurol* 1993;50:873–880.

70. D'Alessandro R, Gamberini G, Granieri E, et al. Prevalence of Parkinson's disease in the Republic of San Marine. *Neurology* 1987;37:1679–1682.

71. Danielczyk W. Twenty-five years of amantadine therapy in Parkinson's disease. *J Neural Transm Suppl* 1995;46:399–405.

72. Deiber MP, Pollak P, Passingham R, et al. Thalamic stimulation and suppression of parkinsonian tremor: evidence of a cerebellar deactivation using positron emission tomography. *Brain* 1993;116:267–279.

73. Delalande I, Destee A, Hache JC, et al. Visual evoked potentials and spatiotemporal contrast sensitivity changes in idiopathic Parkinson's disease and multiple system atrophy. *Adv Neurol* 1996;69:319–325.

74. DeLong MR. Primate models of movement disorders of basal ganglia origin. *Trends Neurosci* 1990;13:281–285.

75. De Michele C, Filla A, Volpe G, et al. Environmental and genetic risk factors in Parkinson's disease: a case control study in southern Italy. *Mov Disord* 1996; 11:1723.

76. Dethy S, Laute MA, Luxen A, et al. Effect of pergolide on endogenous and exogenous L-Dopa metabolism in the rat striatum: a microdialysis study. *J Neural Transm* 1995;101:1–11.

77. Dexter DT, Wells FR, Lees AJ, et al. Increased nigral iron content and alterations in other metal ions occurring in brain in Parkinson's disease. *J Neurochem* 1989;52:1830–1836.

78. DiDonato S, Zeviani M, Giovannini P, et al. Respiratory chain and mitochondrial DNA in muscle and brain in Parkinson's disease patients. *Neurology* 1993; 43:2262–2268.

79. Domino EF, Sheng J. Relative potency and efficacy of some dopamine agonists with varying selectivities for D1 and D2 receptors in MPTP-induced hemiparkinsonian monkeys. *J Pharmacol Exp Ther* 1993; 265:1387–1391.

80. Doty RL, Singh A, Tetrud J, et al. Lack of major olfactory dysfunction in MPTP-induced parkinsonism. *Ann Neurol* 1992;32:97–100.

81. Doty RL, Stern MB, Pfeiffer C, et al. Bilateral olfactory dysfunction in early stage treated and untreated idiopathic Parkinson's disease. *J Neurol Neurosurg Psychiatry* 1992;55:138–142.

82. Dubinski RM, Jankovic J. Progressive supranuclear palsy and a multi-infarct state. *Neurology* 1987; 37:570–576.

83. DuPont E, Anderson A, Boris J, et al. Sustained release Madopar HBS compared to standard release Madopar HBS in the long-term treatment of de novo parkinsonian patients. *Acta Neurol Scand* 1996;93:14–20.

84. Durif F, Uidailhet M, Bonnet A, et al. Levodopa-induced dyskinesias are improved by fluoxetine. *Neurology* 1995;45:1855–1858.

85. Duvoisin RC, Eldridge R, Williams A, et al. Twin study of Parkinson's disease. *Neurology* 1981;31:77–80.

86. Duvoisin RC, Yahr MD. Encephalitis and parkinsonism. *Arch Neurol* 1965;12:227–239

87. Ebmeier KP, Calder SA, Crawford JR, et al. Parkinson's disease in Aberdeen: survival after 3.5 years. *Acta Neurol Scand* 1990;813:294–299.

88. Ebmeier KP, Mutch WJ, Calder SA, et al. Does idiopathic parkinsonism in Aberdeen follow intrauterine influenza? *J Neurol Neurosurg Psychiatry* 1989; 52:911–913.

89. Economo CV. Encephalitis lethargica. *Wien Klin Wochenschr* 1917;30:581–585.

90. Eidelberg D, Moeller JR, Ishikawa T, et al. Regional metabolic correlations of surgical outcome following unilateral pallidotomy for Parkinson's disease. *Ann Neurol* 1996;39:450–459.

91. Esmonde T, Giles E, Gibson M, et al. Neuropsychological performance, disease severity, and depression in progressive supranuclear palsy. *J Neurol* 1996; 243:638–643.

92. Fabrini G, Mouradian MM, Juncos JL, et al. Motor fluctuations in Parkinson's disease: central pathophysiologic mechanisms. *Ann Neurol* 1988;24:366–371.

93. Fahn S, Elton RL, members of the UPDRS Development Committee. Unified Parkinson's Disease Rating Scale. In: Fahn S, Marsden CD, Calne DB, Goldstein M, eds. *Recent developments in Parkinson's disease,* vol 2. Florham Park, NJ: Macmillan Health Care Information, 1987:153–164.

94. Fahn S, Isgreen W. Long term evaluation of amantadine and levodopa combination in parkinsonism by double blind crossover analysis. *Neurology* 1975; 25:695–700.

95. Fearnley TM, Lees AJ. Aging and Parkinson's disease: substantia nigra regional selectivity. *Brain* 1991; 114:2283–2301.

96. Felten, DL, Felten SY, Fuller RW, et al. Chronic dietary pergolide preserves nigrostriatal neuronal integrity in aged Fisher 344 rats. *Neurobiol Aging* 1992; 13:339–351.

97. Fici GJ, Wu H, VonVoigtlander PF, et al. D1 dopamine receptor activity of antiparkinsonian drugs. *Life Sci* 1997;60:1597–1603.

98. Fischer P, Danieloxyk W, Simani M, et al. Dopaminergic psychosis in advanced Parkinson's disease. *Adv Neurol* 1990;53:391–397.

99. Fitzgerald PM, Jankovic J. Lower body parkinsonism: evidence for a vascular etiology. *Mov Disord* 1989; 4:249–260.

100. Forno LS, Sternberger LA, Sternberger NH, et al. Reaction of Lewy bodies with antibodies to phosphorylated and non-phosphorylated neurofilaments. *Neurosci Lett* 1986;64:253–258.

101. Fowler JS, Volkow ND, Wang GJ, et al. Inhibition of monoamine oxidase B in the brains of smokers. *Nature* 1996;379:733–736.

102. Friedman DI, Jankovic J, McCrary JA. Neuroophthalmic findings in progressive supranuclear palsy. *J Clin Neurol Ophthalmol* 1992;12:104–109.

103. Freidman JH, Lannon MC. Clozapine in the treatment of psychosis in Parkinson's disease. *Neurology* 1989;39:1219–1221.

104. Friedman JH, Lannon MC. Clozapine-responsive tremor in Parkinson's disease. *Mov Disord* 1990; 5:225–229.

105. Galasko D, Katzman R, Salmon DP, et al. Clinical and neuropathological findings in Lewy body dementias. *Brain Cogn* 1996;31:166–175.

106. Gassen M, Glinka Y, Pinchasi B, et al. Apomorphine is a highly potent free radical scavenger in rat brain mitochondrial fraction. *Eur J Pharmacol* 1996;308:219–225.

107. Gerfen CR, Engber TM, Mahan LC, et al. D1 and D2 dopamine receptor regulated gene expression of striatonigral and striatopallidal neurons. *Science* 1990; 250:1429–1432.

108. Ghika J, Tennis M, Hoffman E, et al. Idazoxan treatment in progressive supranuclear palsy. *Neurology* 1991;35:619–621.

109. Gibb WRC. Idiopathic Parkinson's disease and the Lewy body disorders. *Neuropathol Appl Neurobiol* 1986;12:223–234.

110. Gibb WRG, Lees AJ. The significance of the Lewy body in the diagnosis of idiopathic Parkinson's disease. *Neuropathol Appl Neurobiol* 1989;15:27–44.

111. Gibb WR, Scott T, Lees AJ. Neuronal inclusions of Parkinson's disease. *Mov Disord* 1991;6:2–11.

112. Ginsberg MD. Delayed neurological deterioration following hypoxia. *Adv Neurol* 1979;26:21–43.

113. Giorguieff-Chesselet MF, Kemel ML, Wandscheer D, et al. Regulation of dopamine release by presynaptic nicotine receptors in rat striatal slices: effect of nicotine in a low concentration. *Life Sci* 1979;25:1257–1262.

114. Godwin-Austin RB, Lee PN, Marmot MG, et al. Smoking and Parkinson's disease. *J Neurol Neurosurg Psychiatry* 1982;45:577–581.

115. Goetz CG. New strategies with dopaminergic drugs: modified formulations of levodopa and novel agonists. *Exp Neurol* 1997;144:17–20.

116. Goetz CG, Lutge W, Tanner C. Autonomic dysfunction in Parkinson's disease. *Neurology* 1986;36:73–75.

117. Goetz CG, Stebbins GT. Risk factors for nursing home placement in advanced Parkinson's disease. *Neurology* 1993;43:2227–2229.

118. Golbe LI. The epidemiology of progressive supranuclear palsy. *Adv Neurol* 1996;69:25–31.

119. Golbe LI. The genetics of Parkinson's disease: a reconsideration. Neurology 1990;40[suppl 3]:7–14.

120. Golbe LI, Davis PH. Prevalence and natural history of progressive supranuclear palsy. *Neurology* 1988; 38:1031–1034.

121. Golbe LI, Di Iorio C, Bonavita V, et al. A large kindred with autosomal dominant Parkinson's disease. *Ann Neurol* 1990;27:276–282.

122. Golbe LI, Di Iorio G, Sanges G, et al. Clinical analysis of Parkinson's disease in the Contursi kindred. *Ann Neurol* 1996;40:55–63.

123. Golbe LI, Farrell TM, Davis PH. Follow up study of early life protective and risk factors in Parkinson's disease. *Mov Disord* 1990;5:66–70.

124. Golbe LI, Lazzarini AM, Schwartz KO, et al. Autosomal dominant parkinsonism with benign course and typical Lewy-body pathology. *Neurology* 1993; 43:2222–2227.

125. Golbe LI, Rubin RS, Cody RP, et al. Follow-up study of risk factors in progressive supranuclear palsy. *Neurology* 1996;47:148–154.

126. Gomez Arevalo G, Jorge R, Garcia S, et al. Clinical and pharmacological differences in early versus late onset Parkinson's disease. *Mov Disord* 1997;12:277–284.

127. Gotham AM, Brown RG, Marsden CD. Depression in Parkinson's disease: a quantitative and qualitative analysis. *J Neurol Neruosurg Psychiatry* 1986; 49:381–389.

128. Goto A. A long duration follow-up study of encephalitis japonica. *Folia Psychiatry Neurol Jpn* 1963; 17:326–334.

129. Gouider-Khouja N, Vidailhet M, Bonnet AM, et al. "Pure" striatonigral degeneration and Parkinson's disease: a comparative clinical study. *Mov Disord* 1995;10:288–294.

130. Grafman J, Litvan I, Stark M. Neuropsychological features of progressive supranuclear palsy. *Brain Cogn* 1995;28:311–320.

131. Grafton ST, Waters C, Sutton J, et al. Pallidotomy increases activity of the motor association cortex in Parkinson's disease: a positron emission tomographic study. *Ann Neurol* 1995;37:776–783.

132. Granata R, Wenning GK, Jolkkonen J, et al. Effect of repeated administration of dopamine agonists on striatal neuropeptide mRNA expression in rats with a unilateral nigral 6-hydroxydopamine lesion. *J Neural Transm* 1996;103:249–260.

133. Grandinetti A, Morens DM, Reed D, et al. Prospective study of cigarette smoking and the risk of developing idiopathic Parkinson's disease. *Am J Epidemiol* 1994; 139:1129–1138.

134. Granieri E, Carreras M, Casetta I, et al. Parkinson's disease in Ferrara, Italy, 1967 through 1987. *Arch Neurol* 1991;48:854–857.

135. Grelack RP, Clark R, Stump JM, et al. Amantadine–dopamine interaction: possible mode of action in parkinsonism. *Science* 1970;169:203–204.

136. Grondin R, Bedard PJ, Britton, DR, et al. Potential therapeutic use of the selective dopamine D1 receptor agonist, A-86929. *Neurology* 1997;49:421–426.

137. Guttman M. Double blind comparison of pramipexole and bromocriptine treatment with placebo in advanced Parkinson's disease. *Neurology* 1997; 49:1060–1065.

138. Hall ED, Andrus PK, Oostveen JA, et al. Neuroprotective effects of the dopamine D2/D3 agonist pramipexole against postischemic or methamphetamine-induced degeneration of nigrostriatal neurons. *Brain Res* 1996; 742:80–88.

139. Hao R, Ebadi M, Pfeiffer RF. Selegeline protects dopaminergic neurons in culture from toxic factors present in the cerebrospinal fluid of patients with Parkinson's disease. *Neurosci Lett* 1995;200:77–80.

140. Hao R, Norgren RB, Lau YS, et al. Cerebrospinal fluid of Parkinson's disease patients inhibits the growth and function of dopaminergic neurons in culture. *Neurology* 1995;45:138–142.

141. Harada H, Nishikawa S, Takahashi K. Epidemiology of Parkinson's disease in a Japanese city. *Arch Neurol* 1983;40:151–154.

142. Harris JP, Calvert JE, Phillipson OT. Processing of spatial contrast in peripheral vision in Parkinson's disease. *Brain* 1992;115:1447–1457.

143. Haug BA, Trenkwalder C, Arden GB, et al. Visual thresholds to low-contrast pattern displacement, color contrast, and luminance contrast stimuli in Parkinson's disease. *Mov Disord* 1994;9:563–570.

144. Hauw JJ, Daniel SE, Dickson D, et al. Preliminary NINDS neuropathologic criteria for Steele-Richardson-Olszewski syndrome (progressive supranuclear palsy). *Neurology* 1994;44:2015–2019.

145. Hazrati LN, Parent A. Projection from the external pallidum to the reticular thalamic nucleus in the squirrel monkey. *Brain* 1994;550:142–146.

146. Heikkila RE, Manzino L, Cabbat FS, et al. Protection against the dopaminergic neurotoxicity of 1-methyl-

affinal-tetrahydropyridine by monoamine oxidase inhibitors. *Nature* 1984;311:467–469.

147. Henderson JM, Yiannikas C, Morris JGL, et al. The postural tremor of Parkinson's diseases. *Clin Neuropharmacol* 1994;17:277–285.

148. Hertzman C, Wiens M, Bowering D, et al. Parkinson's disease: a case-control study of occupational and environmental risk factors. *Am J Ind Med* 1990;17:349–355.

149. Hirano A, Zimmerman HM. Alzheimer's neurofibrillary changes: a topographic study. *Arch Neurol* 1962; 7:227–242.

150. Hirsch EC, Mouatt A, Faucheux B, et al. Dopamine, tremor, and Parkinson's disease [Letter]. *Lancet* 1992;340:125–126.

151. Ho SC, Woo J, Lee CM. Epidemiologic study of Parkinson's disease in Hong Kong. *Neurology* 1989; 39:1314–1318.

152. Holt WL. Epidemic encephalitis: a follow-up study of two hundred and sixty-six cases. *Arch Neurol Psychiatry* 1937;38:1135–1144.

153. Hornykiewicz O. Parkinson's disease and its chemotherapy. *Biochem Pharmacol* 1975;24:1061–1065.

154. Horstink MW, Zijimans JCM, Pasman JW, et al. Severity of Parkinson's disease is a risk factor for peak-dose dyskinesia. *J Neurol Neurosurg Psychiatry* 1990; 53:224–226.

155. Hubble JP, Cao T, Hassanein RES, et al. Risk factors for Parkinson's disease. *Neurology* 1993;43:1693–1697.

156. Hubble JP, Koller WC, Cutler NR, et al. Pramipexole in patients with early Parkinson's disease. *Clin Neuropharmacol* 1995;18:338–347.

157. Hutchison WD, Lozano AM, Davis KD, et al. Differential neuronal activity in segments of globus pallidus in Parkinson's disease patients. *Neuroreport* 1994; 5:1533–1537.

158. Hutton JT; Morris JL, Elias JW. Levodopa improves spatial contrast sensitivity in Parkinson's disease. *Arch Neurol* 1993;50:721–724.

159. Hutton JT, Morris JL, Elias JW, et al. Spatial contrast sensitivity is reduced in bilateral Parkinson's disease. *Neurology* 1991;41:1200–1202.

160. Ikebe S, Tanaka 191, Ozawa T. Point mutations of mitochondrial genome in Parkinson's disease. *Mol Brain Res* 1995;28:281–295.

161. Ikeguchi K, Kuroda A. Mianserin treatment of patients with psychosis induced by antiparkinsonian drugs. *Eur Arch Psychiatry Clin Neurosci* 1995;244:320–324.

162. Inzelberg R, Nissipeanu P, Rabey JM, et al. Comparison of cabergoline and bromocriptine in Parkinson's disease patients with motor fluctuations. *Neurology* 1996;47:785–788.

163. Ishikawa A, Miyatake T. Effects of smoking in patients with early-onset Parkinson's disease. *J Neurol Sci* 1993;117:28–32.

164. Isozaki E, Naito A, Horiguchi S, et al. Early diagnosis and stage classification of vocal cord abductor paralysis in patients with multiple system atrophy. *Clin Neuro* 1996;60: 399–402.

165. Iwasaki Y, Ikeda K, Shiojima T, et al. Deprenyl and pergolide rescue spinal motor neurons from axotomy-induced neuronal death in the neonatal rat. *Neurol Res* 1996;18:168–170.

166. Jankovic J, Hiner B, Brown D, et al. Neurogenic orthostatic hypotension: a double blind, placebo controlled study with midodrine. *Am J Med* 1993;95:38–48.

167. Jankovic J, Ben-Aire L, Schwartz K, et al. Movement time and reaction time following GPi pallidotomy. *Ann Neurol* 1997;42:408 (abst).

168. Jankovic J, Friedman DI, Pirozzolo FJ, et al. Progressive supranuclear palsy: motor, neurobehavioral, and neuro-ophthalmic findings. *Adv Neurol* 1990;53: 293–304.

169. Jankovic J, Linfante I, Dawson LE, Contant C. Young-onset versus late onset Parkinson's disease: clinical features and disease progression. *Ann Neurol* 1997;42: 448 (abst).

169a. Jankovic J, Marsden CD. Therapeutic strategies in Parkinson's disease. In: Jankovic J, Tolosa E, eds. *Parkinson's disease and movement disorders*, 3rd ed. Baltimore: Williams & Wilkins, 1998:191–220.

170. Javoy-Agid F, Ruberg M, Pique L, et al. Biochemistry of the hypothalamus in Parkinson's disease. *Neurology* 1984;34:672–675.

171. Jenkins IH, Fernandez W, Playford ED, et al. Impaired activation of the supplementary motor area in Parkinson's disease is reversed when akinesia is treated with apomorphine. *Ann Neurol* 1992;32:749–757.

172. Jenner P, Olanow CW. Pathological evidence for oxidative stress in Parkinson's disease and related degenerative disorders. In: Olanow CW, Jenner P, Youdim MHB, eds. *Neurodegeneration and neuroprotection in Parkinson's disease*. London: Academic Press, 1996: 24–45.

173. Jimenez-Jimenez FJ, Mateo D, Gimenez-Roldan S. Exposure to well-water and pesticides in Parkinson's disease: a case-control study in the Madrid area. *Mov Disord* 1992;7:149–152.

174. Jimenez-Jimenez FJ, Mateo D, Gimenez-Roldan S. Premorbid smoking, alcohol consumption, and coffee drinking habits in Parkinson's disease: a case-control study. *Mov Disord* 1992;7:339–344.

175. Jimenez-Jimenez FJ, Molina JA, Morano A. Parkinson's disease etiology: risk factors and protection. *Neurologia* 1993;8:256–266.

176. Joel D, Weiner I. The organization of the basal ganglia-thalamocortical circuits: open interconnections rather than closed segregation. *Neuroscience* 1994;63:363–379.

177. Johnson WC, Hedge SE, Duvoisin RC. Twin studies and the genetics of Parkinson's disease: a reappraisal. *Mov Disord* 1990; 5:187–194.

178. Johnston B, Castell J, Stumacher S, et al. Comparison of swallowing function in Parkinson's disease and progressive supranuclear palsy. *Mov Disord* 1997; 12:322–327.

179. Jolkkonen J, Jenner P, Marsden CD. L-DPA reverses altered gene expression of substance P but not enkephalin in the caudate-putamen of common marmosets treated with MPTP. *Mol Brain Res* 1995;32:297–307.

180. Jost WH, Schimrigk K. Constipation in Parkinson's disease. *Klin Wochenschr* 1991;69:906–909.

181. Juncos JL, Engber TM, Raisman R, et al. Continuous and intermittent levodopa differentially affect basal ganglia function. *Ann Neurol* 1989;25:473–478.

182. Kalra S, Bergeron C, Lang AK. Lewy body disease and dementia: a review. *Arch Intern Med* 1996; 156: 487–593.

183. Kempster PA, Wahlqvist ML. Dietary factors in the management of Parkinson's disease. *Nutr Rev* 1994; 52:51–58.

184. Kessler II. Epidemiologic studies of Parkinson's disease: a community-based survey. *Am J Epidemiol* 1972;96:242–254.

185. Kessler II, Diamond EL. Epidemiologic studies of Parkinson's disease: smoking and Parkinson's disease: a survey and explanatory hypothesis. *Am J Epidemiol* 1971;94:16–25.

186. Klatka LA, Louis ED, Schiffer R B. Psychiatric features in diffuse Lewy body disease: a clinicopathologic study using Alzheimer's disease and Parkinson's disease comparison groups. *Neurology* 1996;47:1148–1152.

187. Klawans HL, Bergen D, Bruyn GW. Prolonged drug induced parkinsonism. *Confin Neurol* 1973;35: 368–377.

188. Koller W, Pahwa R, Busenbark K, et al. High-frequency unilateral thalamic stimulation in the treatment of essential and parkinsonian tremor. *Ann Neurol* 1997;42:292–299.

189. Koller WC, Vetere-Overfield B, Barter R. Tremor in early Parkinson's disease. *Clin Neuropharmacol* 1989; 12:293–297.

190. Koller W, Vetere-Overfield B, Gray C, et al. Environmental risk factors in Parkinson's disease. *Neurology* 1990;40:1218–1221.

191. Kondo K, Watanabe K. Lifestyles, risk factors, and inherited predispositions in Parkinson's disease: preliminary report of a case-control study. *Adv Neurol* 1993; 60:346–351.

192. Korczyn A. A double blind study comparing ropinirole and bromocriptine in patients with early Parkinson's disease. *Neurology* 1996;46[suppl]:A159 (abst).

193. Korczyn AD, Goldberg GJ. Extrapyramidal effects of neuroleptics. *J Neurol Neurosurg Psychiatry* 1976; 39:866–869.

194. Kosaka K, Iseki E. Dementia with Lewy bodies. *Curr Opin Neurol* 1996;9:971–975.

195. Kostic V, Przedborski S, Flaster E, et al. Early development of levodopa induced dyskinesias and response fluctuations in young-onset Parkinson's disease. *Neurology* 1991;41:202–205.

196. Kriege D, Carroll MT, Cooper JM, et al. Platelet mitochondrial function in Parkinson's disease. *Ann Neurol* 1992;32:782–788.

197. Kuln W, Muller T, Nastos I, et al. The neuroimmune hypothesis in Parkinson's disease. *Rev Neurosci* 1997;8:29–34.

198. Kurth MC, Adler CH, St. Hilaire M, et al. Tolcapone reduces levodopa requirement in patients with Parkinson's disease experiencing motor fluctuations. *Neurology* 1997;48:81–87.

199. Lance J W, Schwab RS, Peterson EA. Action tremor and the cogwheel phenomenon in Parkinson's disease. *Brain* 1963;86:95–110.

200. Lang A, Lozano A, Tasker R, et al. Neuropsychological and behavioral changes and weight gain after medial pallidotomy. *Ann Neurol* 1997;41:834–835.

201. Lang AK, Curran T, Provias J, et al. Striatonigral degeneration: iron deposition in putamen correlates with the slit-like void signal of magnetic resonance imaging. *Can J Neurol Sci* 1995;22:73–74.

202. Lang AK, Lozano A, Montgomery E, et al. Posteroventral medial pallidotomy in advanced Parkinson's disease. *N Engl J Med* 1997;337:1036–1042.

203. Lange KW, Rausch WD, Gsell W, et al. Neuroprotection by dopamine agonists. *J Neural Trans Suppl* 1994;43:183–201.

204. Langston J W, Ballard P, Tetrud JW, et al. Chronic parkinsonism in humans due to a product of meperidine-analog synthesis. *Science* 1983;219:979–980.

205. Langston J W, Widner H, Goetz CG, et al. Core Assessment Program for Intracerebral Transplantations (CAPIT). *Mov Disord* 1992;7:2–13.

206. Lapchak PA. Therapeutic potentials for glial cell linederived neurotrophic factor (GDNF) based upon pharmacologic activities in the CNS. *Rev. Neurosci* 1996; 7:165–176.

207. Lavoie B, Parent A. Pedunculopontine nucleus in the squirrel monkey: projections to the basal ganglia as revealed by anterograde tract tracing methods. *J Comp Neurol* 1994;344:210–231.

208. Lazzari A M, Myers RH, Zimmerman TR, et al. A clinical genetic study of Parkinson's disease: evidence for dominant transmission. *Neurology* 1994;44:493–506.

209. Le W D, Rowe DB, Xie WJ, et al. Tumor necrosis factor is elevated in the cerebrospinal fluid of patients with Parkinson's disease. *Mov Disord* 1997;12:840 (abst).

210. Lee MS, Marsden CD. Neurological sequelae following carbon monoxide poisoning: clinical course and outcome according to clinical types and brain computed tomography scan findings. *Mov Disord* 1994;9: 550–558.

211. Leenders K L, Palmer AJ, Quinn N, et al. Brain dopamine metabolism in patients with Parkinson's disease measured by positron emission tomography. *J Neurol Neurosurg Psychiatry* 1986;49:853–860.

212. Lees A J. Comparison of therapeutic effects and mortality data of levodopa and levodopa combined with selegeline in patients with early, mild Parkinson's disease. *BMJ* 1995;311:1602–1607.

213. Lehrner J, Brucke T, Kryspin-Exner I, et al. Impaired olfactory function in Parkinson's disease. *Lancet* 1995;345:1054–1055.

214. Lepore F. Visual loss as a causative factor in visual hallucinations associated with Parkinson's disease. *Arch Neurol* 1997;54:799.

215. Levi S, Cox M, Lugon M, et al. Increased energy expenditure in Parkinson's disease. *BMJ* 1990;301: 1256–1257.

216. Levin BE, Tomer R, Rey G. Cognitive impairment in Parkinson's disease. *Neurol Clin* 1992;10:471–485.

217. Lewy FH. Zur pathologischen Anatomie der Paralysis agitans. *Csch Z Nernenheilkd* 1914;50:50–55.

218. Liberman A, Imke S, Muenter M, et al. Multicenter study of cabergoline, a long acting dopamine receptor agonist, in Parkinson disease patients with fluctuating responses to levodopa/carbidopa. *Neurology* 1993;43:1981–1984.

219. Lieberman A, Ranhosky A, Korts D. Clinical evaluation of pramipexole in advanced Parkinson's disease. *Neurology* 1997;49:162–168.

220. Liou HH, Tsai MC, Chen CJ, et al. Environmental risk factors and Parkinson's disease. *Neurology* 1997; 48:1583–1588.

221. Litvan I, Agid Y, Goetz C, et al. Accuracy of the clinical diagnosis of corticobasal degeneration: a clinicopathologic study. *Neurology* 1997;48:119–125.

222. Litvan I, Agid Y, Jankovic J, et al. Accuracy of clinical criteria for the diagnosis of progressive supranuclear palsy (Steele-Richardson-Olszewski syndrome). *Neurology* 1996;46:922–930.

223. Litvan I, Campbell G, Mangone CA, et al. Which clinical features differentiate progressive supranuclear palsy (Steele-Richardson-Olszewski syndrome) from related disorders? A clinicopathological study. *Brain* 1997;120:65–74.

224. Litvan I, Mangone CA, McKee A, et al. Natural history of progressive supranuclear palsy (Steele-Richardson-Olszewski syndrome) and clinical predictors of survival: a clinicopathological study. *J Neurol Neurosurg Psychiatry* 1996;60:615–620.

225. Litvan I, Mega MS, Cummings JL, et al. Neuropsychiatric aspects of progressive supranuclear palsy. *Neurology* 1996;47:1184–1189.

226. Lopez-Talavera JC, Cadelina G, Olchowski J, et al. Thalidomide inhibits tumor necrosis factor alpha, decreases nitric oxide synthesis, and ameliorates the hyperdynamic circulatory syndrome in portal-hypertensive rats. *Hepatology* 1996;23:1616–1621.

227. Louis ED, Fahn S. Pathologically diagnosed diffuse Lewy body disease and Parkinson's disease: do the parkinsonian features differ? *Adv Neurol* 1996; 69:311–314.

228. Louis ED, Klatka LA, Liu Y, et al. Comparison of extrapyramidal features in 31 pathologically confirmed cases of diffuse Lewy body disease and 34 pathologically confirmed cases of Parkinson's disease. *Neurology* 1997;48:376–380.

229. Louis ED, Marder K, Cote H, et al. Mortality from Parkinson's disease. *Arch Neurol* 1997;54:260–264.

230. Low P, Gilden J, Freeman R, et al. Efficacy of midodrine vs placebo in neurogenic orthostatic hypotension. *JAMA* 1997;277:1046–1051.

231. Magazanik LG, Antonov AM, Lukomakaya NA, et al. Blockade of glutamate- and cholinergic ion channels by amantadine derivatives. *Neurosci Behav Phys* 1996; 26:1322.

232. Mann VM, Cooper JM, Krige D, et al. Brain, skeletal muscle and platelet homogenate mitochondrial function in Parkinson's disease. *Brain* 1992;115:333–342.

233. Maraganore DM, Harding AK, Marsden CD. A clinical and genetic study of familial Parkinson's disease. *Mov Disord* 1990;6:205–211.

234. Marconi R, Lefebure-Caparros D, Bonnet AM, et al. Levodopa induced dyskinesias in Parkinson's disease: phenomonology and pathophysiology. *Mov Disord* 1994;9:212.

235. Marder K, Tang MX, Mejia H, et al. Risk of Parkinson's disease among first degree relatives. *Neurology* 1996;47:155–160.

236. Marek K, Friedman J, Hauser R, et al. Phase II evaluation of rasagaline mesylate (TVP-1012), a novel antiparkinsonian drug, in parkinsonian patients not using carbidopa/levodopa. *Mov Disord*. 1998 (*in press*).

237. Markus HS, Cox M, Tomkins AM. Raised resting energy expenditure in Parkinson's disease and its relationship to muscle rigidity. *Clin Sci* 1992;83:199–204.

238. Marsden CD, Tarsy D, Baldessarini RJ. Spontaneous and drug induced movement disorders. In: Benson DF, Blumer D, eds. *Psychiatric aspects of neurologic disease*. Orlando: Grune & Stratton, 1975.

239. Marttila RI, Arstila P, Nikoskelainen J, et al. Viral antibodies in the sera from patients with Parkinson's disease. *Eur Neurol* 1977;15:25–33.

240. Marttila RJ, Kalimo KOK, Ziola BR, et al. Herpes simplex virus subunit antibodies in patients with Parkinson's disease. *Arch Neurol* 1978;35:668–671.

241. Massman PJ, Kreiter KT, Jankovic J, et al. Neuropsychological functioning in cortical-basal ganglionic degeneration. *Neurology* 1996;46:720–726.

242. Masson G, Mestre D, Thin O. Dopaminergic modulation of visual sensitivity in man. *Fundam Clin Pharmacol* 1993;7:449–463.

243. Matison R, Mayeux R, Rosen J, et al "Tip-of-the-tongue" phenomenon in Parkinson's disease. *Neurology* 1982;32:567–570.

244. Mayeux R, Denaro J, Hemenegildo N, et al. A population based investigation of Parkinson's disease with and without dementia: relationships to age and gender. *Arch Neurol* 1992;42:492–497.

245. Mayeux R, Tang MX, Marder K, et al. Smoking and Parkinson's disease. *Mov Disord* 1994;9:207–212.

246. McGeer PL, Itagaki S, McGeer KG. Expression of the histocompatibility glycoprotein HLA-DR in neurological disease. *Acta Neuropathol (Berl)* 1988;76:550–557.

247. Mclean DR, Jacobs H, Mielke BW. Methanol poisoning: a clinical and pathological study. *Ann Neurol* 1980;8:161–167.

248. Melamed E, Rosenthal J, Globus M, et al. Suppression of MPTP induced dopaminergic neurotoxicity in mice by nomifensine and L-dopa. *Brain Res* 1985;342: 401–404.

249. Melcon MO, Anderson D, Vergara R, et al. Prevelence of Parkinson's disease in Junin, Buenos Aries Province, Argentina. *Mov Disord* 1997;12:197–205.

250. Mena I, Court I, Fuenzalida S, et al. Modification of chronic manganese poisoning: treatment with levodopa or 5-OH tryptophane. *N Engl J Med* 1970:82:510.

251. Mena I, Marin O, Fuenzalida S, et al. Chronic manganese poisoning: clinical picture and manganese turnover. *Neurology* 1967;17:128–136.

252. Mendez-Alvarez E, Soto-Otero R, Sanchez-Sellero I, et al. Inhibition of brain monoamine oxidase by addicts of 1,2,3,4—tetrahydroisoquinoline with components of cigarette smoke. *Life Sci* 1997;60:1719–1727.

253. Mendis T, Mohr E, George A, et al. Symptomatic relief from treatment induced psychosis in Parkinson's disease: an open label pilot study with remoxipride. *Mov Disord* 1994;9:197–200.

254. Mestre DR, Thin O, van den Brand CL, et al. Effects of L-dopa on spatiotemporal contrast sensitivity in Parkinson's disease. *Neurology* 1996;69:503–511.

255. Min SK. A brain syndrome associated with delayed neuropsychiatric sequelae following acute carbon monoxide intoxication. *Acta Psychiatr Scand* 1986; 73:80–86.

256. Mizuno Y, Kondo T, Narabayashi H, et al. Pergolide in the treatment of Parkinson's disease. *Neurology* 1995;45[suppl 3]:S13–S21.

257. Mizuno Y, Matuda S, Yoshino H, et al. An immuno-histochemical study on α-ketoglutarate dehydrogenase complex in Parkinson's disease. *Ann Neurol* 1989; 35:204–210.

258. Mizuno Y, Suzuki K, Sone N, et al. Inhibition of ATP synthesis by 1—methyl-4-phenylpyridinium ion (MPP$^+$) in isolated mitochondria from mouse brains. *Neurosci Lett* 1987;81:204–208.

259. Mogi M, Harada M, Kondo T, et al. Brain beta 2-microglobulin levels are elevated in the striatum in Parkinson's disease. *J Neural Transm* 1995;9:87–92.

260. Mogi M, Harada M, Narabayashi H, et al. Interleukin (IL)-1 beta, IL-2, IL-4, IL-6 and transforming growth factor-alpha levels are elevated in ventricular cerebrospinal fluid in juvenile parkinsonism and Parkinson's disease. *Neurosci Lett* 1996;211:13–16.

261. Mogi M, Harada M, Riererer P, et al. Tumor necrosis factor (TNF-α) increases both in the brain and in the cerebrospinal fluid from parkinsonian patients. *Neurosci Lett* 1994;165:208–210.

262. Mogi M, Harada M, Riederer P, et al. Tumor necrosis factor-α (TNF-α) increases both in the brain and in the cerebral spinal fluid from parkinsonian patients. *Neurosci Lett* 1994;193:129–132.

263. Moleman P, Janzen G, von Bargan BA, et al. Relationship between age and incidence of parkinsonism in psychiatric patients treated with haloperidol. *Am J Psychiatry* 1986;143:232–234.

264. Molho ES, Factor SA, Weiner WJ, et al. The use of pramipexole, a novel dopamine agonist, in advanced Parkinson's disease. *J Neural Transm Suppl* 1995;45: 225–230.

265. Morens DM, Grandinetti A, Reed D, et al. Smoking and protection from Parkinson's disease: false association or etiologic clue? *Neurology* 1995;45:1041–1051.

266. Morgante L, Rocca WA, Di Rosa A K, et al. Prevalence of Parkinson's disease and other parkinsonisms: a door-to-door survey in three Sicilian municipalities. *Neurology* 1992;42:1901–1907.

267. Mouradian MM, Heuser IJE, Baronti F, et al. Modifications of central dopaminergic mechanisms by continuous levodopa therapy for advanced Parkinson's disease. *Ann Neurol* 1990;27:15–23.

268. Mouradian MM, Juncos J, Fabbrini G, et al. Motor fluctuations in Parkinson's disease: central pathophysiological mechanisms, Part II. *Ann Neurol* 1988;24: 372–378.

269. Muenter MD, Sharpless MS, Tyce GM, et al. Patterns of dystonia ("I-D-I" and "DID") in response to levodopa therapy of Parkinson's disease. *Mayo Clin Proc* 1977;52:163–174.

270. Mulder DW, Parrott M, Thaler M. Sequelae of Western equine encephalitis. *Neurology* 1951;1:318–327.

271. Munschauer FE, Loh L, Bannister G, et al. Abnormal respiration and sudden death during sleep in multiple system atrophy with autonomic failure. *Neurology* 1990;40:677–679.

272. Mutch WJ, Dingwall-Fordyce I, Downie AW, et al. Parkinson's disease in a Scottish city. *Pr Med J* 1986;292:534–536.

273. Nagashama Y, Fukuyama H, Turjanski N, et al. Cerebral glucose metabolism in corticobasal degeneration: comparison with progressive supranuclear palsy and normal controls. *Mov Disord* 1997;12:691–696.

274. Nakagawa-Hattori Y, Hoshino H, Kondo T, et al. Is Parkinson's disease a mitochondrial disorder? *J Neurol Sci* 1992;107:29–33.

275. Nausieda PA, Wiener WJ, Kaplan LR, et al. Sleep disturbances in the course of chronic levodopa therapy: an early feature of the levodopa psychosis. *Clin Neuropharmacol* 1982;5:183–194.

276. Nicklas WJ, Vyas I, Heikkila R E. Inhibition of NADH-linked oxidation in brain mitochondria by 1-methyl-4-phenyl-pyridine, a metabolite of the neurotoxin, 1-methyl-4-phenyl-1,2,5,6 tetrahydropyridine. *Life Sci* 1985;36:2503–2508.

277. Nieforth KA, Golbe LI. Retrospective study of drug response in 87 patients with progressive supranuclear palsy. *Clin Neuropharmacol* 1993;16:338–346.

278. Nishibayashi S, Asanuma M, Kohno M, et al. Scavenging effects of dopamine agonists on nitric oxide radicals. *J Neurochem* 1996;67:2208–2211.

279. Nutt JC. Levodopa induced dyskinesias. *Neurology* 1990;40:340–345.

280. Obeso J, Linazasaro G, Gorospe A, et al. Complications associated with chronic levodopa therapy in Parkinson's disease. In: Olanow CW, Obeso J, eds. *Beyond the decade of the brain*. Kent: Wells Medical, 1997: 11–36.

281. Okada K, Kobayashi S, Tsunematsu T. Prevalence of Parkinson's disease in Izumo City, Japan. *Gerontology* 1990,36:340–344.

282. Olanow CW, Calne D. Does selegeline monotherapy in Parkinson's disease act by symptomatic or protective mechanisms? *Neurology* 1992;42[suppl 4]:13.

283. Olanow CW, Fahn S, Langston J W, et al. Selegeline and mortality in Parkinson's disease. *Ann Neurol* 1996;40:841–845.

284. Olanow CW, Fahn S, Muenter M, et al. A multi-center double-blind placebo-controlled trial of pergolide as an adjunct to Sinemet in Parkinson's disease. *Mov Disord* 1994;9:40–47.

285. Olanow CW, Hauser RA, Gauger L, et al. The effect of deprenyl and levodopa on the progression of Parkinson's disease. *Ann Neurol* 1995;38:771–777.

286. Olanow CW, Jenner P, Tatton NA, Tatton WG. Neurodegeneration and Parkinson's disease. In: Jankovic J, Tolosa E, eds. *Parkinson's disease and movement disorders*, 3rd ed. Baltimore: Williams & Wilkins, 1998: 67–104.

287. Ondo WG, Contant C, Jankovic J. Weight gain following unilateral pallidotomy. *Mov Disord* 1997;12:844 (abst).

288. Ondo WG, Warrior D, Overby AR, et al. Computerized posturography in progressive supranuclear palsy. *Ann Neurol* 1997;42:449 (abst).

289. Otsuka M, Ichlya Y, Kuwabara Y, et al. Differences in the reduced ^{18}F-dopa uptake of the caudate and the putamen in Parkinson's disease: correlations with the three main symptoms. *J Neurol Sci* 1995;136:169–173.

290. Ozawa T, Tanaka M, Ikebe S, et al. Quantitative determination of deleted mitochondrial DNA relative to normal DNA in parkinsonian striatum by a kinetic PCR analysis. *Biochem Biophys Res Commun* 1990;172: 483–489.

291. Pacchetti C, Albani G, Martignoni E, et al. "Off" painful dystonia in Parkinson's disease treated with botulinum toxin. *Mov Disord* 1995;10:333–336.

292. Pahwa R, Lyons K, McGuire D, et al. Comparison of standard carbidopa-levodopa and sustained release carbidopa-levodopa in Parkinson's disease: pharmacokinetics and quality of life. *Mov Disord* 1997; 12:677–681.

293. Papa SM, Chase T. Levodopa induced dyskinesias improved by a glutamate antagonist in parkinsonian monkeys. *Ann Neurol* 1996;39:574–578.

294. Papp MI, Hahn J E, Lantos PK. Glial cytoplasmic inclusions in the CNS of patients with multiple system atrophy. *J Neurol Sci* 1989;94:79–100.

295. Papp MI, Lantos PL. The distribution of oligodendroglial inclusions in multiple system atrophy and its relevance to clinical symptomatology. *Brain* 1994; 117:235–243.

296. Pappolla MA, Shank DL, Alzofon J, et al. Colloid (hyaline) inclusion bodies in the central nervo us system: their presence in the substantia nigra is diagnostic of Parkinson's disease. *Hum Pathol* 1988;19:27–31.

297. Parent A, Hazrati LN. Functional anatomy of the basal ganglia. II. The place of subthalamic nucleus and external pallidum in basal ganglia circuitry. *Brain Res Rev* 1995;20:128–154.

298. Parker SG, Raval P, Yeulet S, et al. Tolerance to peripheral, but not central, effects of ropinirole, a selective dopamine D2-like receptor agonist. *Eur J Pharmacol* 1994;265:17–26.

299. Parker W D, Boyson SJ, Parks JK. Abnormalities of the electron transport chain in idiopathic Parkinson's disease. *Ann Neurol* 1989;26:719–723.

300. Parkes J D, Curzon G, Knott PJ, et al. Treatment of Parkinson's disease with amantadine end levodopa. *Lancet* 1971;1:1083–1086.

301. Parkes J D, Zilkha KJ, Calver DM, et al. Controlled trial of amantadine hydrochloride in Parkinson's disease. *Lancet* 1970;1:259–262.

302. Parkinson J. *An essay on the shaking palsy.* London: Sherwood, Neely & Jones, 1817.

303. Parkinson's Disease Research Group in the United Kingdom. Comparison of therapeutic effects and mortality data from levodopa and levodopa combined with selegeline in patients with early mild Parkinson's disease. *BMJ* 1995;311:1602–1606.

304. Parkinson Study Group. A controlled trial of lazabemide (Ro19-6327) in untreated Parkinson's disease. *Ann Neurol* 1993;33:350–356.

305. Parkinson's Study Group. Effect of tocopherol and deprenyl on the progression of disability in early Parkinson's disease. *N Engl J Med* 1993;328:176.

305a. Parkinson Study Group. Mortality in DATATOP: a multicenter trial in early Parkinson's disease. *Ann Neurol* 1998;43:318–325.

306. Paulson GW. Addiction to nicotine is due to high intrinsic levels of dopamine. *Med Hypotheses* 1992;38:206–207.

307. Paulson GW, Dadmehr N. Is there a premorbid personality typical for Parkinson's disease? *Neurology* 1991;41[suppl 2]:73–76.

308. Paulson H, Stern M. Clinical manifestations of Parkinson's disease. In: Watts R, Koller W, eds. *Movement disorders.* New York: McGraw-Hill, 1996:183–219.

309. Pearce RK, Hawkes CH, Daniel SE. The anterior olfactory nucleus in Parkinson's disease. *Mov Disord* 1995;10:283–287.

310. Perani D, Bressi S, Testa D, et al. Clinical/metabolic correlations in multiple system atrophy: a flourodeoxyglucose F-18 positron emission tomographic study. *Arch Neurol* 1995;52:179–185.

311. Peters H A, Levine R L, Matthews CG, et al. Extrapyramidal and other neurological manifestations associated with carbon disulfide fumigant exposure. *Arch Neurol* 1988;45:537–540.

312. Pezzoli G, Canesi M, Pesenti A, et al. Pergolide mesylate in Parkinson's disease treatment. *J Neural Transm Suppl* 1995;45:203–212.

313. Pezzoli G, Martignoni E, Pacchetti C, et al. A crossover, controlled study comparing pergolide with bromocriptine as an adjunct to levodopa for the treatment of Parkinson's disease. *Neurology* 1995;45 [suppl 3]:S22–S27.

314. Pfeiffer R F. Antiparkinsonian agents: drug interactions of clinical significance. *Drug Safety* 1996;14:343–354.

315. Piercey M F, Hoffmann WE, Smith MW, et al. Inhibition of dopamine neuron firing by premipexole, a dopamine D3 receptor-preferring agonist: comparison to other dopamine receptor agonists. *Eur J Pharmacol* 1996;312:35–44.

316. Pillon B, Gouider-Khouja N, Deweer B, et al. Neuropsychological pattern of striatonigral degeneration: comparison with Parkinson's disease and progressive supranuclear palsy. *J Neurol Neurosurg Psychiatry* 1995;58:174–179.

317. Playford ED, Jenkins IH, Passingham RE, et al. Impaired mesial frontal and putamen activity in Parkinson's disease: a positron emission tomography study. *Ann Neurol* 1992;32:151–161.

318. Poewe WH, Lees AJ, Stern GM. Low dose levodopa therapy in Parkinson's disease: a 6-year follow-up study. *Neurology* 1986;36:1528–1530.

319. Polymeropolis MH, Higgins JJ, Golbe LI, et al. Mapping of a gene for Parkinson's disease to chromosome 4q21 -q74. *Science* 1996;274:1197–1199.

320. Polymeropolis MH, Lavedan C, Leroy E, et al. Mutation of the asynuclein gene identified in families with Parkinson's disease. *Science* 1997;276:2045–2047.

321. Poungvarin N, Prayoonwiwat N, Devahasatin V, et al. An open label trial of pergolide in Thai patients with Parkinson's disease. *J Med Assoc Thai* 1996;79:205–209.

322. Price M J, Feldman RG, Adelberg D, et al. Abnormalities in color vision and contrast sensitivity in Parkinson's disease. *Neurology* 1992;42:887–890.

323. Rajput A H, Fenton ME, Birdi S, et al. Is levodopa toxic to human substantia nigra? *Mov Disord* 1997;12:634–638.

324. Rajput A H, Martin W, Saint-Hilaire H, et al. Tolcapone improves motor function in parkinsonian patients with the "wearing off" phenomenon. *Neurology* 1997;49:1066–1071.

325. Rajput A H, Offord KP, Beard CM, et al. Epidemiology of parkinsonism: incidence, classification, and mortality. *Ann Neurol* 1984;16:278–282

326. Rajput A H, Pahwa R, Pahwa P, et al. Prognostic significance of the onset mode in parkinsonism. *Neurology* 1993;43:829–830.

327. Rajput A H, Rozdilsky B, Hornykiewicz O, et al. Reversible drug-induced parkinsonism: clinicopathologic study of two cases. *Arch Neurol* 1982;39:644–646.

328. Ramsay R R, Dadgar J, Trevor A, et al. Energy-driven uptake of *N*-methyl-4-phenylpyridine by brain mitochondria mediates the neurotoxicity of MPTP. *Life Sci* 1986;39:581–588.

329. Ramsay R R, Singer TP. Energy-dependent uptake of *N*-methyl-4-phenylpyridinium, the neurotoxic metabolite of 1-methyl-4-phenyl-1,2,3,6-tetrahydropyridine, by mitochondria. *J Biol Chen* 1986;261:7585–7587.

330. Rascol O, Lees AJ, Senard JM, et al. Ropinirole in the treatment of levodopa-induced motor fluctuations in patients with Parkinson's disease. *Clin Neuropharmacol* 1996;19:234–245.

331. Rascol O, Sabatini U, Chollet F, et al. Supplementary and primary sensory motor area activity in Parkinson's disease: regional cerebral blood flow changes during finger movements and the effects of apomorphine. *Arch Neurol* 1992;49:144–148.

332. Reef H E. Prevalence of Parkinson's disease in a multiracial community. *Int Congr Ser* 1977;427:125.

333. Richard IH, Kurlan R, Tanner C, et al. Serotonin syndrome and the combined use of deprenyl and an antidepressant in Parkinson's disease: Parkinson study group. *Neurology* 1997;48:1070–1077.

334. Rinne JO, Lee MS, Thompson PD, et al. Corticobaal degeneration: a clinical study of 36 cases. *Brain* 1994;117:1183–1196.

335. Rinne KM. Treatment of "de novo" parkinsonian patients: the role of cabergoline. Presented at the Fourth International Congress of Movement Disorders, Vienna, 1996.

336. Rinne UK. Early dopamine agonist therapy in Parkinson's disease. *Mov Disord* 1989;4[suppl 1]:S86–S94.

337. Rinne UK, Rinne OG. Madopar HBS in the treatment of early Parkinson's disease. In: Agroli A, Campanella C, eds. *New developments in the treatment of Parkinson's disease*. Rome: Libbey, 1991:17–21.

338. Robbins TW, James M, Lange KW, et al. Cognitive performance in multiple system atrophy. *Brain* 1992; 115:271–291.

339. Roos RAC, Vredevoogd CB, Vandervelde ER. Response fluctuations in Parkinson's disease. *Neurology* 1990;40:1344–1346.

340. Rosati G, Granieri E, Pinna L, et al. The risk of Parkinson disease in Mediterranean people. *Neurology* 1980;30:250–255.

341. Rosenberg NL, Myers JA, Wayne WR. Cyanide-induced parkinsonism: clinical, MRI, and 6-flouorodopa PET studies. *Neurology* 1989;39:142–144.

342. Routtinen HM, Rinne UK. Entacapone prolongs levodopa response in a one month double blind study in parkinsonian patients with levodopa related fluctuations. *J Neurol Neurosurg Psychiatry* 1996;60:36–40.

343. Saint-Cyr JA, Taylor AK, Lang AK. Neuropsycholgal and psychiatric side effects in the treatment of Parkinson's disease. *Neurology* 1993;43[suppl 6]:S47–S52.

344. Saitoh T. Suppression of 1-methyl-4-phenyl-1,2,3,6-tetrahydropyridine (MPTP) induced dopaminergic neurotoxicity in mouse brain by pirocheptine and trihexyphenidyl. *J Neurol Sci* 1988;83:161–166.

345. Savoiardo M, Girotti F, Strada L, et al. Magnetic resonance imaging in progressive supranuclear palsy and other parkinsonian disorders. *J Neural Trans in Suppl* 1994;42:93–110.

346. Sayler ME, Street JS, Bosomworth JC, et al. Analysis of mortality in pergolide treated patients with Parkinson's disease. *Neuroepidemiology* 1996;15:26–32.

347. Schapira AHV, Cooper JM, Dexter D, et al. Mitochondrial complex I deficiency in Parkinson's disease. *J Neurochem* 1990;54:823–827.

348. Schapira AHV, Cooper JM, Dexter D, et al. Mitochondrial complex I deficiency in Parkinson's disease. *Lancet* 1989;1:1269.

349. Schenck CH, Bundlie SR, Mahowald MW. Delayed emergence of a parkinsonian disorder in 38% of 29 older men initially diagnosed with idiopathic rapid eye movement sleep behavior disorder. *Neurology* 1996; 46:388–393.

350. Schneider. JS, Pope A, Simpson K, et al. Recovery from experimental parkinsonism in primates with GMI ganglioside treatment. *Science* 1992;256:843–846.

351. Schoenberg BS, Anderson DW, Haerer AF. Prevalence of Parkinson's disease in the biracial population of Copiah County, Mississippi. *Neurology* 1985;35: 841–845.

352. Schuh LA, Bennett JP. Suppression of dyskinesias in advanced Parkinson's disease: continuous intravenous levodopa shifts dose response for production of dyskinesias but not for relief of parkinsonism in patients with advanced Parkinson's disease. *Neurology* 1993; 43:1545–1550.

353. Schultz DR, Barthal JS, Garrett C. Western equine encephalitis with rapid onset of parkinsonism. *Neurology* 1977;27:1095–1096.

354. Schwab RS, England AC. Projection technique for evaluating surgery in Parkinson's disease. In: Gillingham FJ, Donaldson MC, eds. *Third symposium on Parkinson's disease*. Edinburgh: E.& S. Livingstone, 1969.

355. Schwab RS, Poskanzer DC, England AC, et al. Amantadine in Parkinson's disease: review of more than two years experience. *JAMA* 1972;222:792–795.

356. Schwartz J, Elizan TS. Search for viral particles and virus-specific products in idiopathic Parkinson's disease brain material. *Ann Neurol* 1979;6:261–263.

357. Scott WK, Stajich J, Yamaoka L, et al. Genetic complexity and Parkinson's disease. *Science* 1997;277: 387–389.

358. Semchuk KM, Love EJ, Lee RG. Parkinson's disease: a test of the multifactorial etiologic hypothesis. *Neurology* 1993;43:1173–1180.

359. Semchuk K, Love EJ, Lee RG. Parkinson's disease and exposure to agricultural work and pesticide chemicals. *Neurology* 1992;42:1328–1335.

360. Shahi GS, Moochhala SM. Smoking and Parkinson's disease—a new perspective. *Rev Environ Health* 1991;9:123–136.

361. Shi Y. Study on the prevalence of Parkinson's disease in Hongkou District, Shanghai. *Chin J Epidemiol* 1987;4:205–209.

362. Shiosaki K, Jenner P, Asin KE, et al. ABT:431: The diacetyl prodrug of A-86929, a potent and selective dopamine D1 receptor agonist: in vitro characterization and effects in animal models of Parkinson's diease. *J Pharmacol Exp Ther* 1996;276:150–160.

363. Sofic E, Riederer F, Heinsen H, et al. Increased iron (III) and total iron content in post mortem substantia nigra of parkinsonian brain. *J Neural Transm* 1988; 74:199–205.

364. Spellman GC. Report of familial cases of parkinsonism. *JAMA* 1962;179:160–162.

365. Spillantini MG, Schmidt ML, Lee VMY, et al. Alpha-synuclein in Lewy bodies. *Nature* 1997;338:839–840.

366. Steiner J, Hamilton G, Ross D, et al. Neurotrophic immunophilin ligands stimulate structural and functional recovery in neurodegenerative animal models. *Proc Natl Acad Sci USA* 1997;94:2019–2024.

367. Stern MB, Doty RL, Dotti M, et al. Olfactory function in Parkinson's disease subtypes. *Neurology* 1994;44: 266–268.

368. Stern MB. Head trauma as a risk factor for Parkinson's disease. *Mov Disord* 1991;6:95–97.

369. Stern M, Dulaney E, Gruber SB, et al. The epidemiology of Parkinson's disease: a case-control study of young-onset and old-onset patients. *Arch Neurol* 1991; 48:903–907.

370. Stocchi F, Quinn NP, Barbato L, et al. Comparison between a fast and a slow release preparation of levodopa and a combination of the two: a clinical and a pharmacokinetic study. *Clin Neuropharmacol* 1994;17:38–44.

371. Stone TW. Evidence for a non-dopaminergic action of amantadine. *Neurosci Lett* 1977;4:343–346.

372. Svenson LW. Regional disparities in the annual prevalence rates of Parkinson's disease in Canada. *Neuroepidemiol J* 1991;10:205–210.

373. Tanner CM. The role of environmental toxins in the etiology of Parkinson's disease. *Trends Neurosci* 1989; 12:49–54.

374. Tanner CM, Chen B, Wang W, et al. Environmental factors and Parkinson's disease: a case-control study in China. *Neurology* 1989;9:660–664.

375. Tanner CM, Chen B, Wang W, et al. Environmental factors in the etiology of Parkinson's disease. *Can J Neurol Sci* 1987;419–423.

376. Tanner CM, Grabler P, Goetz CC. Occupation and the risk of Parkinson's disease: a case-control study in young onset patients. *Neurology* 1990;40[suppl 1]: 422.

377. Tanner C, Hubble J, Chan P. Epidemiology and genetics of Parkinson's disease. In: Watts R, Koller W, eds. *Movement disorders*. New York: McGraw-Hill, 1996; 137–152.

378. Tarvonen-Schroder S, Roytta M, Raiha I. Clinical features of leuko-ariosis. *J Neurol Neurosurg Psychiatry* 1996;60:431–436.

379. Tatton WG, Ju WY, Holland DP, et al. (−)-Deprenyl reduces PC12 cell apoptosis by inducing new protein synthesis. *J Neurochem* 1994;63:1572–1575.

380. Tatton WG, Seniuk NA. Trophic-like actions of deprenyl on neurons and astroglia. *Recent Adv Treat Neurodegen Dis Cogn Disord* 1994;7:238.

381. Tatton WG, Wadia JS, Ju WY, et al. (−)-Deprenyl reduces neuronal apoptosis and facilitates neuronal outgrowth by altering protein synthesis without inhibiting monoamine oxidase. *J Neural Transm Suppl* 1996; 48:45–59.

382. Teravainen IT, Calne DB. Action tremor in Parkinson's disease. *J Neurol Neurosurg Psychiatry* 1980;43: 257–263.

383. Tetrud JW, Langston JW. The effect of deprenyl (selegeline) on the natural history of Parkinson's disease. *Science* 1989;245:519–522.

384. Thompson PD, Marsden CD. Gait disorder of subcortical arteriosclerotic encephalopathy: Binswanger's disease. *Mov Disord* 1989;2:1–8.

385. Timberlake WH, Vance MA. Four year treatment of patients with parkinsonism using amantadine alone or with levodopa. *Ann Neurol* 1978;3:119–128.

386. Toth MJ, Fishman PS, Poehiman ET. Free-living daily energy expenditure in patients with Parkinson's disease. *Neurology* 1997;48:88–91.

387. Uitti RJ, Rajput AH, Ahiskog JE, et al. Amantadine treatment is an independent predictor of survival in Parkinson's disease. *Neurology* 1996;46:1551–1556.

388. Uitti RJ, Rajput AH, Ashenhurst EM, et al. Cyanide induced parkinsonism: a clinicopathologic report. *Neurology* 1985;35:921–925.

389. Verhagen Metman L, Locatelli ER, Bravi D, et al. Apomorphine response in Parkinson's disease and the pathogenesis of motor complications. *Neurology* 1997; 48:369–372.

390. Vierregge P, Heberlein I. Increased risk of Parkinson's disease in relatives of patients. *Ann Neurol* 1995; 37:685.

391. Vinerhoets FJG, Schulzer M, Calne D, et al. Which clinical sign of Parkinson's disease best reflects the nigrostriatal lesion. *Ann Neurol* 1997;41:58–64.

392. Von Voigtlander PF, Moore K. Dopamine: release from the brain in vivo by amantadine. *Science* 1971; 174:408–410.

393. Walker J, Potvin A, Tourtellotte W, et al. Amantadine and levodopa in the treatment of Parkinson's disease. *Clin Pharmacol Ther* 1972;13:28–36.

394. Walters JH. Post-encephalitic Parkinson syndrome after meningoencephalitis due to coxsackie virus B, type 2. *N Engl J Med* 1960;263:744–747.

395. Wang SJ, Fuh JL, Liu CY, et al. Parkinson's disease in Kin-Hu, Kinmen: a community survey by neurologists. *Neuroepidemiology* 1994;13:69–74.

396. Ward CD, Duvoisin RC, Ince SE, et al. Parkinson's disease in 65 pain of twins and in a set of quadruplets. *Neurology* 1983;33:815–824.

397. Waters CH, Kirth M, Bailey P, et al. Tolcapone in stable Parkinson's disease. *Neurology* 1997;49:665–671.

398. Waters CH, Miller CA. Autosomal dominant Lewy body parkinsonism in a four generation family. *Ann Neurol* 1994;35:59–64.

399. Watts R. The role of dopamine agonists in early Parkinson's disease. *Neurology* 1997;49[suppl 1]: S34–S38.

400. Watts RL, Mandir AS. Quantitative methods of evaluating Parkinson's disease. In: Olanow W, Lieberman AN, eds. *The scientific basis for the treatment of Parkinson's disease*. Park Ridge: Parthenon Publishing Group, 1992:13–33.

401. Webster DD. Critical analysis of the disability in Parkinson's disease. *Mod Treat* 1968;5:257–282.

402. Wechsler LS, Checkoway H, Franklin GM, et al. A pilot study of occupational and environmental risk factors for Parkinson's disease. *Neurotoxicology* 1991;12: 387–392.

403. Weiden PJ, Mann JJ, Hass G, et al. Clinical nonrecognition of neuroleptic induced movement disorders: a cautionary study. *Am J Psychiatry* 1987;144: 1148–1153.

404. Wenning GK, Ben-Shlomo Y, Magalhaes M, et al. Clinical features and natural history of multiple system atrophy: an analysis of 100 cases. *Brain* 1994;117: 835–845.

405. Wenning GK, Shephard B, Hawkes C, et al. Olfactory function in atypical parkinsonian syndromes. *Acta Neurol Scand* 1995;91:247–250.

406. Wetmur JG, Schwartz J, Elizan TS. Nucleic acid homology studies of viral nucleic acids in idiopathic Parkinson's disease. *Arch Neurol* 1979;36:462–464.

407. Wichman T, DeLong M. Functional and pathophysiological models of the basal ganglia. *Curr Opin Neurobiol* 1996;6:751–758

408. Williams GR, Kurland LT, Goldberg ID. Morbidity and mortality with parkinsonism. *J Neurosurg* 1966; 24:138–143.

409. Winikates J, Jankovic J. Vascular progressive supranuclear palsy. *J Neurol Transm Suppl* 1994;42:189–201.

410. Wolters EC, Hurwitz TA, Mak E, et al. Clozapine in the treatment of parkinsonian patients with dopaminergic psychosis. *Neurology* 1990;40:832–834.

411. Wolters EC, Jansen ENH, Tuynman-Qua HG, et al. Olanzapine in the treatment of dopaminomimetic psychosis in patients with Parkinson's disease. *Neurology* 1996;47:1085–1097.

412. Wolters EC, Tissingh G, Bergmans PL, et al. Dopamine agonists in Parkinson's disease. *Neurology* 1995; 45[suppl 3]:S28–S34.

413. Yagashita A, Oda M. Progressive supranuclear palsy: MRI and pathological findings. *Neuroradiology* 1996; 38[suppl 1]: 560–566.

414. Yahr MD, Duvoisin RC, Schear MJ. Treatment of parkinsonism with levodopa. *Arch Neurol* 1969; 21:343–354.

415. Yamada M, Ohno S, Okayasu I, et al. Chronic manganese poisoning: a neuropathological study with de-

termination of manganese distribution. *Acta Neuropathol (Wien)* 1976;71:1101.

416. Yamada T, Calne DB, Akiyama H, et al. Further observations on au-positive glia in brains with progressive supranuclear palsy. *Acta Neuropathol (Wien)* 1993; 85:308–315.

417. Yoshino H, Nakagawa-Hattori Y, Kondo T, et al. Mitochondrial complex I and II activities of lymphocytes and platelets in Parkinson's disease. *J Neural Transm* 1992;4:27–34.

418. Young V W, Perry TL. Monoamine oxidase B, smoking, and Parkinson's disease. *J Neurol Sci* 1986;72: 265–272.

419. Zayed J, Ducic S, Campanella G, et al. Environmental factors in the etiology of Parkinson's disease. *Can J Neurol Sci* 1990;17:286–291

420. Zhang X X, Jin GZ, Wei Y F. Agonistic actions of pergolide on firing activity of dopamine neurons in substantia nigra compacta area. *Acta Pharmacol Sin* 1995; 16:423–427.

421. Zoldan J, Friedberg G, Weizman A, et al. Ondansetron, a 5-HT3 antagonist for visual hallucinations and paranoid delusional disorder associated with chronic levodopa therapy in advanced Parkinson's disease. *Adv Neurol* 1996;69:541–544.

Pallidal Surgery for the Treatment of Parkinson's Disease and Movement Disorders, edited by
J. K. Krauss, R. G. Grossman, and J. Jankovic.
Lippincott-Raven Publishers, Philadelphia © 1998.

6

Clinical Assessment and Study Design for Pallidal Surgery

Andres M. Lozano and *Anthony E. Lang

*Division of Neurosurgery, Department of Surgery, and *Division of Neurology, Department
of Medicine, The University of Toronto and The Toronto Hospital Neuroscience Centre,
Toronto, Ontario M5T 2S8, Canada*

Pallidal surgery can provide striking benefits to appropriately selected patients with movement disorders (1,3,7,10,12). As with any novel medical or surgical therapy there is an initial exuberant enthusiasm that is usually tempered once a proper appraisal has taken place. There is therefore a need for a detailed assessment of the effects and complications of this newly reintroduced surgical approach. Such an evaluation is necessary to establish the indications for pallidotomy, its contraindications, its associated deleterious effects, the potential placebo effects of surgery, the correlation between target selection, lesion volume, and clinical effect, and determination of the temporal profile of the effects of surgery. The objective of this chapter is to review methods to rate parkinsonian disability clinically and to provide some guidelines for the design of studies to evaluate the consequences of pallidotomy.

CLINICAL ASSESSMENT

The clinical evaluation of Parkinson's disease (PD) can be enigmatic. The signs and symptoms are multiple and can be complex. Regardless of the assessment instrument, clinicians must control for the wide changes in motor function that can occur over time, particularly those that are treatment-related. To address the treatment-related changes in function specifically, evaluations are obtained repeatedly at specified and uniform time points in relation to medication administration.

The spectrum of currently used instruments to assess PD ranges from sophisticated quantitative physiological measures of parkinsonian disability, to evaluator-derived assessments, to patient-reported subjective appraisals of the severity of symptoms. Several objective quantitative physiological measures of bradykinesia, reaction time, movement time, rigidity, tremor, gait, balance, and postural reflexes have been developed (see ref. 16 for review). These techniques have the advantage of providing precise and reproducible numerical measures of parkinsonian disability and allowing rigorous statistical analysis. They are also less prone to interrater variability than the clinical scales commonly in use. These mechanical devices are usually costly and demand a high level of technical expertise. In addition, they require a strong commitment to maintain the equipment in proper order to ensure the reliability of the results. Although ideal in certain research settings, these considerations often make this type of assessment impractical in the clinical arena, which is why most clinical studies rely instead on clinical rating scales.

The ideal PD rating scale has the following properties: (a) ease of administration: short time to administer, minimal technical skill required: (b) low intrarater and interrater variability; (c) highly valid, reliable, and sensitive; and (d) predictive of impairment. To be considered valid, that is, a truly useful, efficacious instrument, the clinical rating tool should possess four principal properties (13): (a) reliability or high reproducibility of the results, both intrarater (test–retest) and between observers; (b) validity, the extent to which the scale measures the parameter it is designed to measure; (c) sensitivity, the ability to distinguish small changes in the parameter that is being measured; and (d) internal consistency, the general pattern of agreement and correlation between test items as a function of disease stage.

Many clinical rating scales have been developed, studied, and applied (see ref. 13 for review). The Core Assessment Program for Intracerebral Transplantation (CAPIT), reported in 1992 (11), has been among the most useful and utilized protocols in surgical trials. CAPIT represented an important step toward standardizing the diagnosis and evaluation of patients with PD. The CAPIT committee proposed the program in recognition of the need for uniformity in diagnostic criteria and clinical outcome measures when surgical trials of transplantation for PD were being conducted by a large number of centers. Since that time, CAPIT has been applied to a large number of surgical therapies for PD, and many granting agencies and sponsors have adopted it as the "gold standard" of PD evaluation. The CAPIT committee itself acknowledged the need for future refinements. It is convenient to use the framework of the CAPIT protocol, modify or supplement it where required, and apply it to pallidotomy trials.

The CAPIT program incorporates the Hoehn and Yahr staging, the Unified Parkinson's Disease Rating Scale (UPDRS), and a dyskinesia rating scale, each in the "best-on" and the practically defined "worst-off" states. We have used each of these scales to assess the results of our surgical series (10,12). The best-on and worst-off conditions have been defined as the condition that both the patient and the physician agree represents the maximum therapeutic benefit or is about as severe as the patient's parkinsonism ever gets. It is convenient to define a practically defined "off" state, after a 12-hour overnight period without medication, to be representative of the patient's worst motor performance. From a practical standpoint, patients are evaluated after an overnight 12-hour drug-free period (practically defined worst-off) and again 1 hour after receiving their morning dose (practically defined best-on). There may be a need to incorporate a further evaluation to better assess the worst dyskinesias, which often occur later in the day.

Hoehn and Yahr Staging

Hoehn and Yahr developed a staging measure for PD that is useful and rapidly administered (HY staging). The original scale was seen as having an overweighing of postural instability. The modified version (Appendix 1) deemphasizes postural stability. This staging system provides an important and informative starting point for classifying the severity of parkinsonism for patients entering surgical trials. However, this staging is not an adequate evaluation of parkinsonism, and it now serves as a supplement to more detailed scales, such as the UPDRS.

United Parkinson's Disease Rating Scale

The United Parkinson's Disease Rating Scale (UPDRS), contained within CAPIT, provides an extensive, objective and subjective assessment of the cardinal features of PD, the complications of treatment, the impact of treatment on patients' mood, mentation, and behavior, and activities of daily life (Appendix 2). Although the UPDRS has undergone a number of validation studies resulting in several recommendations (5,6,14,15), the current 3.0 version is still widely used. The UPDRS evaluates four components: (a) mentation behavior and mood, (b) activities of daily living (ADL); (c) motor examination; and (d) complications of therapy (during the past week). Scores range from 0 (normal) to 199 (worst clinical state). The first two subsections contain extensive information that cannot be evaluated blindly, as much of it is historical. The ADL scores are determined for both the on and off states. The 14 assessments in the motor section of UPDRS are the components administered both in the practically defined worst-off state and in the on-state. Except for rigidity, which cannot be assessed visually, the entire motor examination of the UPDRS can be videotaped in the off and on states and rated by a blinded evaluator.

The ability to secure a videotaped record of the motor examination offers important advantages for randomizing the sequence of the examinations (e.g., the possibility of evaluating postoperative off drugs before preoperative on drugs) and blinding the evaluations of surgical outcomes. Patients are videotaped wearing a hospital gown and hat to blind the evaluator, who may otherwise guess, by the length of hair for example, the temporal relation between the videotaping and the operation.

Dyskinesia Scale Score

The CAPIT committee recommended using a dyskinesia scale (Appendix 3) adopted from Obeso (11). Subsequent to the development of the CAPIT, Goetz and his colleagues tested and calibrated a revised version of the Obeso scale (4). An important component of this new scale is the addition of standardized tasks (drinking from a cup in each hand, putting on a coat, doing up the buttons, undoing them and removing the coat, walking) designed to accentuate the severity of the dyskinesias and to provide an evaluation of the degree to which they interfere with function. Our group has utilized this scale but applied it to each side of the body separately to evaluate the effect of unilateral surgical procedures (10,12).

Self-Reporting

The CAPIT protocol also recommends hour-by-hour self-reporting and a timed test of motor function. For self-reporting patients are required to record one of five conditions: complete on (A), on with dyskinesias (D), partial on (P), complete off (F), and sleep (S). We have not systematically used patient self-reporting because of the uncertain reliability of such data in certain patients.

Timed Maneuvers

The timed maneuvers of CAPIT consist of four tests administered in the worst-off and best-on states. They include arm pronation-supination, hand/arm movement between two points, finger dexterity, and stand-walk-sit tests. We are concerned about the uncritical administration of the originally proposed timed testing assessments of CAPIT (9). A timed assessment of walking is important, and the method chosen in CAPIT appears appropriate. Similarly, the time required to complete 20 successive taps of the right or left hand between two points placed 30 cm apart is a robust measure. The two other evaluations are problematical. They rely on the rater's assessment of what constitutes a complete and accurate pronation-supination cycle or finger tap. The time required for patients with PD with reduced amplitude of movement to complete a cycle of pronation-supination or finger apposition may be difficult to evaluate. When rating the timed test of finger dexterity, for example, one cannot assign an appropriate score to the patient who, because of hypokinesia, can only run the thumb across the fingers perhaps rapidly versus the one who has full-amplitude appositions of the thumb to each finger. The same objection arises when comparing small, incomplete but rapid pronation/supination of the arm versus slower but full-range movements. Other confounding factors are the associated severe tremor, rigidity, the level of the patient's motivation and fatigue, and, in the on state, task-interfering dyskinesias.

Schwab and England Scale

The Schwab and England activity of daily living scale (Appendix 4) assigns a value in increments of 10%, from 100% (totally normal) to 0% (total impairment, bedridden, loss of vegetative functions). This scale can be modified to allow scoring in 5% increments if the level of disability falls between two 10% definitions. Scores for the patients best-on and worse-off should be obtained. The Schwab and England scale is easy and rapid to administer and shows good inter-rater reliability while providing close correlation between the independent scores of examiners and patients with mild PD (8).

STUDY DESIGN

Although pallidal surgery is being increasingly utilized for treatment of advanced Parkinson's disease, studies to demonstrate the safety and efficacy of these procedures are only now being completed. Initial reports have shown considerable discrepancies in the benefits and complications of pallidotomy. There are multiple sources for this variability. First, patient selection criteria may differ among centers. Second, procedural variations, with resultant discrepancies in lesion location and size, may contribute to differences in outcomes. Centers differ in the use of imaging modalities [magnetic resonance imaging (MRI), computed tomography (CT), MRI/CT co-registration, ventriculography]; stereotactic localization systems (e.g., Leksell, Codman-Roberts-Wells, Laitinen stereoadapter); physiological techniques for final lesion selection (impedance monitoring, macrostimulation, semimicroelectrode recording, high-impedance microelectrode recording and stimulation); target selection [the recommended coordinates of Laitinen et al. (7), direct targeting of the medial pallidum based on MRI, or the use of microelectrode recording to determine the location of the sensorimotor portion of the internal segment of the globus pallidus, GPi]; and parameters used for final lesion creation (electrode diameter and exposed tip length; temperature and duration of lesion, number of lesions, interlesion spacing, and the use of somatotopy to select the location, volume, and shape of the lesion). Finally, there are significant differences among centers in the selection of pre- and postoperative assessment tools and the manner by which the data are collected (e.g., prospective versus retrospective, blinded versus nonblinded assessments). Herein lies the importance of standardizing the clinical assessment and the reports of outcome measures.

These sources of variability can account for significant intercenter differences in outcome results and make comparisons of results across centers difficult. Furthermore, inadequate assessment techniques make arguments for the validity of pallidotomy in the treatment of PD prone to criticism similar to that responsible for the demise of procedures that were prematurely advocated as efficacious for PD (e.g., adrenal medullary transplantation). Failure to apply valid and reliable target identification techniques and outcome measures in studies of the results of pallidotomy also impairs the ability to make scientifically sound conclusions about the role of specific regions of the internal portion of the globus pallidus (GPi) in the pathophysiology of Parkinson's disease.

STUDY DESIGN FOR PALLIDAL SURGERY

To compare results across centers, accurately, carefully designed, prospective studies are needed. This type of study design should enable many of the outstanding issues related to pallidal surgery indications, procedures, and outcomes to be addressed. Some of the important caveats for the design of surgical trials of PD are listed in Table 6-1.

When assessing the value of therapies or interventions, the available data are classified into one of three categories according to certain defined

TABLE 6-1. *Study design caveats*

1. Patients should be evaluated by a multidisciplinary team that includes neurologists, neuropsychologists, and neurosurgeons. The diagnosis of idiopathic PD should be confirmed. Other parkinsonian syndromes should be identified using clinical criteria and radiological investigations
2. The study should be prospective.
3. The most powerful study design is a prospective double-blind trial in which patients are randomized to surgery or to simulated surgery.
4. The number of patients enrolled must be sufficient to allow a statement of the utility and complications of pallidotomy.
5. In those instances where no benefit is found, a power analysis should confirm that the conclusion is valid and that a type II statistical error has been avoided.
6. Evaluations should be performed at baseline and at intervals after surgery in both the on and off states.
7. Because of the day-to-day variations in PD, particularly for treated patients experiencing fluctuations, a minimum of two baseline evaluations should be obtained.
8. Because changes in medication dosages may confound preoperative versus postoperative comparisons, dosages should be changed as little as possible throughout the course of the study. This may not be possible but nevertheless is highly desirable.
9. Evaluations should be randomized and blinded. Videotaping of motor evaluations greatly facilitates this study design.
10. Patients should be followed for a minimum of 1 year. A subset of patients should be evaluated at longer follow-up times to assess the long-term effects of surgery.

criteria (Table 6-2) (2). The gold standard of any "drug" study is the placebo-controlled, randomized, double-blind design with between-subjects comparisons (class I evidence). For a number of reasons, such a design is usually difficult or even impossible when evaluating surgical therapies because an adequate placebo group may not be available. For a surgical treatment, it would require a simulated operation. Because pallidal surgery is performed with awake patients and take approximately 4 hours for mapping, it would in fact involve an elaborate process with "sham" microelectrode recordings, which is practically difficult. A nonoperated group may be used instead of a placebo group. However, patients would need to be randomized into treatment or nontreatment arms, and the nonoperated group would not be subject to the "nonspecific" benefits of surgery. Furthermore, it may be difficult to find patients willing to be randomly assigned to surgical or nonsurgical therapies. A crossover design could help in this respect where patients who were initially randomized to medical therapy could cross over to the surgical arm at a defined time. The use of a control, nonoperated group collected without randomization introduces selection bias into the analysis.

We have opted for a prospective within-subjects design, comparing patients before and after GPi pallidotomy (10,12). A model study flow chart is included in Table 6-3. We have evaluated patients

TABLE 6-3. *Pallidal surgery study flow chart*

1. Patients undergo neurological, neurosurgical, and neuropsychological evaluation.
2. Does the patient fulfill the inclusion exclusion criteria?
3. Medications are optimized and stable. If possible, antiparkinsonian medications are maintained as constant as possible throughout the study.
4. Patient gives informed consent to enter the study.
5. Patients are videotaped wearing a hospital gown and hat to facilitate blinding.
6. Evaluations are repeated at 1 week (deemed not necessary after the first 27 patients), 3 months, 6 months, 1 year, and yearly after surgery.
7. Videotapes are randomized and scored by a neurologist experienced in the use of the above scales and who was not involved in the patient's pre- or postoperative care.

using the H&Y, UPDRS, dyskinesia scale, a single timed tapping test, and the S&E scale (all in best-on and worse-off) at baseline (mean of at least two evaluations) and at specified times after surgery. The utility of these widely used scales for assessing the results of surgery is that they provide a means by which results can be compared among centers. Individual scores from the UPDRS motor examination on both the ipsilateral and contralateral sides can be analyzed. In addition, motor items can be grouped to quantitate effects on the cardinal signs of PD, total akinesia (UPDRS items 23 to 26), total tremor (UPDRS items 20 + 21), total rigidity (UPDRS item 22), and a composite postural instability/gait score (UPDRS items 13 + 14 + 15 + 29 + 30). Evaluations of drug-induced dyskinesias were also obtained, with separate scores for right and left sides as well as a total score that includes axial involvement.

In our first report of 14 patients (12) we used videotaped recordings of the neurological evaluations to blind the examiners to: (a) "on" or "off" states, (b) pre- or postoperative status, and (c) time after surgery. During videotaping all patients wore hospital gowns and caps to mask pre- and postoperative status. Certain aspects of the clinical examination that require examiner–patient contact (e.g., rigidity) could not be assessed in this manner. When reporting our initial results, items of the motor section of UPDRS that did not require examiner–patient contact (i.e., all except

TABLE 6-2. *Class of evidence when evaluating studies*

Class	Evidence
I:	Prospective randomized controlled trials (PRCT)—the gold standard of clinical trials, although some may be poorly designed, lack sufficient patient numbers, or suffer from other methodological inadequacies.
II:	Clinical studies in which the data were collected prospectively, and retrospective analyses that were based on clearly reliable data. Included in this class are case-control studies.
III:	Most studies based on retrospectively collected data. Evidence used in this class indicates clinical series, databases or registries, case reviews, case reports, and expert opinions.

rigidity) were randomly and blindly evaluated from videotape records of patients examined in "on" and "off" states. Raters were not directly involved in the care of the patients. This type of study provided class II evidence (Table 6-2).

We attempted to keep the dosage of antiparkinsonian drugs constant for the duration of the study period to avoid confounding the results. Total L-dopa (and peripheral decarboxylase inhibitor) equivalents was calculated by adding the total dose of standard L-dopa (milligrams) + 0.75 × the dose of the controlled—release (CR) preparation (milligrams) + 10 times the bromocriptine (milligram) dose and 100 times the pergolide (milligram) dose. When converted in this fashion, there was a small but significant decrease in medications 6 months after pallidotomy (12).

CONCLUSION

We have made blinded assessments, using videotaped examinations, to document the postoperative improvements in the cardinal signs of Parkinson's disease following microelectrode-guided stereotactic GPi pallidotomy. Independent examiners familiar with the evaluation scales blindly and randomly (vis-á-vis preoperative versus postoperative videotapes and on versus off medications) scored those items in the motor subscale of the UPDRS amenable to blinded evaluation. Using this methodology, which we believe removes as much bias as possible in the context of the surgical nature of the intervention, we have demonstrated clear alleviation of akinesia, tremor, and dyskinesia on the contralateral side to the surgery during the "off" state. More modest improvements were demonstrated on the ipsilateral side off-period akinesia and ipsilateral on-period dyskinesias. These results were corroborated by nonblinded assessments and extended to include rigidity, which could not be evaluated in a blinded fashion. The timed tapping test used also demonstrated improvements both contralaterally and, more modestly, ipsilaterally. This was the only measure, other than dyskinesia, that was improved during the "on" state.

Given the variability of the course of PD, surgical variations, and day-to-day fluctuations in patient performances, and the effects of patient and physician expectations on clinical evalua-

tions, we recommend the adoption of a blinded, randomized study design. Because of the practical difficulties associated with a randomized, placebo-controlled blinded pallidotomy trial, we have opted for randomized and blinded assessments of videotaped UPDRS examinations for evaluating the outcome of surgical interventions for PD. The elimination of as many sources of bias as possible is necessary for critical evaluation of these interventions. Although more time-consuming in the short run, ultimately the use of defined, blinded study designs will lead to the generation of data that are less ambiguous. This will lead to more rapid acceptance (or rejection) of new surgical procedures by the medical and scientific communities, patient groups, and health management organizations.

Acknowledgments. This work was supported by the Parkinson's Foundation of Canada (A.M.L.) and the National Parkinsons Foundation (A.E.L.). A.M.L. is a Medical Research Council of Canada Clinician-Scientist.

REFERENCES

1. Baron MS, Vitek JL, Bakay RA, et al. Treatment of advanced Parkinson's disease by posterior GPi pallidotomy: 1-year results of a pilot study. *Ann Neurol* 1996; 40:355–366.
2. Bullock R, Chesnut RM, Clifton G, et al. *Guidelines for the management of severe head injury.* American Association of Neurological Surgeons, 1995:1–3.
3. Dogali M, Fazzini E, Kolodny E, et al. Stereotactic ventral pallidotomy for Parkinson's disease. *Neurology* 1995;45:753–761.
4. Goetz CG, Stebbins GT, Shale HM, et al. Utility of an objective dyskinesia rating scale for Parkinson's disease: inter- and intrarater reliability assessment. *Mov Disord* 1994;9:390–394.
5. Hely MA, Chey T, Wilson A, et al. Reliability of the Columbia scale for assessing signs of Parkinson's disease. *Mov Disord* 1993;8:466–472.
6. Henderson L, Kennard C, Crawford TJ, et al. Scales for rating motor impairment in Parkinson's disease: studies of reliability and convergent validity. *J Neurol Neurosurg Psychiatry* 1991;54:18–24.
7. Laitinen LV, Bergenheim AT, Hariz MI. Leksell's posteroventral pallidotomy in the treatment of Parkinson's disease. *J Neurosurg* 1992;76:53–61.
8. Lang AE. Clinical rating scales and videotape analysis. In: Koller WC, Paulsen G, eds. *Therapy of Parkinson's disease.* New York: Marcel Dekker, 1990:3–30.
9. Lang AE, Benabid AL, Koller WC, et al. The core assessment program for intracerebral transplantation [letter; comment]. *Mov Disord* 1995;10:527–528.
10. Lang AE, Lozano AM, Montgomery EB, et al. Posteroventral pallidotomy in Parkinson's disease: two year experience. *N Engl J Med* 1997 (in press).

11. Langston JW, Widner H, Goetz CG, et al. Core assessment program for intracerebral transplantations (CAPIT). *Mov Disord* 1992;7:2–13.
12. Lozano AM, Lang AE, Gàlvez-Jiménez N, et al. GPi pallidotomy improves motor function in patients with Parkinson's disease. *Lancet* 1995;346:1383–1387.
13. Martinez-Martin P. Rating scales in Parkinson's disease. In:Jankovic J, ed. *Parkinson's disease and movement disorders.* Baltimore: Williams & Wilkins, 1993:281–292.
14. Martinez-Martin P, Gil-Nagel A, Gracia LM, et al. Unified Parkinson's disease rating scale characteristics and structure: the Cooperative Multicentric Group. *Mov Disord* 1994;9:76–83.
15. Van Hilten JJ, van der Zwan AD, Zwinderman AH, et al. Rating impairment and disability in Parkinson's disease: evaluation of the Unified Parkinson's Disease Rating Scale. *Mov Disord* 1994;9:84–88.
16. Watts RL, Glatt SL, Koller WC. Objective measures of motor disability. In: Koller WC, Paulsen G, eds. *Therapy of Parkinson's disease.* New York: Marcel Dekker, 1990;31–62

APPENDIX 1: MODIFIED HOEHN AND YAHR STAGING OF PARKINSON'S DISEASE

Note: This material was taken from Lang (8), with permission.

Stage 0   No signs of disease
Stage 1   Unilateral disease
Stage 1.5   Unilateral disease plus axial involvement
Stage 2   Bilateral disease, without impaired balance
Stage 2.5   Bilateral disease, with recovery on pull test
Stage 3   Mild to moderate bilateral disease; some postural instability; physically independent
Stage 4   Severe disability; still able to walk or stand unassisted
Stage 5   Wheelchair-bound or bedridden unless aided

APPENDIX 2: UNIFIED PARKINSON DISEASE RATING SCALE

Note: This material is modified from Langston et al. (11).

I. Mentation, behavior, mood

1. *Intellectual impairment*
   0   None
   1   Mild (consistent forgetfulness with partial recollection of events with no other difficulties)
   2   Moderate memory loss with disorientation and moderate difficulty handling complex problems
   3   Severe memory loss with disorientation to time and often place; severe impairment with problems
   4   Severe memory loss with orientation only to person; unable to make judgments or solve problems

2. *Thought disorder*
   0   None
   1   Vivid dreaming
   2   "Benign" hallucination with insight retained
   3   Occasional to frequent hallucination or delusions without insight, could interfere with daily activities
   4   Persistent hallucination, delusions, or florid psychosis

3. *Depression*
   0   Not present
   1   Periods of sadness or guilt greater than normal, never sustained for more than a few days or a week
   2   Sustained depression for 1 week
   3   Vegetative symptoms (insomnia, anorexia, abulia, weight loss)
   4   Vegetative symptoms with suicidality

4. *Motivation/initiative*
   0   Normal
   1   Less assertive than usual, more passive
   2   Loss of initiative or disinterest in elective (nonroutine) activities
   3   Loss of initiative or disinterest in day-to-day (routine) activities
   4   Withdrawn, complete loss of motivation

MAXIMUM: 16 points

II. Activities of daily living (determine for "on/off")

5. *Speech*
   0   Normal
   1   Mildly affected, no difficulty being understood
   2   Moderately affected, may be asked to repeat

3   Severely affected, frequently asked to repeat

4   Unintelligible most of time

6. *Salivation*

0   Normal

1   Slight but noticeable increase; may have nighttime drooling

2   Moderately excessive saliva; may have minimal drooling

3   Marked drooling

7. *Swallowing*

0   Normal

1   Rare choking

2   Occasional choking

3   Requires soft food

4   Requires nasogastric or gastric tube

8. *Handwriting*

0   Normal

1   Slightly small or slow

2   All words small but legible

3   Severely affected; not all words legible

4   Most words illegible

9. *Cutting food, handling utensils*

0   Normal

1   Somewhat slow and clumsy but no help needed

2   Can cut most foods but some help needed

3   Food must be cut but can feed self

4   Needs to be fed

10. *Dressing*

0   Normal

1   Somewhat slow; no help needed

2   Occasional help with buttons or arms in sleeves

3   Considerable help required but can do something alone

4   Helpless

11. *Hygiene*

0   Normal

1   Somewhat slow but no help needed

2   Needs help with shower or bath or very slow in hygienic care

3   Requires assistance for washing, brushing teeth, going to bathroom

4   Helpless

12. *Turning in bed and adjusting bed clothes*

0   Normal

1   Somewhat slow no help needed

2   Can turn alone or adjust sheets but with great difficulty

3   Can initiate but not turn or adjust alone

4   Helpless

13. *Falling (unrelated to freezing)*

0   None

1   Rare falls

2   Occasional, fewer than one per day

3   Average of once per day

4   Falls more than once daily

14. *Freezing When Walking*

0   Normal

1   Rare; may have start hesitation

2   Occasional falls from freezing

3   Frequent freezing; occasional falls

4   Frequent falls from freezing

15. *Walking*

0   Normal

1   Mild difficulty; may drag legs or decrease arm swing

2   Moderate difficulty; requires no assistance

3   Severe disturbance; requires assistance

4   Cannot walk at all even with assistance

16. *Tremor*

0   Absent

1   Slight and infrequent; not bothersome to patient

2   Moderate; bothersome to patient

3   Severe; interferes with many activities

4   Marked; interferes with many activities

17. *Sensory complaints related to parkinsonism*

0   None

1   Occasionally has numbness, tingling, and mild aching

2   Frequent but not distressing

3   Frequent painful sensation

4   Excruciating pain

MAXIMUM: 52 points

III. Motor examination

18. *Speech*

0   Normal

1   Slight loss of expression, diction, volume

2   Monotone; slurred but understandable; moderately impaired

3   Markedly impaired; difficult to understand

4   Unintelligible

19. *Facial expression*

0   Normal

1   Slight hypomimia; could be poker-faced

2   Slight but definite abnormal diminution in expression

3   Moderate hypomimia; lips parted some of time

4   Masked or fixed face; lips parted one-quarter inch or more with complete loss of expression

20. *Tremor at rest*

Face

0   absent

1   Slight and infrequent

2   Mild and present most of time

3   Moderate and present most of time

4   Marked and present most of time

Right upper extremity (RUE)

0   Absent

1   Slight and infrequent

2   Mild and present most of time

3   Moderate and present most of time

4   Marked and present most of time

Left upper extremity (LUE)

0   Absent

1   Slight and infrequent

2   Mild and present most of time

3   Moderate and present most of time

4   Marked and present most of time

Right lower extremity (RLE)

0   Absent

1   Slight and infrequent

2   Mild and present most of time

3   Moderate and present most of time

4   Marked and present most of time

Left lower extremity (LLE)

0   Absent

1   Slight and infrequent

2   Mild and present most of time

3   Moderate and present most of time

4   Marked and present most of time

21. *Action or postural tremor*

RUE

0   Absent

1   Slight; present with action

2   Moderate; present with action

3   Moderate; present with action and posture holding

4   Marked; interferes with feeding

LUE

0   Absent

1   Slight; present with action

2   Moderate; present with action

3   Moderate; present with action and posture holding

4   Marked; interferes with feeding

22. *Rigidity*

Neck

0   Absent

1   Slight or only with activation

2   Mild moderate

3   Marked but full range of motion

4   Severe

RUE

0   Absent

1   Slight or only with activation

2   Mild to moderate

3   Marked but full range of motion

4   Severe

LUE

0   Absent

1   Slight or only with activation

2   Mild to moderate

3   Marked but full range of motion

4   Severe

RLE

0   Absent

1   Slight or only with activation

2   Mild to moderate

3   Marked but full range of motion

4   Severe

LLE

0   Absent

1   Slight or only with activation

2   Mild to moderate

3   Marked but full range of motion

4   Severe

23. *Finger taps*

Right

0   Normal

1   Mild slowing; reduction in amplitude; or both

2   Moderate impaired; definite and early fatiguing; may have occasional arrests

3   Severely impaired; frequent hesit-
    tions and arrests
4   Can barely perform
Left
0   Normal
1   Mild slowing; reduction in ampli-
    tude; or both
2   Moderate impaired; definite and
    early fatiguing; may have occa-
    sional arrests
3   Severely impaired; frequent hesita-
    tions and arrests
4   Can barely perform

24. *Hand movements* (open and close hands in
    rapid succession with widest amplitude
    possible)
    Right
    0   Normal
    1   Mild slowing; reduction in ampli-
        tude; or both
    2   Moderate impaired; definite and
        early fatiguing; may have occa-
        sional arrests
    3   Severely impaired; frequent hesita-
        tions and arrests
    4   Can barely perform
    Left
    0   Normal
    1   Mild slowing; reduction in ampli-
        tude; or both
    2   Moderately impaired; definite and
        early fatiguing; may have occa-
        sional arrests
    3   Severely impaired; frequent hesita-
        tions and arrests
    4   Can barely perform

25. *Rapid alternating movements* (pronate and
    supinate hands)
    Right
    0   Normal
    1   Mild slowing; reduction in ampli-
        tude; or both
    2   Moderately impaired; definite and
        early fatiguing; may have occa-
        sional arrests
    3   Severely impaired; frequent hesita-
        tions and arrests
    4   Can barely perform

Left
0   Normal
1   Mild slowing; reduction in ampli-
    tude; or both
2   Moderately impaired; definite and
    early fatiguing; may have occa-
    sional arrests
3   Severely impaired; frequent hesita-
    tions and arrests
4   Can barely perform

26. *Leg agility* (tap heel on ground: amplitude
    should be 3 inches)
    Right
    0   Normal
    1   Mild slowing; reduction in ampli-
        tude; or both
    2   Moderately impaired; definite and
        early fatiguing; may have occa-
        sional arrests
    3   Severely impaired; frequent hesita-
        tions and arrests
    4   Can barely perform
    Left
    0   Normal
    1   Mild slowing; reduction in ampli-
        tude; or both
    2   Moderately impaired; definite and
        early fatiguing; may have occa-
        sional arrests
    3   Severely impaired; frequent hesita-
        tions and arrests
    4   Can barely perform

27. *Arising from chair* (patient arises with arms
    folded across chest)
    0   Normal
    1   Slow; may need more than one at-
        tempt
    2   Pushes self up from arms or seat
    3   Tends to fall back; may need multiple
        tries but can arise without assistance
    4   Unable to arise without help

28. *Posture*
    0   Normal erect
    1   Slightly stooped, could be normal for
        older person
    2   Definitely abnormal; moderately
        stooped, may lean to one side
    3   Severely stooped with kyphosis

    4   Marked flexion with extreme abnormality of posture

29. *Gait*

    0   Normal

    1   Walks slowly; may shuffle with short steps; no festination or propulsion

    2   Walks with difficulty; little or no assistance needed; some festination; short steps or propulsion

    3   Severe disturbance; frequent assistance needed

    4   Cannot walk

30. *Postural stability* (retropulsion test)

    0   Normal

    1   Recovers unaided

    2   Would fall if not caught

    3   Falls spontaneously

    4   Unable to stand

31. *Body bradykinesia and hypokinesia*

    0   None

    1   Minimal slowness; could be normal; deliberate character

    2   Mild slowness and poverty of movement; definitely abnormal; decreased amplitude of movement

    3   Moderate slowness, poverty, small amplitude of movement

    4   Marked slowness; poverty; or small amplitude of movement

MAXIMUM: 108 points

IV. Complications of therapy (during the past week)

    A. Dyskinesias

32. *Duration:* What proportion of the waking day are dyskinesias present? (historical information)

    0   None

    1   1–25% of day

    2   26–50% of day

    3   51–75% of day

    4   76–100% of day

33. *Disability:* How disabling are the dyskinesias? (historical information, may be modified by office examination)

    0   Not disabling

    1   Mildly disabling

    2   Moderately disabling

    3   Severely disabling

    4   Completely disabling

34. *Painful dyskinesias:* How painful are the dyskinesias?

    1   Not painful

    1   Slightly

    2   Moderately

    3   Severely

    4   Markedly

35. *Presence of early morning dystonia* (historical information)

    0   No

    1   Yes

B. Clinical fluctuations

36. *"Off" periods:* Are any predictable as to timing after a dose of medication?

    0   No

    1   Yes

37. *"Off" periods:* Are any unpredictable as to timing after a dose of medication?

    0   No

    1   Yes

38. "Off" periods: Do any come on suddenly (e.g., over a few seconds)?

    0   No

    1   Yes

39. *"Off" periods:* What proportion of the waking day is the patient "off" on average?

    0   None

    1   1–25% of day

    2   26–50% of day

    3   51–75% of day

    4   76–100% of day

C. Other complications

40. *Does the patient have anorexia, nausea, or vomiting?*

    0   No

    1   Yes

41. *Does the patient have any sleep disturbances* (e.g., insomnia or hypersomnolence)?

    0   No

    1   Yes

42. *Does the patient have symptomatic orthostasis?*

    0   No

    1   Yes

MAXIMUM: 23 points

TOTAL SCORE 199

APPENDIX 3: DYSKINESIA SCALE SCORE

Note: This material is modified from Goetz et al. (4) and Langston et al. (11).

Severity Rating Code

0   Absent.
1   Minimal severity; patient is not aware of dyskinesia.
2   Patient is conscious of the presence of dyskinesias, but there is no interference with voluntary motor acts (or completion of the motor acts of the rated task).
3   Dyskinesias may impair voluntary movements, but the patient is normally capable of undertaking most motor tasks (or completion of the motor acts of the rated task).
4   Intense interference with motor control (or completion of the motor acts of the rated task), and daily life activities are greatly limited.
5   Violent dyskinesias, incompatible with any motor task.

Duration

0   Absent
1   Present only when carrying out motor tasks
2   Present for 25% to 50% of waking hours
3   Present for 51% to 75% of waking hours
4   Present for 76% to 99% of waking hours
5   Continuous throughout the day: 100%

APPENDIX 4: SCHWAB AND ENGLAND ACTIVITIES OF DAILY LIVING SCALE

Note: This material is modified from Lang (8). Rating can be assigned by rater or by patient.

100%   Completely independent. Able to do all chores without slowness, difficulty, or impairment.
90%   Completely independent. Able to do all chores with some slowness, difficulty, or impairment. May take twice as long.
80%   Independent in most chores. Takes twice as long. Conscious of difficulty and slowing.
70%   Not completely independent. More difficulty with chores. Takes three to four times as long on chores for some. May take large part of day for chores.
60%   Some dependence. Can do most chores but very slowly and with much effort. Errors, some impossible.
50%   More dependent. Needs help with one-half of chores. Difficulty with everything.
40%   Very dependent. Can assist with all chores but can do few alone.
30%   With effort can now and then do a few chores alone or begin alone. Much help needed.
20%   Can do nothing alone. Can give some slight help with some chores. Severe invalid.
10%   Totally dependent, helpless.
0%   Vegetative functions, such as swallowing and bladder and bowel function are not present. Bedridden.

Pallidal Surgery for the Treatment of Parkinson's Disease and Movement Disorders, edited by
J. K. Krauss, R. G. Grossman, and J. Jankovic.
Lippincott-Raven Publishers, Philadelphia © 1998.

7

Indications for Pallidal Surgery for Parkinson's Disease

Eugene C. Lai and *†Joachim K. Krauss

*Departments of Neurology and *Neurosurgery, Baylor College of Medicine, Houston, Texas 77030, USA; and †Department of Neurosurgery, Inselspital, University of Berne, 3010 Berne, Switzerland*

Parkinson's disease (PD) is characterized by progressive symptoms of cogwheel rigidity, bradykinesia, resting tremor, and postural instability. Associated symptoms often also include micrographia, hypophonia, and gait disturbance. In the early stages of the disease, these symptoms can be adequately ameliorated by treatment with medications, especially levodopa. However, as the disease progresses, medical therapy typically becomes less and less effective. Other symptoms, such as freezing, falling, swallowing difficulty, painful spasms, depression, and dementia, add to disturbances of the activities of daily living. In addition, the adverse effects of long-term levodopa therapy, which include levodopa-induced dyskinesias and motor fluctuations, often disable patients with advanced disease. Until recent years there has been no effective treatment for these debilitating symptoms, and patients often deteriorate helplessly to incapacitation and total care. The encouraging results of posteroventral pallidotomy (PVP), reported by Laitinen et al. in 1992 (19), have sparked marked interest in the use of PVP as a treatment option for advanced PD (5,16,24,25). Several groups have since confirmed the favorable results of PVP.

EFFICACY OF PVP

Lang et al. (20,23) followed 40 PD patients who underwent PVP. Some of the patients were examined 2 years after surgery. These authors con-

cluded that for late-stage PD pallidotomy significantly reduced levodopa-induced dyskinesias and off-period disability. Much of the benefit was sustained at 2 years, although some improvements, such as those on the ipsilateral side and in the axial symptoms, waned within the first year.

Baron et al. (1) studied the effect of pallidotomy in 15 patients after 1 year and found that it significantly alleviated all cardinal parkinsonian motor signs and reduced drug-induced dyskinesias and motor fluctuations. The improvements occurred predominantly contralateral to the lesion but were also present ipsilaterally. Surgery resulted in little morbidity, including a lack of significant deficits on neuropsychological and psychiatric testing. The benefits were sustained at 1 year after PVP.

Fazzini and colleagues (3,6) followed 11 patients suffering from PD for up to 4 years after unilateral pallidotomy. They observed persistent contralateral improvement and unexpected ipsilateral improvement of motor symptoms. There was protracted relief of contralateral dyskinesias and maintenance of relatively stable levodopa dosage. Other groups have reported similar benefits of PVP (8,12–14,29).

BAYLOR COLLEGE OF MEDICINE EXPERIENCE

Altogether 42 patients (22 women, 20 men) with advanced PD underwent unilateral, microelectrode-guided PVP between August 1995 and October 1996. They represent our first group of consecutive patients who completed a 3-month postoperative evaluation (18). PVP was typically performed contralateral to the more affected side of the body; and if both sides were similarly affected, the procedure aimed to alleviate symptoms for the dominant side. Thirty-one of these patients also completed their 12-month evaluation.

At the beginning of the study, patients were considered eligible for pallidotomy if (a) their clinical findings were consistent with idiopathic PD; (b) they had a history of response to levodopa therapy; (c) they had evidence of advanced disease (disabling motor fluctuations, dopa-induced dyskinesia, or freezing; and Hoehn and Yahr stage 3 or above during their "off" period); (d) their antiparkinsonian medications were optimized and held constant for at least 1 month prior to surgery; (e) their ages were between 18 and 75 years; and (f) they agreed to return for scheduled follow-up evaluations (15,18,26). Exclusion criteria were (a) marked cerebral atrophy or ischemic changes on magnetic resonance (MR) scans of the brain; (b) the presence of features suggestive of atypical Parkinson's syndromes; (c) major depression or other psychiatric disorder; (d) moderate to advanced dementia (Mini-Mental State Examination score less than 20); (e) alcohol or drug abuse within the past 12 months; (f) Hoehn and Yahr stage 5 during their "on" period; (g) serious medical illness that would increase the risk of surgically related complications; (h) orthostatic hypotension defined by a drop of systolic blood pressure of more than 30 mm Hg from supine to standing; (i) neurosurgical procedures within the past 3 months; and (j) poor response to prior pallidotomy or thalamotomy.

At their 3-month post-PVP clinical evaluation, patients were asked to rate their improvement relative to their parkinsonian symptoms since PVP as marked, moderate, slight, none, or worse. Thirty-seven patients (88%) reported marked or moderate improvement, and none became worse. When patients were asked to report the most notable postoperative changes, alleviation of slowness, stiffness, and drug-induced involuntary movements were cited most often. For patients with disabling dyskinesia, relief of that symptom was judged to be the greatest benefit of PVP. The percent of time during the day that patients were awake and in the "on" state improved from 52.1% to 75.6% (Fig. 7-1). They were also more independent and functional during this period as evidenced by an improvement of the Modified Schwab and England Activities of Daily Living

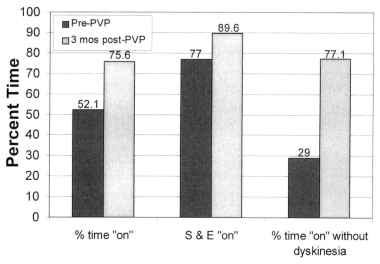

FIG. 7-1. Comparison of percent "on" period during awake time, the modified Schwab and England Activity of Daily Living scale during "on" period, and percent "on" period without levodopa-induced dyskinesia in patients prior to posteroventral pallidotomy and 3 months postoperatively (*n* = 42).

scale (27) from 77.0% to 89.6%. Significantly, their time "on" without dyskinesia increased from 29.0% to 77.1%.

The mean Unified Parkinson's Disease Rating Scale (UPDRS) (4) total activities of daily living (ADL) score in the "off" state improved from 31.21 ± 5.86 preoperatively to 18.40 ± 5.35 at 3 months after PVP (41.0% improvement, $p < 0.001$). In the "on" state the mean score also dropped from 16.40 ± 4.51 to 8.33 ± 3.63 (49.2% improvement, $p < 0.001$). The mean UPDRS total motor score in the "off" state improved from a preoperative value of 56.83 ± 13.21 to 34.0 ± 11.66 at 3 months after PVP (40.2% improvement, $p < 0.001$). The mean score in the "on" state changed from 29.79 ± 9.75 to 15.83 ± 8.16 (46.9% improvement, $p < 0.001$). Features of motor functioning that were most alleviated by PVP were rigidity, bradykinesia, and tremor (Fig. 7-2). The side of the body contralateral to the PVP lesion showed significantly more improvement. During the "off" period the UPDRS rigidity scores (item 22) improved 58.8% on the contralateral side and 25.9% on the ipsilateral side. The change was even more impressive dur-

ing the "on" period: 75% on the contralateral side and 32.6% on the ipsilateral side. Impairment in rapid movements (UPDRS items 23–26) was significantly lessened. The "off" period improvement was 49.6% contralaterally and 24% ipsilaterally, and the "on" period improvement was 61.4% and 19.6%, respectively. The UPDRS tremor score (items 20–21) was markedly better at 3 months after PVP. During the "off" period the tremor score improved 72.6% contralaterally and 29.8% ipsilaterally. During the "on" period it improved 95.3% contralaterally and 55.3% ipsilaterally. Thirty-one patients completed their 12-month post-PVP evaluation. The extent of alleviation of parkinsonian signs and symptoms noted at their 3-month evaluation was maintained at 12 months. Adverse experiences were infrequent and relatively minor. There were no persistent side effects.

Therefore microelectrode-guided unilateral PVP is a safe, effective treatment for advanced PD if the lesion is placed accurately. This procedure is most efficacious in alleviating symptoms on the contralateral side. It significantly reduces levodopa-induced dyskinesias, rigidity, bradykinesia,

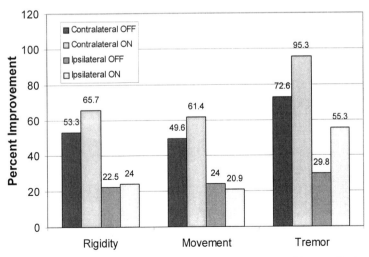

FIG. 7-2. Percent improvement in mean scores of Unified Parkinson's Disease Rating Scale (UPDRS) for rigidity, rapid movement, and tremor 3 months after posteroventral pallidotomy (*n* = 42). Scores for the contralateral (*contra OFF* and *contra ON*) and ipsilateral (*ipsi OFF* and *ipsi ON*) sides to the PVP lesion were assessed separately during both "off" and "on" periods prior to posteroventral pallidotomy and 3 months postoperatively.

tremor, and motor fluctuations. It enhances the patient's baseline activities of daily living.

SPECIFIC INDICATIONS FOR PALLIDOTOMY

Results from our group and others have demonstrated that PVP is effective for treatment of PD, especially rigidity, bradykinesia, and tremor (Fig. 7-2). Nevertheless, it is an invasive procedure, and its potential benefits should be weighed against its associated risks and cost. Adverse experiences such as stroke, intracerebral hemorrhage, seizures, cognitive impairment, or mental confusion may occur; but most groups agree that the procedure is relatively safe, and adverse events are uncommon (1,3, 6,8,12–14,18,20,29). Our experience performing pallidal surgery and following more than 100 patients postoperatively has helped us propose the following guidelines for indications and contraindications for PVP (Table 7-1).

Parkinson's disease is a progressive disease, and patients become more disabled with time. There is a substantial decline in well-being and quality of life when symptoms can no longer be adequately controlled by medications. It is reasonable to consider PVP treatment for patients whose Hoehn and Yahr stage is 3 or more during their "off" period that occupies more than 25% of their awake time despite optimal medical management.

TABLE 7-1. *Indications and contraindications for pallidotomy*

Indications
    Advanced PD with rigidity and bradykinesia that are refractory to medical therapy
    Dopa-induced dyskinesia
    "On–off" motor fluctuation
    Painful cramps and dystonia
    Intolerance to side effects of antiparkinsonian medications
Contraindications
    No history of responsiveness to levodopa treatment
    Previous history of stroke or intracranial lesion
    Severe cerebral atrophy
    Severe deconditioning and physical disabilities that prevent rehabilitation
    Severe dementia

Levodopa is presently the most effective drug for symptomatic treatment of PD. After chronic use, however, patients often develop complications, particularly dyskinesias and motor fluctuations (11). Dyskinesias commonly present as choreiform movements of the head, trunk, and limbs. Dystonia, tremor, or myoclonus can also occur. Peak dose dyskinesias are more common, but biphasic symptoms may also be observed. They may cause severe disability and pain, preventing the use of higher doses of levodopa. The effect of PVP on incapacitating dyskinesias is impressive (10). We followed 31 patients with levodopa-induced dyskinesias for 1 year or more after PVP (Fig. 7-3), and the dyskinesias were substantially alleviated. After PVP, daily levodopa dosage either remained unchanged or was increased to optimize functioning. At 3 months after PVP the duration of dyskinesia declined by 47%, disability by 63%, and pain by 87%. These symptom improvements were maintained at 12 months after PVP (18). Dyskinesias were reduced bilaterally by PVP, but the contralateral side benefited more. PVP can be especially helpful to young-onset PD patients because they are particularly likely to develop levodopa-induced dyskinesias early in the course of therapy. "On-off" motor fluctuations are signs of advanced PD and known complications of long-term levodopa use. Latency of action and duration of benefit after levodopa ingestion becomes unpredictable. Medication effects can wear off suddenly, causing abrupt deterioration in mobility and function. These symptoms are distressing to patients because from hour to hour they cannot foretell whether they can perform even the basic activities of daily living. These symptoms may be reduced somewhat by adjusting the levodopa dosage and timing and by the use of dopaminergic agonists. Unfortunately, medical treatment becomes ineffective eventually. When this situation is reached, PVP can further alleviate the motor fluctuations. After PVP, patients typically reported that their daily "on" period increased and activities of daily living, according to the Modified Schwab and England ADL scale, improved. It was due to a more predictable response to levodopa and a longer duration of therapeutic action with the drug.

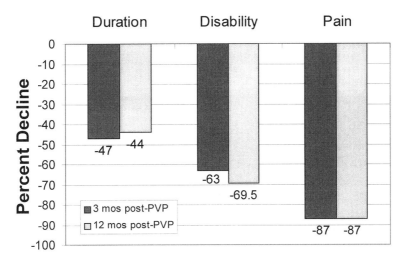

FIG. 7-3. Percent decline in levodopa-induced dyskinesia duration, disability, and pain in patients at 3 and 12 months after posteroventral pallidotomy compared to preoperatively (*n* = 31).

Pain and aching are disturbing symptoms and can substantially affect patients' quality of life. They occur with advanced PD, mostly as morning or nocturnal painful muscle cramps in the limbs, especially affecting the feet, during "off" periods. Other patients experience pain during "on" periods with excessive levodopa-induced dyskinesia and dystonic posturing. In addition, some of them suffer diphasic responses to levodopa and have painful dystonia or dyskinesia at the beginning and end of a dose. Medical treatments of these conditions are unsatisfactory because of the side effects of muscle relaxants and anxiolytics. Common analgesics typically do not help much. PVP is effective in relieving these aggravations. In our study, pain from dyskinesia was reduced by 87% up to 12 months after PVP (Fig. 7-3). In many patients, painful symptoms were completely eliminated.

Many PD patients remain active and functional for many years by treatment with available medications, but some are not as fortunate. Their treatment benefits are limited by substantial side effects from medications, such as stomach upset, nausea, hallucinations, dizziness, drowsiness, headache, loss of appetite, and vision changes. Others develop levodopa-induced dyskinesias early in their course of therapy and cannot be adequately treated. These patients are good candidates for PVP, which may be the only effective way to diminish their parkinsonian symptoms.

SPECIFIC CONTRAINDICATIONS FOR PALLIDOTOMY

Posteroventral pallidotomy has been shown to be effective treatment for advanced symptoms of idiopathic PD. To ensure beneficial results, patients should have a history of levodopa responsiveness so a correct diagnosis is more certain. Patients whose parkinsonian symptoms have never been improved by levodopa treatment may have other forms of parkinsonism, such as multiple system atrophy, progressive supranuclear palsy, corticobasal ganglionic degeneration, vascular parkinsonism, and other parkinsonism-plus syndromes (28). These conditions have not yet been demonstrated to benefit from PVP, and surgical treatment for symptomatic improvement, in general, is not recommended at this time. Some centers experienced in PVP are starting to conduct studies to investigate additional movement disorders that may benefit from PVP (17,22,30), but results are preliminary so far.

The PVP creates a permanent lesion of the globus pallidus internus (GPi). In the rare case, small cerebral ischemic infarctions and hemorrhages occur during exploration of the GPi or when placing the lesion. Most frequently, these lesions remain asymptomatic. In our initial series of 42 patients, one patient experienced a small ischemic infarction in the corona radiata and the periventricular white matter resulting in transient dysphasia. Another patient had an ischemic lesion that had a similar appearance, but he was completely asymptomatic and the lesion was discovered only by routine postoperative MR imaging (15,18). Isolated and small intracerebral lesions such as these generally do not appear to cause permanent motor or sensory deficits. However, if a patient has had previous strokes, a mass lesion, or intracranial surgery, the risk of exacerbating old deficits and giving rise to new ones may be increased (21). An extra lesion may damage other critical parts of the brain and worsen cerebral function. Dramatic deficits may result in performances that are mostly bilaterally innervated (e.g., bulbar functions and cognition) if the opposite side of the brain is already affected by previous injury. Therefore such patients might have a higher risk for complications after PVP.

On the other hand, we have shown that the presence of mild to moderate degrees of periventricular lucencies and deep white matter changes did not have significant adverse effects on the clinical outcome of PVP (2). Patients with status cribriformis and lacunes did have a higher risk of transient side effects, but they benefited from PVP as much as other patients in the long term. Therefore they should be counseled appropriately but not be denied treatment. Mild to moderate cortical atrophy or ventriculomegaly that is compatible with age also has no adverse effect on the clinical outcome of PVP (2). Severe cerebral atrophy, however, may be the source for technical difficulties for the stereotactic procedure. First, an atrophic brain is more likely to shift within the cranium with different head positions and with loss of cerebrospinal fluid, making precise location of the lesion target more difficult. Moreover, the shape of the brain may be more irregular and its compliance upon insertion of the electrode may be less predictable. Successful PVP is more of a challenge under such circumstances.

Severe deconditioning and physical disabilities often affect patients with advanced PD. Orthope-dic problems, such as degenerative disease of the spine or joints and bone fractures or deformities, can cause pain and immobility that do not improve with PVP. Often in a severely disabled patient physical therapy is needed after PVP to optimize beneficial effects. When the patient is unable to participate owing to physical limitations, post-PVP improvements are adversely affected. Our experience suggests that if patients are wheelchair-bound or bedridden during "on" periods before PVP, it is unlikely that they will be able to walk unassisted after PVP. These patients should have realistic expectations and be counseled about the potential benefits versus the risks of PVP. In general, such patients are not ideal candidates for the procedure.

Patients with severe dementia usually require total care and have limited quality of life. They do not have sufficient judgment and insight to perceive the risk versus benefit ratio of PVP. They are more at risk for complications that may cause further cognitive and physical deterioration. In this context it is important to point out that advanced PD often is associated with mild cognitive deficits that are not considered a contraindication to PVP. In our initial series of 42 patients, 6 patients had Mini-mental state examination (MMSE) (7) scores below 27 (mean 23.8, range 20–26) before PVP. At 3 months after PVP their mean MMSE score was improved to 26.5 (range 21–30, $p = 0.019$). Hence PVP may even have additional beneficial effects in patients with mild dementia.

ADDITIONAL FACTORS FOR CONSIDERATION

Age is not an important factor when determining clinical outcome after PVP. Rather, a patient's general health is more relevant. Of our 42 patients, 10 were 70 years of age or older (range 70–74 years) at the time of surgery (18). Their mean UPDRS motor scores improved by 36.1%, which was comparable to the mean scores (40.2%) of the whole group. However, improvement of their mean UPDRS ADL scores was less: 30.3% compared to 41.0% for the entire group. Patients with serious systemic or psychiatric diseases are less appropriate candidates for PVP, but the determination should be individualized. Major systemic diseases may cause a higher risk of complications and impede recovery after PVP. Psychiatric illnesses may be a contraindication to PVP if the patient lacks adequate insight into the severity of the symptoms or has grossly unrealistic expectations from the procedure.

Severe intractable tremor can be treated by pallidotomy or thalamotomy. Our results indicate that patients with parkinsonian tremor, during both "off" and "on" periods, benefited greatly from PVP (Fig. 7-2). Thalamotomy is highly effective treatment for severe tremor and dyskinesias, but it has less or no effect on other parkinsonian symptoms (9). Therefore if a patient has disabling parkinsonian features in addition to tremor, PVP might be preferred over thalamotomy. Some symptoms of advanced PD are difficult to treat with levodopa therapy, including speech and swallowing difficulties, such as hypokinetic dysarthria, stuttering, dysphagia, and drooling. Frequent freezing is another symptom. Unfortunately, these features are alleviated only slightly by PVP, and the effects are generally more short-lived.

Gait and balance problems are common with advanced PD. These symptoms are distressful because they are often associated with falls, immobility, and greater dependence during activities of daily living. Although improved by unilateral PVP, the benefits are usually less remarkable and more transient. Walking requires the support and coordination of both legs, and it is possible that improving the contralateral limb by PVP is not sufficient to reduce severe disabilities. Many patients can improve further over time with intensive physical therapy. However, patients whose gait and balance difficulties are their most severe symptoms should expect less dramatic improvement from unilateral PVP.

Only unilateral PVP has been discussed in this chapter so far. Several groups have reported that simultaneous bilateral PVP increased the complication rate for undesirable neurological deficits, such as worsening of speech, cognition, or gait (24). Therefore most centers do not perform such procedures. We think that previous pallidotomy or thalamotomy is not a contraindication for contralateral PVP, in general, unless the patient responded poorly or had notable complications from prior surgery. Our preliminary experience shows that PVP to the opposite GPi may be considered at 6 to 12 months after the first procedure if a patient shows progressive deterioration of symptoms on the ipsilateral side. Staged PVP appears to be safe and effective if the indications and contraindications for the first procedure are similarly followed. Nevertheless, it remains unclear at this time whether these patients are at a higher risk to develop speech difficulties or cognitive deficits more frequently.

CHRONIC PALLIDAL STIMULATION

The experiences with chronic pallidal stimulation are limited so far. It appears that basically the indications are similar to those for pallidotomy. Chronic pallidal stimulation might be preferable to pallidotomy in certain groups of patients. The risk of side effects might be lower in patients with significant vascular encephalopathy or cerebral atrophy. In our experience this method is also preferable with regard to technical aspects during the operative procedure in patients who are barely able to cooperate owing to severe akinesia in the "off" state. It might also be more beneficial in patients with limited capabilities to cooperate because of dementia. Chronic pallidal stimulation might also be considered an alternative in patients who previously underwent contralateral pallidotomy or thalamotomy. According to our preliminary experience, simultaneous bilateral chronic pallidal stimulation is not associated with a higher rate of side effects than unilateral stimulation. We have noted even improvement of speed in individual patients.

CONCLUSIONS

Posteroventral pallidal surgery is a highly effective, relatively safe treatment for advanced symptoms of PD. If performed properly, it is especially useful for alleviating rigidity, bradykinesia, levodopa-induced dyskinesia, "on-off" motor fluctuations, and pain symptoms. However, it cannot be considered a panacea, and patients should have realistic expectations. The indications for posteroventral pallidal surgery

include (a) advanced PD with rigidity and bradykinesia that are refractory to medical therapy;
(b) levodopa-induced dyskinesia; (c) "on-off"
motor fluctuation; (d) painful cramps and dystonia; and (e) intolerance to the side effects of antiparkinsonian medications.

Acknowledgment. We thank the M. R. Bauer
Foundation for its support.

REFERENCES

1. Baron MS. Vitek JL, Bakay RA., et al. Treatment of advanced Parkinson's disease by posterior GPi pallidotomy: 1-year results of a pilot study. *Ann Neurol* 1996;
   40:355–366.
2. Desaloms JM, Krauss JK, Lai, EC, Jankovic J, Grossman
   RG. Posteroventral medial pallidotomy for Parkinson's
   disease: preoperative magnetic resonance imaging features and clinical outcome. *J Neurosurg* 1998;89 (in
   press).
3. Dogali M, Fazzini E, Kolodny E, et al. Stereotactic ventral pallidotomy for Parkinson's disease. *Neurology*
   1995;45:753–761.
4. Fahn S, Elton RL, Members of the UPDRS Development
   Committee. Unified Parkinson's Disease Rating Scale.
   In: Fahn S, Marsden CD, Calne DB, Goldstein M, eds.
   Recent developments in Parkinson's disease, vol 2.
   Florham Park, NJ: Macmilan Health Care Information,
   1987;153–164.
5. Favre J, Taha JM, Nguyen TT, Gildenberg PL, Burchiel
   KJ. Pallidotomy: a survey of current practice in North
   America. *Neurosurgery* 1996;39:883–892.
6. Fazzini E, Dogali M, Sterio D, Eidelberg D, Beric A.
   Stereotactic pallidotomy for Parkinson's disease: a long-
   term follow-up of unilateral pallidotomy. *Neurology*
   1997;48:1273–1277.
7. Folstein MF, Folstein SE, McHugh PR. Mini-mental
   state: a practical guide for grading the mental state of patients for the clinician. *J Psychiatr Res* 1975;12:189–198.
8. Iacono RP, Lonser RR, Kuniyoshi S. Unilateral versus
   bilateral simultaneous posteroventral pallidotomy in
   subgroups of patients with Parkinson's disease. *Stereotact Funct Neurosurg* 1995;65:6–9.
9. Jankovic J, Cardoso F, Grossman RG, Hamilton WJ.
   Outcome after stereotactic thalamotomy for parkinsonian, essential, and other types of tremor. *Neurosurgery*
   1995;37:680–686.
10. Jankovic J, Lai E, Krauss J, Grossman R. Surgical treat-
    ment of levodopa induced dyskinesia. In: Stern G, ed.
    Parkinson's disease, XIIth International Symposium on
    Parkinson's Disease, London. Philadelphia: Lippincott-
    Raven (in press).
11. Jankovic J, Marsden CD. Therapeutic strategies in
    Parkinson's disease. In: Jankovic J, Tolosa E, eds. *Parkin-
    son's disease and movement disorders*, 2nd ed. Balti-
    more: Williams & Wilkins, 1993:115–144.

12. Johansson F, Malm J, Nordh E, Hariz M. Usefulness of
    pallidotomy in advanced Parkinson's disease. *J Neurol
    Neurosurg Psychiatry* 1997;62:125–132.
13. Kishore A, Turnbull IM, Snow BJ, et al. Efficacy, sta-
    bility and predictors of outcome of pallidotomy for
    Parkinson's disease; six-month follow-up with addi-
    tional 1-year observations. *Brain* 1997;120:729–737.
14. Kopyov O, Jacques D, Duma C, et al. Microelectrode-
    guided posteroventral medial radiofrequency pallidotomy
    for Parkinson's disease. *J Neurosurg* 1997;87: 52–59.
15. Krauss JK, Desaloms JM, Lai EC, King DE, Jankovic J,
    Grossman RG. Microelectrode-guided posteroventral
    pallidotomy for treatment of Parkinson's disease: post-
    operative magnetic resonance imaging analysis. *J Neu-
    rosurg* 1997;87:358–367.
16. Krauss JK, Jankovic J. Surgical treatment of Parkinson's
    disease. *Am Fam Physician* 1996;54:1621–1629.
17. Krauss JK, Jankovic J, Lai EC, Rettig GM, Grossman RG.
    Posteroventral medial pallidotomy in levodopa-unrespon-
    sive parkinsonism. *Arch Neurol* 1997;54:1026–1029.
18. Lai EC, Jankovic J, Krauss JK, et al. Efficacy of uni-
    lateral, microelectrode-guided, posteroventral pallidot-
    omy in the treatment of advanced Parkinson's disease.
    (*submitted*).
19. Laitinen LV, Bergenheim AT, Hariz MI. Leksell's pos-
    teroventral pallidotomy in the treatment of Parkinson's
    disease. *J Neurosurg* 1992;76:53–61.
20. Lang AE, Lozano AM, Montgomery E, Duff J, Tasker
    R, Hutchinson W. Posteroventral medial pallidotomy in
    advanced Parkinson's disease. *N Engl J Med* 1997;337:
    1036–1042.
21. Lim JY, De Salles AAF, Bronstein J, Masterman DL,
    Saver JL. Delayed internal capsule infarctions follow-
    ing radiofrequency pallidotomy. *J Neurosurg* 1997;87:
    955–960.
22. Lozano AM, Kumar R, Gross RE, Giladi N, Hutchison
    W, Dostrovsky JO, Lang AE. Globus pallidus internus
    pallidotomy for generalized dystonia. *Mov Disord* 1997;
    12:865–876.
23. Lozano AM, Lang AE, Galvez-Jimeniz N, et al. Effect
    of GPi pallidotomy on motor function in Parkinson's
    disease. *Lancet* 1995;346:1383–1390.
24. Obeso JA, Guridi J, DeLong M. Surgery for Parkinson's
    disease. *J Neurol Neurosurg Psychiatry* 1997;62:2–8.
25. Olanow CW. GPi pallidotomy—have we made a dent in
    Parkinson's disease. *Neurology* 1996;40:341–343.
26. Ondo W, Jankovic J, Lai EC, et al. Assessment of motor
    function after stereotactic pallidotomy. *Neurology* 1998;
    50:266–270.
27. Schwab RS, England AC. Projection technique for eval-
    uating surgery in Parkinson's disease. In: Fillingham FJ,
    Donaldson IML, eds. *Third symposium on Parkinson's
    disease*. Edinburgh: E. & S. Livingstone, 1969;152–157.
28. Stacy M, Jankovic J. Differential diagnosis of Parkin-
    son's disease and the parkinsonism plus syndromes.
    Neurol Clin 1992;10:341–359.
29. Sutton JP, Couldwell W, Lew MF, et al. Ventroposterior
    medial pallidotomy in patients with advanced Parkin-
    son's disease. *Neurosurgery* 1995;36:1112–1117.
30. Vitek JL, Bakey RA. The role of pallidotomy in Parkin-
    son's disease and dystonia. *Curr Opin Neurol* 1997;10:
    332–339.

*Pallidal Surgery for the Treatment of Parkinson's
Disease and Movement Disorders,* edited by
J. K. Krauss, R. G. Grossman, and J. Jankovic.
Lippincott-Raven Publishers, Philadelphia © 1998.

8

Operative Techniques for Pallidal Surgery

*†Joachim K. Krauss and †Robert G. Grossman

°*Department of Neurosurgery, Inselspital, University of Berne, 3010 Berne, Switzerland; and*
†Department of Neurosurgery, Baylor College of Medicine, Houston, Texas 77030, USA

Since its reintroduction into clinical practice by Laitinen et al., pallidotomy has been rapidly readopted by a number of neurosurgical centers (31). Pallidal surgery has been performed most often within the framework of clinical studies in academic hospitals, but it is now becoming almost already a "routine procedure" that is performed in various settings. The variety of surgical techniques has been exemplified by a survey of the current practice of pallidotomy in North America (10). Pallidotomy may be performed in many ways using basic localization techniques for target confirmation or more sophisticated methods such as microelectrode recording. There is no "best" or most convenient surgical technique, and minor technical variations are evident even among surgeons who agree on the same conceptual rationales and technical requirements. Depending on the methods used, the operative time for pallidal surgery may range from 2 to 10 hours.

This chapter gives an overview of current techniques used for pallidal surgery. We describe our operative method and refer to the various principles or technical variations used by other groups. Clinical results are presented elsewhere in this book. Knowledge of different techniques and the pitfalls of pallidal surgery may be helpful for avoiding intraoperative or postoperative complications. Comparison of various techniques at this time with regard to complications and results are possible only to a limited extent. For learning and adopting the technique of pallidotomy it is advis-

able to visit one of the major centers with surgical expertise. Recently, also, courses and educational programs conveying the major principles of the procedure are being offered.

STEREOTACTIC FRAME SYSTEMS AND INSTRUMENTATION

Stereotactic surgery is based on a cartesian coordinate system that implies that any point in space can be determined by three coordinates (x, y, and z), which are defined with regard to three intersecting orthogonal planes (Fig. 8-1). Various stereotactic frame systems, instruments, and software packages are being offered for functional stereotactic operations (11). "Semistereotactic" approaches for pallidotomy as performed by Cooper during the 1950s are no longer used because of their inaccuracy (6). So far, the precision of frameless stereotactic systems has not been sufficient to allow its application to basal ganglia lesioning for the treatment of movement disorders. The stereotactic frame serves not only as a reference base for calculating the stereotactic coordinates, it also provides rigid fixation of the skull. The mechanical accuracy of current frames is in the range of less than 1 mm. Translational types of stereotactic devices and arc-centered systems may be used. It is important, however, to note the differences in the trajectories when multiple parallel pathways are obtained for microelectrode recording with these two systems. Generally, it is advantageous to use

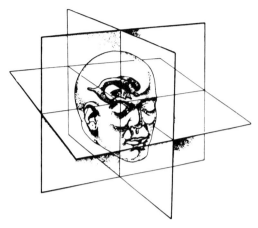

FIG. 8-1. Cartesian coordinate system showing the three orthogonal intersecting planes used to define the coordinates in stereotactic surgery. (*From* ref. 47, with permission.)

systems with relatively shorter instruments (guiding cannulas and electrodes) during functional stereotactic surgery, as there is less risk of deviation at the target site than with longer instruments. The length of the probes of systems used frequently for such purposes, such as the Leksell system or the Riechert-Mundinger system (with the Zamorano-Dujovny semiarc), is 19 cm, equaling the distance from the arc to the target. Console software or software packages for target calculation are commercially available, although many surgeons use additional software or their own software for this purpose.

PREOPERATIVE PREPARATION OF THE PATIENT

Formal neurological assessments should be performed within days preoperatively. We obtain nonstereotactic magnetic resonance imaging (MRI) routinely in all patients. With regard to the cost of the hospital stay and the current practice of reimbursement of health insurance carriers in the United States, patients are often admitted on the same day the surgery is performed. Most protocols require that antiparkinsonian medication be stable for at least 1 month preoperatively. For patients who have difficulty sleeping a short-acting benzodiazepine not interfering with par-

kinsonian symptoms may be administered the evening before surgery. It is obvious that patients must be off coumarin derivates, and coagulation parameters are corrected prior to pallidal surgery. Medications interfering with thrombocyte aggregation, such as aspirin, should be stopped at least 10 days before surgery. Cooperation of the patient is needed during the surgical procedure to guide placement of the lesion, so it is important that patients are informed in detail about each step of the procedure.

It is feasible to perform pallidotomy while the patient is off levodopa medication. We advise patients to take the last levodopa dose not later than 12 hours prior to surgery, as being off levodopa allows more easy monitoring of the efficacy of the lesioning on parkinsonian target symptoms, such as bradykinesia, rigidity, and tremor, which may guide the decision whether a lesion should be enlarged or additional lesions be made. Furthermore, dyskinesias during the "on" state may interfere with fixation of the stereotactic head frame and stereotactic imaging, and they can cause artifacts during microelectrode recording.

Pallidotomy for treatment of Parkinson's disease is usually performed under local anesthesia. General anesthesia is reserved for rare conditions; for example, it may be necessary in bilateral procedures for severe dystonic or hyperkinetic syndromes in children (29). In particular, under such circumstances intraoperative microelectrode recording is clearly advantageous. Intraoperative communication and neurological assessment is crucial during neurophysiological confirmation of the target and lesion-making. We do not administer "premedication" or sedating or centrally acting analgesic drugs prior to or during any phase of the procedure. Laitinen administers a combination of pethidine and atropine 15 minutes before mounting the stereotactic device (30). Some groups use sedation for fixating the stereotactic head frame by intravenous administration of propofol or short half-life benzodiazepines (13,44). Propofol is not ideally suited for this purpose, as it may elicit abnormal movements and can interfere with parkinsonian symptoms (26). It has also been shown that propofol may suppress the firing of human pallidal neurons (17).

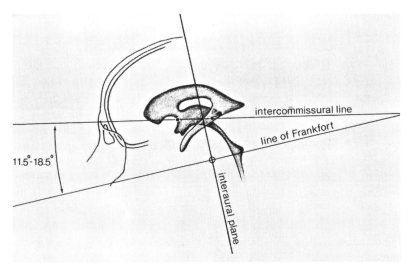

FIG. 8-2. Relation between the intercommissural line and the "*Frankfurter horizontale*" (orbitomeatal line). Usually the intercommissural line is angled at 11.5 to 18.5 degrees above the orbitomeatal line (49).

The perioperative use of prophylactic anticonvulsants is controversial. Occasionally, preoperative "loading" with relatively high doses contributes to postoperative lethargy and confusion. Corticosteroids are given intravenously before starting the procedure to reduce edema along the trajectory and around the lesion. There are no scientific data with regard to the efficacy of this prophylaxis or the doses needed. We routinely administer a bolus of 20 mg dexamethasone or 100 mg prednisolone. Intravenous antibiotic prophylaxis is given prior to the procedure and may be maintained for 24 hours. We use third-generation cephalosporins, such as cefuroxime or cefotiam.

We place both an intravenous line and an arterial line to obtain accurate measurement of arterial blood pressure. Careful intraoperative and perioperative monitoring of the blood pressure is helpful for immediately recognizing and counteracting blood pressure rises or hypotension. Arterial hypertension may occur any time during the procedure, in particular when not using sedation. Presumably, the risk of intracerebral hemorrhage is reduced when hypertension is corrected promptly. Occasionally, arterial hypotension is seen during the procedure. In one patient before we routinely placed arterial lines we had to abort the operation because of the occurrence of a vasovagal syncope during macrostimulation. Monitored care by an anesthesiologist experienced in functional stereotactic surgery has proved valuable in our practice. Indwelling urinary catheters can be helpful in elderly patients. A mixture of a short-acting and a long-acting local anesthetic is injected locally when fixating the stereotactic frame to the patient's skull. The frame is attached to the patient's head, avoiding any rotation or tilt of the head relative to the frame axes. The base line (*y*-axis) should be as nearly parallel to the intercommissural line as possible; hence the stereotactic frame is usually tilted slightly above the orbitomeatal line (Fig. 8-2). When using the Leksell G frame, the earbars are helpful for this purpose.

STEREOTACTIC TARGETING AND STEREOTACTIC ATLASES

Traditionally, the target coordinates in functional stereotactic surgery are extrapolated with regard to landmarks of the third ventricle (39,40). For contemporary pallidotomy the pallidal target coordinates, in general, are referred to the intercommissural line—the line between the anterior commissure (AC) and the posterior commissure (PC). The commissures may be identified with various imaging methods including stereotactic ventriculography (13), computed tomography (CT) (3,23,27,30), or MRI (3,20,25,32). As indicated by Lozano et al., a potential source of error derives from the stereotactic atlas that is used for reference (32). Human stereotactic brain atlases present mean values for the three-dimensional location of a target and show exemplary anatomical specimens. Pallidal coordinates differ remarkably between the Schaltenbrand-Bailey atlas and its newer edition, the Schaltenbrand—Wahren atlas (39,40). The lateral coordinates differ by 1 to 2 mm and the vertical coordinates by 2 to 3 mm. According to Lozano et al. the coordinates in the Schaltenbrand-Wahren edition match more closely with physiological mapping, which is in accordance with our experience. The AC-PC based atlas-derived coordinates should be corrected in patients with shorter or longer AC—PC lines or widening of the third ventricle (14).

STEREOTACTIC IMAGE ACQUISITION

There are divergent opinions among groups with regard to which stereotactic imaging method is most suitable for pallidal surgery. For decades, stereotactic ventriculography was used to identify the AC and the PC. To avoid parallax effects, ventriculography was ideally performed with fixed x-ray tubes with long projection lines. Although ventriculography allows precise identification of the commissures, direct visualization and confirmation of the pallidal target is not possible. Occasionally, intraventricular application of contrast medium is not well tolerated. In recent years ventriculography has been increasingly replaced by stereotactic CT or MRI. It has been demonstrated that CT- and MRI-guided localization of the commissures is accurate and may even be superior to ventriculography (1,15).

We use stereotactic CT guidance to identify the commissures. Contiguous 1-mm axial scans through the third ventricle with the indicator panels carrying the fiducials mounted on the frame are obtained on a GE 9800 CT scanner or a helical CT scanner (General Electric Medical Systems, Milwaukee, WI, USA). The imaging data are transferred to a GE Advantage Windows work station, where the axial scans and coordinated simultaneous reformatted sagittal and coronal images are displayed. The simultaneous and multiplanar display allows accurate localization of the commissures. The most posterior margin of the AC and the most anterior margin of the PC is determined. When the commissures are present on more than one axial scan, the images displaying the largest diameter of the AC and the PC are selected, respectively. Additionally, the CT image coordinates of the frame center are determined. For the tentative location of the target in the posteroventral globus pallidus internus (GPi) we use the following AC-PC based coordinates: 19 to 21 mm lateral to the midline, 4 to 5 mm below the AC-PC line, and 2 to 3 mm anterior to the midcommissural point (Fig. 8-3).

Misalignment correction for the target calculation must be applied when the AC-PC line is not in perfect alignment with the three orthogonal axes of the stereotactic frame. Tilting of the AC—PC line relative to the y-axis is encountered most frequently with the AC and the PC shown on different axial images. The AC-PC line may also be slightly rotated, or the head may be tilted laterally in relation to the frame. Infrequently the latter has been a problem in our experience. Various methods have been used to correct for misalignment (38,42). We have developed a computerized misalignment correction algorithm that has been implemented on a personal computer with a spreadsheet program (28). Basically, this algorithm corrects for deviations of the axis of the AC-PC line in relation to the stereotactic frame by rotating the target vector by various angles. The frame coordinates of the preliminary target are then retranslated to CT coordinates, and the position is checked on multiplanar images with the interactive software for its proximity to the internal capsule and the choroidal fissure. If the target appears to be too close to these structures it is moved farther away, by 1 or 2 mm. The target coordinates are calculated independently by the neurosurgeon directly from the imaging data and by the neuroradiologist using the programmed algorithm. The pallidal target may also be defined with the help of work stations with computer-resident digitized stereotactic atlases with maps that can be shrunk or stretched to fit the patient's individual anatomy (22).

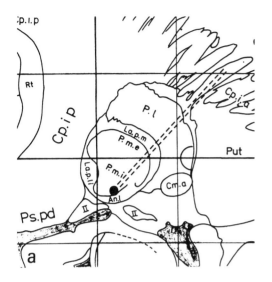

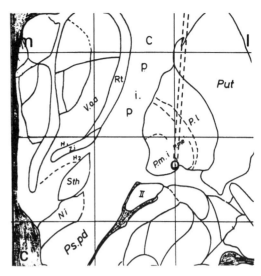

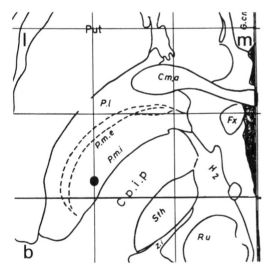

FIG. 8-3. Location of the preliminary target in the posteroventral lateral globus pallidus internus and the trajectory to the target on (a) sagittal, (b) axial, and (c) coronal diagrams: (a) right side = rostral, (b) right side = medial, (c) left side = medial. Stereotactic coordinates for the pallidal target: *x*, 20 mm lateral to the intercommissural line; *y*, 2 mm anterior to midcommissural point; *z*, 4 mm below the intercommissural line. *Gray areas*, cerebrospinal fluid; *0*, preliminary target; *An.l*, ansa lenticularis; *Cm.a*, anterior commissure; *Cp.ia*, anterior limb of internal capsule; *Cp.ip*, posterior limb of internal capsule; *Fx*, fornix; *H1*, Forel's field H1; *H2*, Forel's field H2; *La.p.li*, lamina pallidi limitans; *La.p.m*, lamina pallidi medialis; *Ni*, substantia nigra; *P.l*, globus pallidus lateralis (sive externus); *P.m.e*, globus pallidus medialis (sive internus)—external segment; *P.m.i*, globus pallidus medialis (sive internus)—internal segment; *Ps.pd*, pes pedunculi; *Put*, putamen; *Rt*, nucleus reticulatus thalami; *Ru*, nucleus ruber; *Sth*, subthalamic nucleus; *V.oa*, nucleus ventralis oralis anterior thalami; *Zi*, zona incerta.(Modified from ref. 40, with permission.)

Stereotactic MR imaging allows direct identification of the pallidal target and the bordering internal capsule (32). Nevertheless, most surgeons consider the spatial relation of the pallidal target to the commissures as well when calculating the frame coordinates. There are still concerns about the accuracy of stereotactic MR imaging because of the possibility of image distortion (51). More sophisticated techniques and MR sequences that

minimize geometrical distortion are being developed. Magnetic distortions are due to both gradient field nonlinearities and resonance offsets, including field inhomogeneities and chemical shift. There are several techniques to reduce MR image distortion. Three-dimensional data sets with magnetization prepared rapid gradient echoes have been shown to be of particular advantage (8). Advances in methods to correct gradient and mag-

netic field inhomogeneities have yielded a geo-
metric accuracy of about 1 mm, comparable to
that of CT scanning.

SURGICAL TECHNIQUE

Usually the pallidal operation is performed immediately once the frame coordinates have been
calculated. With the use of Laitinen's stereo
adapter, the procedure may also be done another
day (30). In the operating room the patient is positioned comfortably in a semisitting position.
The stereotactic frame is fixed to the table with a
Mayfield adapter (Fig. 8-4). This position avoids
leakage of cerebrospinal fluid (CSF) intraoperatively and reduces the possibility of "brain shift."
It is sufficient to shave only a small amount of
hair in the frontal region at the site of the planned
longitudinal incision, which is prepared with an
antiseptic and infiltrated with local anesthetic.
We place a burr hole 7 to 9 cm above the orbital
rim and 2 cm lateral to the midline. Thus, we usually achieve an angle of 40 to 45 degrees between
the trajectory to the target and the AC-PC line in
the sagittal plane. Dogali et al. approached the

pallidal target in their initial patients with angles
as low as 28 degrees (9). Others place the burr
hole at the level of the coronal suture (30). The
cranial opening may also be made with a twist
drill. Usually 3-mm twist drills are used (9). Microelectrode recording may be performed via a
single twist drill hole or via separate twist drill
holes for each pathway (32,46). A burr hole allows better visualization and subsequent preservation of cortical vessels. The dura is coagulated
and incised in a cruciate fashion. Any coagulation of even small bridging veins should be
avoided, as it may result in venous infarctions
(Fig. 8-5). A guiding cannula that allows passing
of microelectrodes and "macroelectrodes" is inserted into the brain at the crown of a gyrus after
coagulation and incision of the arachnoid.

Physiological Localization:
Is Microelectrode Recording Necessary?

Physiologic confirmation of the target is considered mandatory during functional stereotactic
neurosurgery. Methods used for pallidal surgery
include microelectrode recording, "semi"—mi-

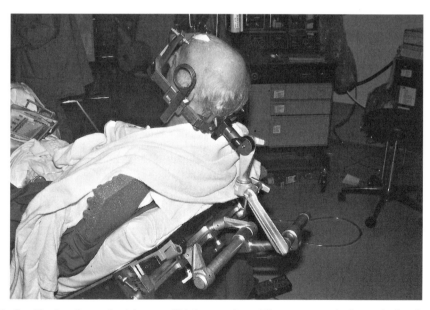

FIG. 8-4. Positioning the patient for a pallidal procedure. The stereotactic frame is fixed to a Mayfield adapter, with the patient in a semisitting position. The location for the burr hole is indicated by
the white patch.

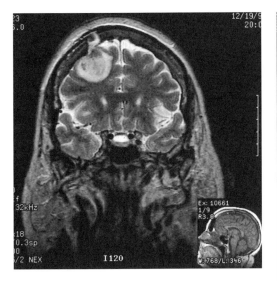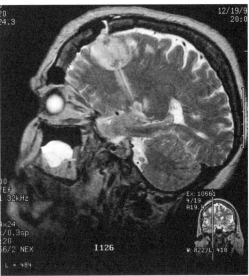

FIG. 8-5. Coronal and sagittal T2-weighted MR sequences from a 61-year-old woman 2 days after a right-sided pallidotomy. Note the incidental finding of an asymptomatic frontal venous infarction.

croelectrode recording, microstimulation, photic stimulation, impedance recording, and macrostimulation. It is debated at the present time which neurophysiological methods should be considered the "gold standard" of pallidal surgery. Microelectrode recording and stimulation have not replaced macrostimulation but, in general, are considered complementary methods. Although several surgeons regard microelectrode recording important for achieving good clinical outcome at low risk (2,25,32,50), others argue that the results using macrostimulation alone are comparable and thus microelectrode recording is unnecessary (19,23,24,30). Arguments against the use of microelectrode recording frequently include a significant increase of operating time and dependence on a neurophysiologist during the operation. These objections, however, are not necessarily valid. Indeed, microelectrode recording in the frame of scientific neurophysiological studies may be time-consuming. Modified techniques for routine clinical use, however, add little operating time (25,27). The techniques and the interpretation of the signals are easily learned by functional neurosurgeons. Whereas macrostimulation allows us to determine thresholds for assessing the proximity of the neighboring inter-

nal capsule and optic tract, there is no way to determine exactly where the electrode is placed within the pallidum—whether in the GPi or in the globus pallidus externus (GPe).

There is little hope that results from groups who do not use microelectrode recording compared to those who integrate this technique in their surgical armamentarium will allow answers to the question of whether the latter technique is superior. This question may be addressed adequately only with a properly designed prospective study performed by the same surgical team. Nevertheless, microelectrode recording offers a unique opportunity for electrophysiological study of the basal ganglia and their circuitry.

Microelectrode Recording and Microstimulation

The rationales and techniques of microelectrode recording of extracellular single-unit discharges and microstimulation are discussed in detail by Hutchison in Chapter 9 of this book. Here, we concentrate only on some aspects with regard to the surgical procedure and lesion-making. Intraoperative microelectrode recording techniques with high-impedance electrodes have been pioneered in pallidal surgery by groups from Atlanta, New York, and Toronto (18,43,50). Other groups have made several technical modifications.

The Atlanta group uses multiple microelectrode passes (2,50). In the initial patients of their series, 3 to 11 passes (average 6.8) were made to define the "sensorimotor" territory of the GPi and the location of the optic tract and internal capsule (2). Lozano and colleagues explored two to eight electrode tracks in their initial series (33); and Taha and colleagues recorded one to three trajectories, 2 mm apart, for each patient via separate twist-drill holes for each trajectory (46).

We use microelectrode recording to identify the structures along the trajectory and to delineate the borders of the GPi with special emphasis on the ventral border (45). The microelectrode is advanced via the guiding cannula with a hydraulic microdrive, and single-unit recordings are sought from 20 mm above the tentative target to 5 mm below it. The signals are displayed on speakers and on an oscilloscope, and they are analyzed on-line. The relative position of the units with regard to the tentative target is mapped on graph paper, taking into account the firing pattern and frequency. We investigate only a few cells for their response to movement-related activity. We regard such activity as helpful, confirming the validity of the recording; but we do not use this information to guide placement of the lesion. Differentiation of neuronal firing patterns is accomplished based on established criteria (18,43). In patients with tremor, neurons firing in synchrony with the frequency of the tremor may be found in both the GPi and the GPe. After leaving the posteroventral pallidum the background noise diminishes notably. When the optic tract is entered by the microelectrode, occasionally a slight increase in the basal background activity is heard over the speakers. The recording is supplemented by microstimulation 3 to 4 mm below the ventral pallidal border with the room light off. Visual sensations, such as seeing stars or "Christmas lights" in differerent colors, are reported by most but not all patients. At this location we also perform photic stimulation, switching a flashlight on and off in front of the patient's eyes. Frequently this maneuver results in slight changes in the basic firing rate of the optic tract.

When the first trajectory yields satisfactory localization with identification of striatal cells, GPe pausers and bursters, laminar border cells, and abundant high-frequency discharge from GPi cells; in an adequate and proportionate spatial distribution, no additional tracks are made. In most patients only one or two pathways are investigated, although we have explored three to five pathways when necessary.

The Atlanta group and others have also applied microstimulation to identify the location of the corticospinal tract in the internal capsule (3,32). Microstimulation of the corticospinal tract can evoke tetanic contractions of the contralateral extremities.

Some groups use "semi"-microelectrodes with tip diameters of 25 μm or more (13,20,36). Such electrodes do not allow recording of single units, but they do record background mass electrical activity, which has been called "neuronal noise." This technique is simpler than microelectrode recording and requires less-specialized technical equipment. It has been shown to differentiate the putamen, GPe, GPi, internal capsule, and the optic tract in experienced hands (36). It can also be used to detect movement-related discharges in the GPi. The spatial resolution, however, is less accurate than "true" microelectrode recording.

Impedance Recording

Impedance is a complex phenomenon that reflects the resistance of tissue to current flow and the properties of the system by which it is determined. Electrical impedance in tissue is defined as "a measurement of the ratio of the voltage to the resulting current that is generated in the tissue" (5). Most standard radiofrequency lesion generators allow measurement of electrical impedance. The electrical impedance of the brain structures transversed can be measured while the lesioning electrode is forwarded to the target. Nuclear masses such as the basal ganglia can be distinguished easily from subcortical white matter and neuronal bundles, as well as from CSF. Because impedance monitoring is relatively nonspecific it is of limited value. The signal changes can be displayed acoustically with speakers. The change of the impedance upon entering the basal ganglia yields a characteristic signal. Typically, the impedance rises from about 300 ohms to about 600 ohms with the 1.1×3-mm electrode. There are some minor fluctuations when the probe is advanced within the basal ganglia to the pallidal target while traversing the medullar laminae between the external and internal pallidum as well as within the internal pallidum. The impedance abruptly drops when the choroidal fissure is entered. Laitinen has used impedance recording in conjunction with macrostimulation to guide the ventral extension of the pallidal lesion (30). No further lesioning was performed when the impedance dropped below 400 ohms.

Macrostimulation

Impedance recording, macrostimulation, and lesion-making are usually performed with the same macroelectrode. For pallidal surgery we use a 1.1-mm unipolar electrode with a 3-mm uninsulated tip. A *"setzeffekt,"* consisting of some amelioration of contralateral parkinsonian symptoms, is noted occasionally when the tip of the electrode reaches the pallidal target. This effect, in contrast to thalamic surgery, however, is much less consistent and weaker in the pallidum. Most often it is only barely noticeable. Macrostimulation is used to assess the threshold for the spread of current to the optic tract and the internal capsule. The effect of the stimulation depends on a variety of stimulation parameters, which makes it difficult to directly compare thresholds described from different centers.

We apply macrostimulation with a pulse width of 1 ms at various frequencies including 5, 10, 20, 50, and 100 Hz. The voltage is increased incrementally from 0 V to 4 V if no response is elicited at a lower threshold. The occurrence of capsular or optic responses or of any other effects is noted. Capsular responses may consist of muscular twitches at low frequencies or tonic contractions at higher frequencies. Optic responses typically are described as flashing lights in the contralateral visual field. If no capsular or optic responses are evoked below a threshold of 2 V, the final lesion is made at the planned site. Otherwise, we withdraw the electrode in 0.5-mm increments and repeat the stimulation. It is more difficult to evaluate intrinsic pallidal effects from stimulation with the frequencies that are commonly used. Occasionally slight improvement of contralateral parkinsonian symptoms are noted or mild dyskinetic movements are evoked with higher frequencies. An intense feeling of fear and sometimes of impending death can be elicited with stimulation at 100 Hz at a threshold of 3 to 4 V. This effect, which was always obtained when the voltage was increased to the threshold with the electrode properly placed at the final target site appears to be an intrinsic pallidal response possibly related to the stimulation of pallidal neurons or circuitries related to emotion.

Instead of incrementally increasing the voltage during macrostimulation, other surgeons use fixed stimulation parameters. Johansson et al., for example, conduct electrical stimulations with 10 mA at 6 Hz and with 5 mA at 60 Hz (21). It has been noted that low-frequency stimulation at 2–10 Hz may increase muscle tone and tremor (10).

In their pivotal report on posteroventral pallidotomy, in 1992 Laitinen et al. reported postoperative homonymous visual field defects in 14% of patients (31). Subsequent reports using microelectrode recording or macrostimulation alone consistently have noted lower rates of this side effect. Visual evoked potentials have been found to be a helpful adjunct to macrostimulation (4). Monocular stimulation with flash stimuli has been used, alternating epochs between ipsilateral and contralateral eyes.

Radiofrequency Lesioning

In the past, several methods were used for lesioning during functional stereotactic surgery. Apparently, nowadays all centers performing pallidotomy apply thermo-controlled radio frequency lesioning. The lesion is made with the same electrode used for macrostimulation. It is a matter of controversy where the pallidal lesion should be placed. This topic is discussed more thoroughly in Chapter 20. The final decision where the lesion is to be located depends on a variety of factors, in particular on the concept of the optimal target of the surgical team and the methods used for target confirmation.

Some centers perform "test lesions" before the final lesion is made. Such lesions usually are produced by heating the electrode to 45° to 60°C for 10 to 60 seconds. Rarely, higher temperatures limited to a few seconds are applied, for example, 84°C for 10 seconds (46). The rationales for test lesions have been questioned, in particular with regard to the notion that irreversible tissue damage may occur with temperatures as low as 45°C (34).

Here we briefly outline our method of lesion-making for posteroventral lateral GPi pallidotomy-subpallidotomy. Test lesions are not performed. We intend to place the lesion within 1 mm of the ventral border of the lateral GPi according to the microelectrode mapping. In fully cooperative patients the lesion is placed with the tip located 0.5 mm below the area where the last clearly discernible typical GPi cells were recorded in case no phosphenes are elicited by macrostimulation below 2 V. Otherwise, the electrode is withdrawn in 0.5-mm increments, as described above, with repeated macrostimulation until visual responses are no longer evoked below 2 V. In patients who are not cooperating adequately or who do not report consistent responses, and in the rare cases of pallidotomy performed under general anesthesia, the tip of the electrode is placed slightly above the ventral pallidal border to create the lesion. Microelectrode studies have implied that the border between the globus pallidus and the subpallidal fiber bundles is not a sharp boundary (45). Initially we have made two or three lesions spaced apart over a distance of 3 mm with the electrode tip along the same trajectory. The lesions are created with the temperature controlled at 75°C for 60 seconds. More recently we have applied two lesions spaced 1.5 to 2.0 mm apart. During lesioning the strength and mobility of the contralateral arm, speech, and visual fields are monitored, which allows early detection of possible adverse effects. If such effects should occur, the radiofrequency lesioning is discontinued.

Various other techniques are applied by other centers for placement of radiofrequency lesions. It is not always entirely clear from the description of the surgical procedures where exactly in the GPi the lesions are placed, in particular with regard to the most ventral lesion. Some groups perform intraoperative ventriculography

to check the position of the electrode relative to the AC-PC line (20,44). Some noninclusive examples for the differences in lesion placement are as follows. Whereas most groups place subsequent lesions in a ventral to dorsal direction along a single trajectory by withdrawing the electrode, other groups do the reverse (21). Bakay, in contrast, places lesions along different parallel tracts aiming at reducing the activity of the physiologically defined sensorimotor pallidum (2). Taha et al. make three subsequent lesions spaced 2 mm apart along the same trajectory with each lesion created with a 1.3 × 2 mm electrode at 84°C for 60 seconds (46). A fourth lesion is added if kinesthetic or tremor-synchronous cells were recorded more than 6.5 mm above the base of the pallidum. Lozano et al. use a 1 × 3 mm electrode, heating the electrode subsequently from 70° to 80° and finally to 90°C for 60 seconds (32,33). Iacono et al. use a 1.6 × 2 mm electrode to create lesions at 65° to 80°C for 30 to 60 seconds (20). They vary the time of lesioning with regard to the thresholds at which capsular or optic responses were evoked by macrostimulation.

During placement of the lesion or immediately thereafter some patients develop transient involuntary movements. These movements usually are confined to the extremities contralateral to the side of the lesion. Most frequently they have a choreic or choreoathetotic appearance, but dystonic or hemiballistic hyperkinesias may also be observed (33,35). In general, they last for a few minutes up to half an hour. Occasionally minor choreic movements are seen for several hours. Such involuntary movements occur with appropriate placement of the lesion in the pallidum. Their appearance has been considered to predict a more favorable clinical outcome with regard to parkinsonian symptoms (35).

Radiofrequency lesioning is believed superior to all the methods used in the past to create therapeutic lesions during functional stereotactic surgery: It allows better definition of the lesion by varying the parameters, such as the diameter of the electrode, the exposed length of the electrode tip, and modulation of the time and temperature of the lesion-making. The "predictability" of the lesion has been stressed, particularly with regard to experimental studies using egg white (7,16). However, we found a lack of correlation in the volumes of pallidal lesions according to MRI studies during the immediate postoperative period and at a 6-month follow-up in 36 patients who underwent pallidotomy for treatment of advanced Parkinson's disease (27). Although radiofrequency coagulation represents the best lesioning method currently available, it may not be the optimum method for the future. There is renewed interest in chemical lesioning techniques. Convection-enhanced delivery of quinolinic acid to the GPi to specifically lesion neurons expressing the *N*-methyl-D-aspartate (NMDA) receptor in *N*-methyl-4-phenyl-1,2,3,6-tetrahydropyridine (MPTP) parkinsonian monkeys resulted in significant improvement of parkinsonian symptoms (12). Histological examination showed that administration of the excitotoxin had caused selective damage to GPi neurons with complete sparing of surrounding white matter tracts.

Chronic Pallidal Stimulation

Basically the same neurophysiological techniques that are used for defining the target during pallidotomy can be used to determine the optimal site for chronic pallidal stimulation (13,37,41,48). The rationales and principles of deep brain stimulation (DBS) are dealt with in more detail elsewhere in this volume.

Two electrodes are available for this purpose (Fig. 8-6). A quadripolar electrode allows stimulation via different combinations of the four contacts. A monopolar electrode with a single contact may also be used having the advantage of being free of the 1.5-mm deadspace located at the tip of the quadripolar electrode.

The impulse generator may be implanted during the same operative session after induction of general anesthesia, or the electrode may be externalized to perform test stimulations.

Postoperative Care

Dural closure is not necessary, as the burr hole is located close to the vertex. We place a small piece of gelatin, such as Gelfoam, in the dural opening. The burr hole can be covered by a plastic burr hole cover or a miniplate to achieve satisfactory cosmesis (Fig. 8-7).The skin is closed with a two-layer suture. Postoperatively, patients are observed overnight in an intermediate care unit. We reinstitute levodopa medication on the first postoperative day starting with about half of the preoperative dosage. The usual preoperative dosage is given the following day. In general, the total levodopa dosage remains unchanged, but minor adjustments are made. For example, in patients who tolerated only small levodopa doses preoperatively but who had to take such doses frequently, higher doses may be given at greater intervals. We obtain postoperative MRI scans routinely on the second postoperative day to confirm appropriate placement of the pallidal lesion (Fig. 8-7). Patients usually are discharged 2 to 4 days postoperatively.

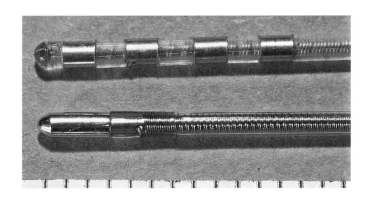

FIG. 8-6. Electrodes used for chronic deep brain stimulation of the pallidum: quadripolar and monopolar electrodes (Medtronic, Minneapolis, MN, USA).

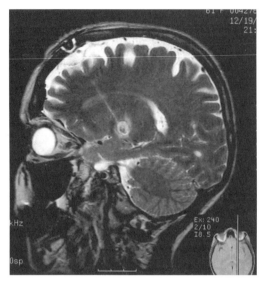

FIG. 8-7. Sagittal T2-weighted MR scan in a 61-year-old woman 2 days postoperatively showing the location of the lesion in the posteroventral lateral globus pallidus internus. Note the electrode track. The burr hole is covered by a plastic burr hole cover for satisfactory cosmesis.

REFERENCES

1. Alterman RL, Kall BA, Cohen H, Kelly PJ. Stereotactic ventrolateral thalamotomy: is ventriculography necessary? *Neurosurgery* 1995;37:717–722.
2. Bakay RAE. Comment on: Sutton JP, Couldwell W, Lew MF, et al. Ventroposterior medial pallidotomy in patients with advanced Parkinson's disease. *Neurosurgery* 1995;36:1116–1117.
3. Baron MS, Vitek JL, Bakay RAE, et al. Treatment of advanced Parkinson's disease by posterior GPi pallidotomy: 1-year results of a pilot study. *Ann Neurol* 1996; 40:355–366.
4. Bonaroti EA, Rose RD, Kondziolka D, Baser S, Lunsford LD. Flash visual evoked potential monitoring of optic tract function during macroelectrode-based pallidotomy. In: Lunsford LD, ed. *Neurosurgical Focus*, vol 3. www.neurosurgery.org. 1997:2.
5. Bullard DE, Nashold BS Jr. Impedance recording in functional neurosurgery. In: Gildenberg PL, Tasker RR, eds. *Textbook of stereotactic and functional neurosurgery*. New York: McGraw-Hill, 1997:949–953.
6. Cooper IS. *Parkinsonism: its medical and surgical therapy*. Springfield, IL: Charles C. Thomas Publisher, 1961.
7. Dieckmann G, Gabriel E, Hassler R. Size, form and structural peculiarities of experimental brain lesions obtained by thermocontrolled radiofrequency. *Confin Neurol* 1965;26:134–142.
8. DiPierro CG, Francel PC, Jackson TR, Kamiryo T, Laws ER Jr. Optimized magnetic resonance image-guided stereotaxis: a technique with validation based on the ante-

rior commissure–posterior commissure line. In:Lunsford LD, ed. *Neurosurgical Focus*, vol 3. www.neurosurgery. org. 1997:2.
9. Dogali M, Fazzini E, Kolodny E, et al. Stereotactic ventral pallidotomy for Parkinson's disease. *Neurology* 1995;45:753–761.
10. Favre J, Taha JM, Nguyen TT, Gildenberg PL, Burchiel KJ. Pallidotomy: a survey of current practice in North America. *Neurosurgery* 1996;39:883–892.
11. Gildenberg PL, Tasker RR, eds. *Textbook of stereotactic and functional neurosurgery*. New York: McGraw-Hill, 1997.
12. Gogate N, Corthesy ME, Lonser RR, Old field EH. Convection-enhanced superselective excitotoxic pallidal lesioning for Parkinson's disease. *Neurosurgery* 1997;41:739.
13. Gross C, Rougier A, Guehl D, Boraud T, Julien J, Bioulac B. High-frequency stimulation of the globus pallidus internalis in Parkinson's disease: a study of seven cases. *J Neurosurg* 1997;87:491–498.
14. Grossman RG, Hamilton WJ. Movement disorders. In: Grossman RG, Hamilton WJ, eds. *Principles of neurosurgery*. Philadelphia: Lippincott-Raven, 1991; 305–317.
15. Hariz MI, Bergenheim AT. A comparative study on ventriculographic and computerized tomography-guided determinations of brain targets in functional stereotaxis. *J Neurosurg* 1990;73:565–571.
16. Hassler R, Mundinger F, Riechert T. *Stereotaxis in Parkinson syndrome*. New York: Springer-Verlag, 1979.
17. Heit G, Murphy G, Jaffe R, Golby A, Silverberg G. Effects of propofol on human globus pallidus neurons: *Stereotact Funct Neurosurg* 1996–1997;67:74.
18. Hutchison WD, Lozano AM, Davis KD, Saint-Cyr JA, Lang AE, Dostrovsky JO. Differential neuronal activity in segments of globus pallidus in Parkinson's disease patients. *Neuroreport* 1994;5:1533–1537.
19. Iacono RP. Stereotactic pallidotomy [Letter]. *J Neurosurg* 1996;85:987–988.
20. Iacono RP, Shima F, Lonser RR, Kuniyoshi S, Maeda G, Yamada S. The results, indications, and physiology of posteroventral pallidotomy for patients with Parkinson's disease. *Neurosurgery* 1995;36:1118–1127.
21. Johansson F, Malm J, Nordh E, Hariz M. Usefulness of pallidotomy in advanced Parkinson's disease. *J Neurol Neurosurg Psychiatry* 1997;62:125–132.
22. Kall BA, Kelly PJ, Goerss BS, Frieder G. Methodology and clinical experience with computed tomography and a computer-resident stereotactic atlas. *Neurosurgery* 1985;17:400–407.
23. Kishore A, Turnbull IM, Snow JB, et al. Efficacy, stability and predictors of outcome of pallidotomy for Parkinson's disease: six-month follow-up with additional 1-year observations. *Brain* 1997;120:729–737.
24. Kondziolka D, Lunsford LD. Stereotactic pallidotomy [Letter]. *J Neurosurg* 1996;85:986–987.
25. Kopyov O, Jacques D, Duma C, et al. Microelectrode-guided posteroventral medial radiofrequency pallidotomy for Parkinson's disease. *J Neurosurg* 1997;87:52–59.
26. Krauss JK, Akeyson EW, Giam P, Jankovic J. Propofol-induced dyskinesias in Parkinson's disease. *Anesth Analg* 1996;83:420–422.
27. Krauss JK, Desaloms JM, Lai EC, King DE, Jankovic J, Grossman RG. Microelectrode-guided posteroventral pallidotomy for treatment of Parkinson's disease: post-

operative magnetic resonance imaging analysis. *J Neurosurg* 1997;87:358–367.

28. Krauss JK, King DE, Grossman RG. Alignment correction algorithm in CT-guided functional neurosurgery. *Stereotact Funct Neurosurg* 1996–1997;67:30.

29. Krauss JK, Mohadjer M, Nobbe F, Mundinger F. Bilateral ballism in children. *Childs Nerv Syst* 1991;7:342–346.

30. Laitinen LV. Pallidotomy for Parkinson's disease. *Neurosurg Clin North Am* 1995;6:105–112.

31. Laitinen LV, Bergenheim AT, Hariz MI. Leksell's posteroventral pallidotomy in the treatment of Parkinson's disease. *J Neurosurg* 1992;76:53–61.

32. Lozano A, Hutchison W, Kiss Z, Tasker R, Davis K, Dostrovsky J. Methods for microelectrode-guided posteroventral pallidotomy. *J Neurosurg* 1996;84:194–202.

33. Lozano AM, Lang AE, Galvez-Jimenez N, et al. Effect of GPi pallidotomy on motor function in Parkinson's disease. *Lancet* 1995;346:1383–1387.

34. Lunsford LD. Comment on: Favre J, Taha JM, Nguyen TT, Gildenberg PL, Burchiel KJ. Pallidotomy: a survey of current practice in North America. *Neurosurgery* 1996;39:890–892.

35. Merello M, Cammarota A, Betti O, et al. Involuntary movements during thermolesion predict a better outcome after microelectrode guided posteroventral pallidotomy. *J Neurol Neurosurg Psychiatry* 1997;63:210–213.

36. Ohye C. Neural noise recording in functional neurosurgery. In: Gildenberg PL, Tasker RR, eds. *Textbook of stereotactic and functional neurosurgery.* New York: McGraw-Hill, 1997:941–947.

37. Pahwa R, Wilkinson S, Smith D, Lyons K, Miyawaki E, Koller WC. High-frequency stimulation of the globus pallidus for the treatment of Parkinson's disease. *Neurology* 1997;49:249–253.

38. Patil AA, Gelber P. Accuracy of thalamotomy target determination using axial images only. *Stereotact Funct Neurosurg* 1991;56:104–108.

39. Schaltenbrand G, Bailey P. *Introduction to stereotaxis with an atlas of the human brain.* Stuttgart: Thieme Medical Publishers, 1959.

40. Schaltenbrand G, Wahren P. *Atlas for stereotaxy of the human brain.* Stuttgart: Thieme Medical Publishers, 1977.

41. Siegfried J, Lippitz B. Bilateral chronic electrostimulation of ventroposterolateral pallidum: a new therapeutic approach for alleviating all parkinsonian symptoms. *Neurosurgery* 1994;35:1126–1130.

42. Spiegelmann R, Friedman WA. Rapid determination of thalamic CT-stereotactic coordinated: a method. *Acta Neurochir (Wien)* 1991;110:77–81.

43. Sterio D, Beric A, Dogali M, Fazzini E, Alfaro G, Devinsky O. Neurophysiological properties of pallidal neurons in Parkinson's disease. *Ann Neurol* 1994;35:586–591.

44. Sutton JP, Couldwell W, Lew MF, et al. Ventroposterior medial pallidotomy in patients with advanced Parkinson's disease. *Neurosurgery* 1995;36:1112–1117.

45. Taha JM, Favre J, Baumann TK. Functional anatomy of the pallidal base in Parkinson's disease. *Neurosurgery* 1996;39:1164–1168.

46. Taha JM, Favre J, Baumann TK, Burchiel KJ. Tremor control after pallidotomy in patients with Parkinson's disease: correlation with microrecording findings. *J Neurosurg* 1997;86:642–647.

47. *Todd-Wells manual of stereotaxic procedures.* Codman and Shurtleff: Randolph; 1967.

48. Tronnier VM, Fogel W, Kronenbuerger M, Steinvorth S. Pallidal stimulation: an alternative to pallidotomy? In: Lunsford LD, ed. *Neurosurgical Focus*, vol 3. www.neurosurgery.org. 1997:2.

49. Van Manen J. *Stereotactic methods and their application in disorders of the motor system.* Assen: van Gorcum, 1967.

50. Vitek JL, Bakay RAE, DeLong MR. Microelectrode-guided pallidotomy for medically intractable Parkinson's disease. *Adv Neurol* 1997;74:183–198.

51. Walton L, Hampshire A, Forster DMC, Kemeny AA. A phantom study to assess the accuracy of stereotactic localization, using T1-weighted magnetic resonance imaging with the Leksell stereotactic system. *Neurosurgery* 1996;38:170–178.

Pallidal Surgery for the Treatment of Parkinson's Disease and Movement Disorders, edited by J. K. Krauss, R. G. Grossman, and J. Jankovic. Lippincott-Raven Publishers, Philadelphia © 1998.

9

Microelectrode Techniques and Findings of Globus Pallidus

William D. Hutchison

Department of Surgery, Division of Neurosurgery and Playfair Neuroscience Unit, The Toronto Hospital (Western Division), Toronto, Ontario, Canada M5T 2S8

The interest in microelectrode techniques during stereotactic procedures is at an unprecedented high due to the resurgence in the number of centers performing pallidotomy in patients with refractory Parkinson's disease and other movement disorders. The usefulness of microelectrode recordings for stereotactic localization of thalamic targets has been recognized for some 35 years, since its introduction by Albe-Fessard and Guiot (1,20), despite major technological advances in other areas of stereotactic neurosurgery such as imaging. On the other hand, the basic technique of extracellular recording has remained relatively unaltered, and general descriptions of the technique are available (19), as are more specific descriptions applied to the human thalamus (14,34,49).

The increasing interest in structures of the basal ganglia as targets for neurosurgical intervention warrants further treatment of the subject. The major purpose here is to give an overview of the equipment and techniques required for extracellular recording in human basal ganglia and describe the neurophysiological features that distinguish these structures and findings that relate to the pathophysiology of Parkinson's disease and other movement disorders.

TECHNIQUES OF MICROELECTRODE RECORDINGS

Microelectrode Construction Methods

There are now several commercial sources for microelectrodes with extensions that make them suitable for use with a stereotactic guide tube. These devices are considerably more expensive (the cost of a box of 10 electrode tips is similar to the price of one prefabricated long electrode), but this may be still the best choice for those (perhaps most) who have neither the time, equipment, nor inclination to make electrodes. There is, however, a considerable measure of confidence obtained when one has personally inspected and tested all electrodes to be used. The electrodes employed in our cases are commercially available paralyene-C insulated tungsten or platinum-iridium. Tungsten electrodes have good tensile strength and remain rigid as thin wire, whereas platinum has the advantage of being a catalyst for the electrolysis of water, so it can dissipate excess negative charge by forming hydrogen and hydroxyl ions instead of eroding metal from the tip. The platinum–platinum chloride (Pt-PtCl) junction is nonpolarizable and "irreversible," making it more durable for microstimulation. Current technique is to plate tungsten electrodes with platinum to obtain these desirable properties. Despite these precautions, with repeated microstimulation (especially with monophasic pulses where there is a net charge transfer) through the tip, there is usually some decrease in the impedance of the electrode tip likely due to loss of insulation at the tip.

The electrodes are available with tip sizes ranging from 15 to 40 μm and initial impedances of 0.5–1.8 MΩ; they are fitted into extension tubes of stainless steel. The manufacturer deposits the insulation on the etched metal from a vapor phase using a sputter technique (38), and uniform tip exposure is produced with a high (2000 V) arc pulse. The tips are fragile and should not be touched or come into contact with any hard material during construction.

Holding the electrode in the middle of the shank with blunt-nosed pliers, the end connector pin is cut off with scissors or fine wire cutters, and the paralyene-C insulation is stripped off by scraping with a scalpel blade or the wire cutters and then sanding any remaining insulation away with fine emery paper. The stripped end, which should take on a shiny appearance, is inserted into the stainless steel tubing (25 gauge and about 30 cm, or 12 inches, long); the wire is carefully crimped (one or two bends) as it is inserted to make good electrical contact with the inner tube. This step requires some manual dexterity, as the tungsten shank is quite brittle and can splinter or break off readily. The last 5 mm or so should be inserted without crimping so the exposed tungsten electrode (about 1–2 cm of the original 7 cm) is rectilinear with the stainless steel extension tube. Kapton tubing insulation is cut to a length just short of the 25-gauge steel tubing and is slid over the distal end of the steel extension tube.

Under 4× magnification, epoxy resin glue is mixed and applied in small amounts to the last 5 mm of the steel shank and over the adjacent insulated portion of the tungsten. The Kapton tubing is then slid down past the portion of the electrode where it joins the extender at a distance of about 2–3 mm, and more epoxy glue is applied to fill the 2- to 3-mm space between the insulated electrode and the Kapton tube. The glue should still be fluid enough to run into the space, which can be assisted by applying negative pressure to draw it into the space by starting with a 1-mm overlap and pulling back on the distal end of the extender tube the remaining 1–2 mm. Excess glue not flowing into the space and remaining on the outside of the Kapton insulation should be removed before it hardens, otherwise it may not fit inside the protective carrier tube.

Electrode Testing and Plating

The electrodes are tested at this point to make sure the junction of the two insulators is patent by taking an impedance measurement at the tip (it should be near or the same as the manufacturer's measurement) and then immersing the junction into the saline. The reading should remain stable in both positions. Direct current (3–5 V) can be applied while the electrode is immersed in saline to observe sites of electrolytic bubble formation [the Hubel-bubble technique (24)], which should be only at the tip if the paralyene insulation has not been scratched during the above procedure and the epoxy glue junction is patent. This method can also be used to clean the electrode tip after use or for prolonged storage to remove oxides from the tip before plating. An IMP-1 impedance tester (Bak Electronics, Germantown, MD) can be used for both measurements and electrolytic testing, as it has a switch and external connector for the DC input.

The preparation of the gold and platinum black plating solutions has been described by Millar (41) and is not repeated here. A low current (10–100 nA) is used for electroplating the electrodes. Old electrophoresis units can be used as the current source for this purpose, but Ohm's law says that you can also obtain 100 nA from a 10-MΩ resistor connected to a 10-V battery. A WPI constant-current stimulator (A360) has also been used at the lowest setting of 0.1 µA; an ammeter in the circuit is a good idea to monitor the current source. The negative lead is attached to the steel extension tube (to attract the positively charged metal cations), and the positive lead is attached to the plating solution. The tip of the electrode is immersed in the gold solution for about 10 seconds at about 50–100 nA (or any combination totaling about 0.5–1.0 microcoulomb) and then in the platinum black solution for an equal amount of time, being careful not to touch the tip to any hard surface. The tip takes on a yellowish or more fuzzy appearance when observed under the high-power objective of the microscope, but the main criterion is a lower impedance measurement after the plating, which is 0.2–0.5 MΩ in our hands. One can be overly zealous with plating because the resistance continues to drop with more electroplating due to build-up of metal at the tip, so it is advisable to examine the tips under a microscope to monitor the procedure at least initially.

The completed electrodes are then inserted backward into 19-gauge protective carrier tubes (about 20 cm long) and held in place with autoclave tape bearing a label indicating an identification number, final impedance, and tip size. The protective carrier tubes serve only to protect the tips during storage and are not part of the final setup, so the length is not important. The electrodes in their protective guide tubes, the inner guide tube, and the leads for attachment to the preamplifier are placed in green cloth in a perforated metal surgical instrument container and sterilized with ethylene oxide gas before use. Electrodes have also been used following a 10-minute cycle in the autoclave. The box is labeled on the outside with names, phone numbers, a description of the contents, and specific instructions to avoid the contents being scrubbed down before gas sterilization. In practice, and depending on the case load, it is recommended that a spare electrode box containing duplicate equipment be available. Current practice is to rotate through three boxes with about six to eight good electrodes in each.

Basic Electronic Equipment

Amplifiers

The basic setup for the amplification, filtering, display, and storage of neuronal signals is depicted in Fig. 9-1. Differential amplifiers (Op amps[1]), which are most often used for biological recordings, amplify the difference between the two inputs. The advantage of amplifying the difference is that any large-amplitude, low-frequency sinusoids (noise) picked up are common to the two leads and are subtracted—a procedure referred to as common mode rejection. The Neuroamp-1 (Axon Instruments, Foster City, CA) has a useful blanking circuit that allows the differential amplifier to be used with the high-voltage stimu-

lation pulses typically required for microstimulation with high-impedance electrodes (up to about 100 V). The blanking circuit feeds a logic pulse to the amplifier equal in duration to the pulse train from the stimulator (Fig. 9-1). During this time the amplifier is in "hold" mode and protects the other amplifiers downstream from being saturated by the stimulus artifact.

Noise, Shielding, and Grounding

Background noise on recordings is mostly a function of the tip size mixed with any AC mains line noise (hum) that has not been eliminated. The other sources of noise, such as the thermal noise of the electrode tip itself and the intrinsic noise in the particular Op amp being used in the headstage preamplifier, can be considered small in comparison. A larger tip size "sees" more action potentials farther away, so the noise difference associated with gray versus white matter on the recordings may be indiscernible with a 15-μm tip but should be clearer with a 40 μm tip. The lead to the microelectrode is a particularly sensitive region for mains pickup, as the combined high impedance of the Op Amp input and the electrode (e.g., 1 MΩ) means that currents induced by stray capacitance as low as 1 nA can give rise to sizable voltages (1 mV).

Two strategies are normally used: The lead to the microelectrode is kept as short as possible, or shielding is provided for the lead and any exposed portion of the microelectrode extension rod (if necessary). In the driven shield arrangement shown in Fig. 9-1, the output from the Op-amp is sent to the shielding, which reduces the capacitive burden of the source signal (neuronal spike) (42). The second and third harmonics of the 60-Hz mains pickup (240 and 480 Hz) can extend well into the spike bandwidth passed by the recording amplifier (200 Hz to 100 kHz). In practice it usually involves turning off noncritical external AC mains, which can be a blood pressure monitor, digital interface, overhead projector, electric-powered patient bed, or anything requiring a low DC voltage conversion from AC mains, as it is often the AC to DC power supply rectifiers that give rise to the noise (41). If the of-

---

[1] These operational amplifiers take their name from the fact that they were originally employed for performing mathematical operations.

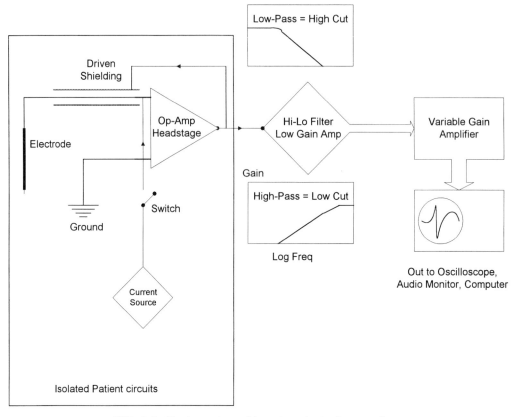

FIG. 9-1. Equipment used for microelectrode recording.

fending instrument has been identified it should be properly shielded, grounded, or moved further away from the microelectrode. Grounding should be to one common point, preferably to the grounded side of the preamplifier using a "star" formation to avoid ground loop problems.

Filters

Filters are normally employed in the circuit to remove unwanted frequencies from the raw biological signal and pass the frequency of interest. A low-pass filter removes high-frequency signals, and a high-pass filter removes low-frequency signals (Fig. 9-1). With extracellular recording, one wishes to see the neuronal spikes on a common stable baseline for spike discrimination. The usual settings cut out everything below 200–300 Hz and everything above about 10 kHz. The high-

pass filter removes the slow-wave component at a lower setting, but removal of any remaining low-frequency hum requires a somewhat higher setting. If this line noise pickup cannot be solved by any logical (or illogical) method, a notch filter can be used to remove specifically the offending 60-Hz (or 50-Hz, depending on the country) frequency from the signal. For recording potentials from the optic tract, the low-frequency component is desirable; hence the high-pass filter must be opened (0.2 Hz) to allow the signal through and the low-pass signal filtered to smooth the trace if desired. A discussion of filter types and design is beyond the scope of this chapter, but a few points are worth noting. The commonly used Butterworth-type filters are good but produce slightly more spike distortion than Bessel-type filters. All filters produce some small time delays, so channels being compared for phase relations should be filtered similarly. To avoid aliasing, the signal should be filtered with a cutoff less than one-fifth to one-tenth the rate at which it is digitized.

Spike Discriminators

Spike discriminators are used to detect the firing of an individual neuron (spike shape) from a group of simultaneously recorded neurons and convert its occurrence in time to a logic pulse output. Small-tipped (15 µm) electrodes frequently record more than one spike, and large-tipped (40 µm) electrodes are almost always comprised of multiunit recordings. The output signal can be split, with one signal sent to a counter/computer and the other used to trigger another oscilloscope after a 0.5- to 5.0-ms delay to superimpose the spikes, or "spike-trigger." A simple level indication is an adequate but not optimal method of counting single spikes in a multiunit recording (Fig. 9-2).

The dual window discriminator with delay (Bak Electronics, Germantown, MD) is the best overall tool for monitoring the multiplexor output; it shows the gates as well as the sweeped-out spike waveform. It can be combined with a digital oscilloscope in a storage mode to hold a sample ("reference") spike shape and compare it to subsequent ones. In this way, one can easily see the relative width of spikes (e.g., the difference between axonal and somatodendritic recordings) and the longer after-potential of the border cells, which gives them their characteristic sound on the audio monitor.

Audio Monitor

An audio monitor designed specifically for the purpose of listening to neuronal recordings is a

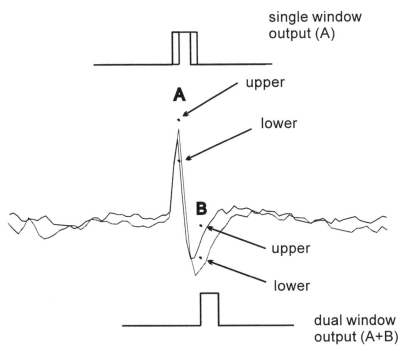

FIG. 9-2. Spike discrimination. Two differently shaped spikes are shown with the corresponding logic pulse output of a single window and a dual (time-amplitude) window discriminator. The single window registers a pulse for both spikes within the two variable voltage levels (window A), whereas the advantage of the dual window (A + B) can be seen separating out, or discriminating, a single spike of similar amplitude but slightly longer duration.

good investment. Aural fatigue can be considerable when listening to noisy signals for prolonged periods, and some monitors are much better at enhancing the sound of small spikes in the recordings and filtering out background noise with noise clipping circuits (Grass Instruments, Quincy, MA). It is useful to have a switch on the front panel to be able to hear both the raw signal and the TTL logic pulse output from the unit being discriminated. This practice can be very instructive during the examination of responses to movements, as changes in the size of the spike due to movement of the tip of the electrode with respect to the neuron being recorded are fairly common in stereotactic recording situations. Changes in spike amplitude also modulate the amplitude of the audio signals, which can be misinterpreted as a neuronal response. By listening only to the square pulse "clicks" produced by the spike discriminator, a change in pulse frequency with limb movement is more readily detected.

Operating Room Setup Procedure

The microelectrode, microdrive, adaptor, and microelectrode guide tube are assembled under sterile conditions. The hydraulic microdrive is sterilized in 2% glutaraldehyde (Cidex) for at least 30 minutes and rinsed with sterile water. The microelectrode arc car adaptor along with a holder and all parts needed for its assembly are autoclaved for 10 minutes and allowed to cool. The hydraulic microdrive is then fastened to the adaptor with a hex-bolt. The microelectrode guide tube is fitted into the arc car adaptor up to the stop-lug and fastened in place with a protruding set-screw. The extruded length of the microelectrode guide tube is the same length as the stereotactic guide tube and fits inside it so the tips are flush. When the microelectrode tip is set to the zero position with respect to the tip of this tube on the sterile table, it is also flush with the known position of the stereotactic guide tube when placed in the brain. The shielded recording/stimulating lead from one side (positive with the Neuroamp-1A; Axon Instruments, Foster City, CA) of the differential amplifier headstage is attached to the electrode; the

other side (negative) is attached to a ground (the protruding set-screw of our microelectrode guide tube), and the indifferent or patient common ground lead is clipped to the guide tube adaptor or stereotactic frame (whichever gives less noise). It is considered good practice not to attach the "patient ground" lead to anything other than the guide tube or the stereotactic frame.

RECORDING IN PALLIDUM AND SURROUNDING STRUCTURES

Striatum/Putamen

In the usual position starting 15 mm from the target, recording starts within the globus pallidus externus (GPe), so striatal units are not normally encountered. Recordings have been made from striatum on occasion, and neurons were found that had properties similar to those studied in nonhuman primates (10,31,45,46). Striatal neurons have low firing rates (1–5 Hz) of fairly large amplitude spikes that may be phasically activated by movements if the recording is from the somatosensory portion of the putamen. Less commonly encountered in nonhuman primates are tonically active units (TANs), which fire in a regular pattern at 5 to 10 Hz and may respond to specific behaviorally relevant sensory stimuli (4,32,33).

Globus Pallidus Externus

Neurons in the GPe show a much higher level of activity than striatal neurons and have been characterized by two "signature" types; the low-frequency discharge-bursting neurons (LFD-B) and the slow-frequency discharge-pausing neurons (SFD-P) (17) (Fig. 9-3). These types are found in human GPe, but there is some variability in firing rates in the GPe from patient to patient. Cells in the GPe respond during voluntary movements with either excitation or inhibition, and sometimes a combination is observed, termed here a biphasic response. During intraoperative examinations about 35% of all cells encountered show responses related to active and passive movements of one or more joints. Some of these cells were additionally tested during a visu-

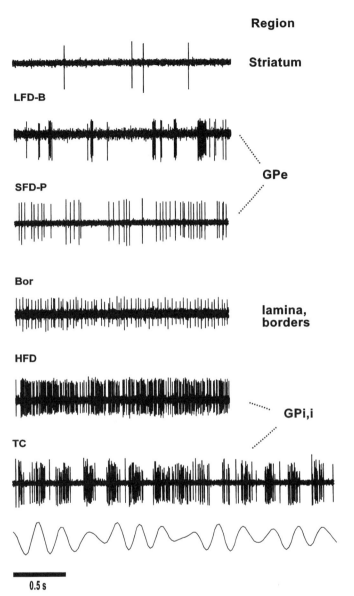

FIG. 9-3. Spontaneous ongoing discharge of typical neurons found in trajectories through various regions of basal ganglia in PD patients. Top trace shows the low firing rate of a striatal neuron. Next two traces are typical patterns of globus pallidus externus (GPe) units. The regular firing pattern of a border cell is shown in the middle trace. The bottom two traces are examples of globus pallidus internus, internal segment (GPi,i) neurons, a high-frequency discharge neuron (*HFD*), and a tremor cell (*TC*). *LFD-B*, low-frequency discharge with bursts; *SFD-P*, slow-frequency discharge with pauses; *Bor*, border cell. Below the tremor cell recording is an accelerometer trace taken from the back of the contralateral hand.

ally cued single reaching task. The patient was requested to reach and depress a button after a "ready" and a "go" signal, repeated five times; the response of the cell was averaged (29). Of 19 GPe cells examined, 14 (74%) showed significant responses during the trials. Of those responding, 64% were excited, 14% were inhibited, and 21% were biphasic.

Internal Lamina and Border Cells

Between the GPe and globus pallidus internus (GPi) is the internal medullary lamina, which can usually be discerned by an absence of recorded cells and relative quiet background noise (see previous section). At the margins of this lamina at the base of the GPe and the top of the GPi may be found so-called border cells, which have a distinctive regular firing pattern compared to the pallidal cells and have longer afterpotentials. The best current estimate from our data of the firing rate of 44 border cells is a mean ($\pm$ SD) of 30.0 ± 14.5 Hz. Border cells are thought to be displaced cells of the substantia innominata of Reichert (12) (nucleus basalis) and probably contain acetylcholine as their transmitter (they stain positively for choline acetyltransferase) (7). We have observed cells of this type sometimes to switch between a regular discharge mode and a burst discharge mode. In our experience, border cells sometimes show small modulations during reaching movements, and the changes in firing pattern appear to occur spontaneously, although a few of the cells have been observed to change from regular firing to burst-mode firing during reaching (unpublished observations).

Globus Pallidus Internus

The GPi consists of an external and internal segment (GPi,e and GPi,i) separated by the internal lamina incompleta or accessory medullary lamina. When the tip of the electrode is advanced into the GPi,e there is usually an increase in the background noise in the recording, signaling that the tip is in a cell-dense region, and neurons are recorded with higher rates of discharge than are usually seen in the GPe. Typ-

ically, these are described as high frequency discharge (HFD) neurons, and no pauses in their activity are discernible (Fig. 9-3). Our current best estimate of the mean background firing rate of GPi,e neurons (± 1 SD) is 67 ± 14 Hz (range 53–81 Hz) (25,28). Most of the time the transition between GPi,e and GPi,i is unremarkable with a few exceptions. In more anteriorly placed trajectories there can be border cells and another small (~1 mm) quiet zone that marks the presence of the internal lamina incompleta. Some patients have higher rates of firing in the more ventral portion of the GPi (GPi,i) when compared to the GPi,e (28) (Fig. 9-4, bottom panel). In some patients with tremor, there appears to be an increased incidence of tremor cells in the more ventral portion of the GPi (27) (Figs. 9-3, 9-5). Whether this is coextensive with the portion of GPi that receives direct input from striatal neurons with motor cortex afferent input or input from the subthalamic nucleus (or both) is not yet known. There is, however, a tendency for neurons with the highest spontaneously ongoing discharges to be found in the GPi,i (28). The average firing rate of GPi,i neurons has been estimated in our series to be 83 ± 25 Hz ($n = 164$), whereas that in the GPi,e is 66 ± 20 Hz ($n = 198$).

Individual neurons can respond to movements (Fig. 9-6). Responses to active and passive movements in the GPi can be excitatory, inhibitory, or both (i.e., biphasic). Responses may be obtained from movements of more than one joint on the contralateral side as well as joints on the ipsilateral side, although the latter is less common. During intraoperative examination, about 34% of GPi cells respond to movements of one or more joints. Responses of GPi neurons on visually cued single reaching tasks have been recorded and averaged over five repeated trials (29). In a sample of 26 cells, 19 (73%) were modulated by the task. Inhibitory responses (10/19, or 53%) and excitatory responses during movements (8/19, or 42%) were encountered, suggesting that both excitation and inhibition of the output neurons of the basal ganglia are involved in movement control, which may function in an inhibitory center and excitatory surround arrangement (18,40).

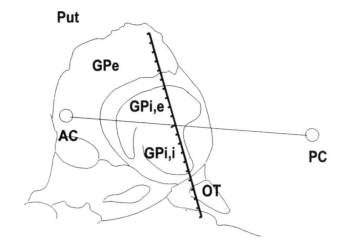

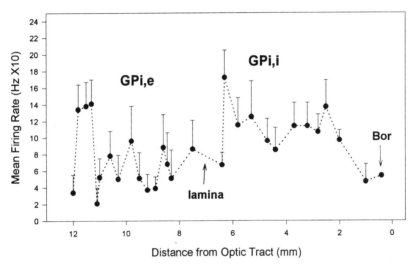

FIG. 9-4. Firing rates of neurons on a typical trajectory path of the microelectrode through the pallidum. **Top.** Sagittal section from the Schaltenbrand and Wahren atlas 20 mm lateral to the midline showing the trajectory (each small division is 1 mm). **Bottom.** Mean firing rate (+ SD) profile of individual neurons encountered in the electrode track shown above, normalized to the distance from the dorsal border of the optic tract. Note that firing rates in most of the globus pallidus internus, external segments (GPi,e) are lower than those in GPi internal segments (GPi,i), and a border cell is shown at the bottom with a low standard deviation of firing owing to the regular firing pattern. The lamina incompleta is distinguishable on this trajectory which is mainly within the GPi. *AC,* anterior commissure; *PC,* posterior commissure; *OT,* optic tract; *Put,* putamen.

Optic Tract

Microstimulation is used to determine the position of the optic tract and the internal capsule (see below). To a large extent the position of the final lesion site is determined in relation to these two eloquent structures to avoid paresis or homonymous hemianopsia. Microstimulation has advantages over macrostimulation techniques in that one can precisely delineate these structures because the current density is highly localized at the tip. Possible mechanical damage to these struc-

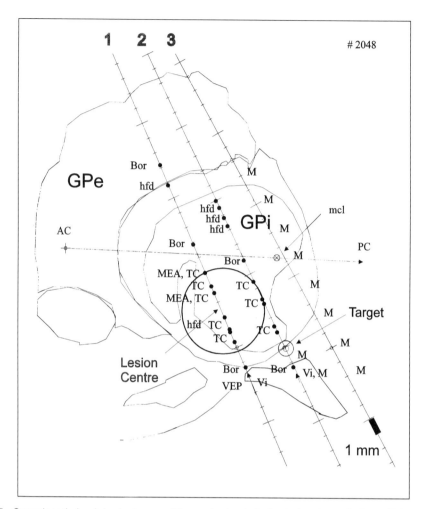

FIG. 9-5. Completed physiological map of three electrode trajectories through the pallidum with physiological data recorded on the sagittal map (20 mm lateral) of the region. Note the location of the optic tract and capsule determined by microstimulation. *Vi,* visual response to microstimulation; *VEP,* visual evoked potential (strobe); *M,* motor response to microstimulation; *mcl,* midcommissural point; *MEA,* movement-evoked activity.

tures is less likely using a fine-diameter (250 μm) microelectrode instead of a large-diameter macroelectrode (2–3 mm). With microelectrodes, the top of the optic tract is routinely mapped with a precision of less than 1 mm in the anterosuperior to posteroinferior trajectories used (Fig. 9-5). The stimulus parameters are a 1-second train at 300 Hz using a 0.2-ms pulse width varying in intensity from 1 to 100 μA. Patients most often report stars or sparkles of light, often in a wedge-shaped portion of the contralateral visual field. The reported

colors are white, yellow, or occasionally red and blue; and increasing the stimulus intensity gives rise to a larger portion of the visual field occupied by the phosphenes and more intense light. Less commonly, scotomas (dark clouds) are reported. The difficulty recognizing scotomas might be the reason a few patients fail to report phosphenes with microstimulation of the optic tract at sites where good recordings of visual-evoked potentials were obtained. This is one hypothesis why this would occur in an otherwise attentive and co-

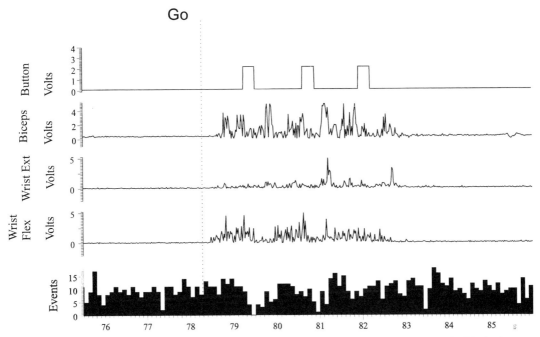

FIG. 9-6. Movement-related activity in the pallidum during a sequential reaching task. Excitation or inhibition can be found in both segments of the pallidum, although inhibition seems to be more common in the inner segment (shown here). Top trace is when the button was depressed, and *Go* refers to the LED visual cue. Rectified surface of the electromyogram (EMG) of the forearm muscles is shown in the middle traces. Firing of the GPi unit is shown in the histogram with a bin width of 100 ms.

operative patient. From a methodological point of view, the fact that it occurs emphasizes the need for microrecording and microstimulation capabilities during stereotactic pallidotomy.

Internal Capsule

As a general rule, trajectories that pass through the internal capsule have recordings that are "quiet" (cell-sparse) compared to the neuronal activity of the pallidum (cell-dense). The occasional recording of axons in the internal capsule is possible with a fine-tipped electrode (15 μm), and the waveforms of large axons can be similar to those of somatodendritic potentials. More often, however, they are monophasic and much shorter in duration (<1 ms) than the latter and are recorded over a short distance in the track (100 μm) compared to the range over which a neuronal soma can be recorded (200–300 μm). During active or passive movements these units can have a large phasic ac-

tivation from a slow background discharge (Fig. 9-7), indicative of their premotoneuronal function. The location of the internal capsule is determined with microstimulation during every stereotactic pallidotomy. Tetanic contraction of the musculature is seen with suprathreshold stimulation; and with increasing current intensity there is an increase in force of contraction and muscles involved: The patient reports a pulling or tugging sensation. With stimulation at or near threshold, the patients may report a paresthesia sensation, and it is not known if it is an orthodromic or antidromic effect of capsule fiber stimulation.

The topographical depiction by Hassler et al. of the homonculus in the posterior limb of the internal capsule (23) is generally true: Head and face responses tend to be located at or close to the genu; arm responses are near the middle third of the posterior limb; and leg responses tend to be located in the posterior one-third of the posterior limb. The topographical organization of pyrami-

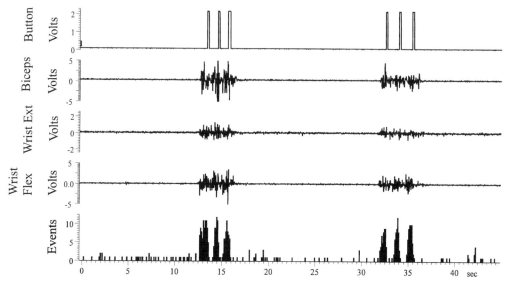

FIG. 9-7. Pyramidal tract axons in the posterior limb of the internal capsule can be recorded and show clear movement-related activation from low ongoing rates of discharge. Task is the same as in Fig. 9-6, with a bin width of 100 ms.

dal tract fibers is not as discrete and finely ordered as Hassler's homunculus depicts. There is a paucity of accurate anatomical data on the organization of pyramidal tract fibers at the level of the capsule, as most clinical studies and stereotactic lesion studies cannot provide histological data (48). One study of fiber degeneration with silver staining techniques in monkeys (11) shows that the foot region of the corticospinal tract is a large, elongated band centered in the middle of the capsule extending to most of the posterior third of the posterior limb, and the thumb region is distinct and located medial and closer to the genu (11). Some of the results with microstimulation of the capsule reflect this organization. With initial target trajectories in a medial sagittal plane near the genu, few pallidal recordings are found, but face motor responses moved to hand responses more posteriorly and inferiorly. In more lateral locations in pallidum, face responses may still be present as well as hand and foot responses more inferoposteriorly; more laterally still, only lower limb responses are found. These findings indicate that the pyramidal tract fasciculi to craniofacial and somatic regions form layers in the anteroposterior plane and in the long axis of the posterior limb. This organi-

zation may be of further use in the initial trajectories of a physiological mapping session to determine their relative mediolateral position early. The organization also indicates that it is necessary to continue with microstimulation mapping several millimeters into the capsule to determine the predominant fiber population in the core of the posterior limb.

Selection of Lesion Site and Lesioning

If a series of three trajectories in the same sagittal plane spaced 3 mm apart all have optic tract responses at the bottom and motor responses are predominantly in the lower limb, the target sagittal plane is too lateral (i.e., 22 or 24 mm). Characteristic findings when the placement is too medial (i.e., 16–18 mm lateral to the midline) are no recordings where GPe cells should be and GPi units that start at about 6 mm above the target, with no optic tract and only head and face motor capsule responses. The current protocol of Lozano and Tasker is to make a single thermocoagulation lesion in the posteroventral region of the GPi 3 mm away from the closest recorded response from the optic tract and internal capsule. This point is typically in cellular areas with high-frequency discharge neurons with large-amplitude spikes having some movement-related activity and tremor cells (if the patient has tremor). Visual and motor function are monitored as the probe tip is incremented from 60°C for 60 seconds to a maximum of 90°C for 90 seconds using a high-frequency (100 kHz) sine wave current generator (OWL Universal RF System, Diros Technology, Toronto, Canada). The lesioning probe has a diameter of 1 mm, and the last 3 mm is uninsulated, which results in a lesion with dimensions of approximately $4 \times 4 \times 6$ mm when visualized on postoperative magnetic resonance imaging (MRI) scans. Further details and discussion of lesion targets and methods have been reported elsewhere (39).

INTRAOPERATIVE OBSERVATIONS DURING MICROELECTRODE RECORDING

As of this writing, 148 patients have undergone microelectrode recording in the basal ganglia (excluding the thalamus) for treatment of idiopathic Parkinson's disease with unilateral pallidotomy, bilateral pallidotomy (dystonia only), unilateral DBS in the GPi (some contralateral to a previous pallidotomy), and bilateral subthalamic DBS. The procedures were done in 139 cases of idiopathic Parkinson's disease (PD), 5 cases of Parkinson-plus syndromes (4 striatonigral degeneration, 1 Shy-Drager), 1 case of idiopathic hemiparkinsonism, 2 patients with primary dystonia, and 1 case of secondary hemidystonia. This diverse patient base has allowed collection of a large amount of neurophysiological data which have been only partially analyzed to yield information on basal ganglia function and dysfunction in movement disorders. The following topics are selected areas of interest that have been examined in some detail, in addition to results already presented that relate directly to techniques of identification and localization of structures.

Elevated Activity of Pallidal Outflow in Parkinsonism

According to models of basal ganglia dysfunction based on work with the neurotoxin 1-methyl-

4-phenyl-1,2,3,6-tetrahydropyridine (MPTP) monkey model of PD, the underlying mechanism of the cardinal symptoms is hyperactivity of the basal ganglia output from the GPi and a hypoactive GPe (2,3,13,22,52; but see ref. 8). Pallidal recordings from 227 neurons in six patients in the "off" state were examined for mean firing rates in segments of the globus pallidus based on reconstruction of trajectories (28). Firing rates were determined from histograms of spontaneous ongoing activity and from the reciprocal of the most common interspike interval to determine the degree of clustering of spikes in the recordings (Fig. 9-8). There were significant differences between the various segments of the globus pallidus. The values in the ventral portion of the GPi in PD patients were higher than those in the GPe or the GPi,e and were similar to firing rates found in monkeys with MPTP-induced parkinsonism (15, 16). On the other hand, the mean firing rates in the GPe in this study were similar to those in control monkeys, supporting other workers' findings suggesting that the GPe is not suppressed in parkinsonism (8). Some patients had low firing rates in the GPe, and others had higher firing rates, which suggests individual differences that may relate to PD symptomatology. Studies using histological indicators of metabolic function indicate patches of elevated activity in the GPe (47), which may also contribute to the increased variation seen in GPe firing rates within subjects.

Apomorphine Effects on Pallidal Cells

To test the models discussed above directly, parkinsonian patients in the off state undergoing microelectrode exploration for pallidotomy were administered apomorphine (APO)[2] while recording neurons in the globus pallidus (25). In 14 patients it was possible to monitor the firing rate of 15 neurons continuously as the effect of APO was observed. Consistent with the above model and studies performed in MPTP monkeys, three of three GPe neurons showed increased firing rates, and 10 of 12 GPi neurons showed decreased activity after APO. In addition, the average firing

---

[2] A nonselective D1, D2 dopamine receptor agonist. The dose was 30–100 μg/kg SC.

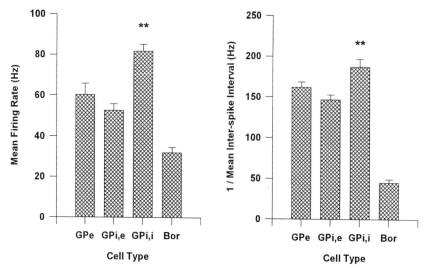

FIG. 9-8. Differential neuronal activity in segments of the globus pallidus revealed by mean firing rates calculated from rate histograms (left) and from the one per interspike intervals (right).

rates of many neurons were determined from single-unit histograms before ($n = 312$) and after ($n = 196$) injection of the drug. The average firing rates before and after APO are shown in Fig. 9-9. Before the drug was given it is evident that the rate in the more ventral portion of the GPi (GPi,i) was higher than that in either the GPi,e or the GPe, a result previously reported in another patient sample (28). At 25 to 35 minutes after APO the mean firing rate of the GPe neurons showed some increase, but more pronounced was the decrease observed in both segments

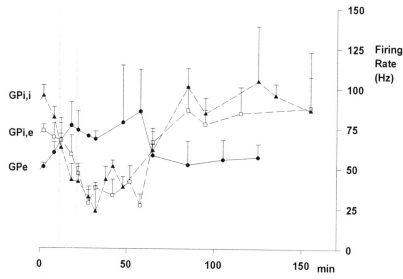

FIG. 9-9. Average firing rates of neurons recorded in the GPe and both segments of the GPi before and after apomorphine administration. Vertical lines indicate the time range when some patients reported they were feeling the effects of the drug (i.e., "on" state).

of the GPi. Although fewer units were recorded 80 minutes after APO, the mean firing rates appeared to recover to values similar to those determined before APO. These results lend strong support to the basic tenets of the models of basal ganglia dysfunction.

Tremor Cells (4–6 Hz)

Cells with oscillations in firing rates at the same frequency as limb tremor (Fig. 9-3, bottom trace) have been observed and studied for some time in the thalamus of monkeys and humans (9,21,35, 36). Early workers made only passing reference to tremor cells in the human pallidum (30,50), but more recent studies have characterized their properties in MPTP primates (5,6,43) and in humans (27). Autocorrelogram analysis of tremor cells in the GPi (Fig. 9-10) has been carried out and showed that there is a variable amplitude of oscillation of pallidal tremor cells that can be graded and compared to the patient tremor scores. Preliminary work on Fourier analysis of tremor cells (26) shows that tremor cell frequency can vary within a patient if tremors in the arm and foot are

of different frequencies. In this case a tremor cell can be identified as partaking in the loop for the "arm" or a "foot" by identifying the matching frequency (Fig. 9-11). All of the tremor cells in this sample of 228 neurons were found to lie in the range of 3.7 to 5.6 Hz. This finding does not support a commonly held theory of tremorgenesis that oscillations at 12 to 14 Hz in the globus pallidus generate tremor in the thalamus via hysteresis in thalamic cell membranes—the thalamic "filter" theory (37, 44; see also ref. 51). In most patients with PD, tremor cells are predominantly located in the ventral portion of the GPi and appear to be rare or absent in the GPe. One reason for the rarity of tremor cells in the GPe may be due to sampling bias if the microelectrode trajectories typically do not pass through the portion of the GPe that corresponds with the sensorimotor GPi. However, movement-related activity is frequently found in this portion of the GPe, so it seems unlikely that they were missed. Tremor cells are found in the subthalamic nucleus of MPTP monkeys, so it may be that the 4- to 6-Hz oscillations are intrinsic or resonant with the direct striatopallidal pathway or the direct cortico-

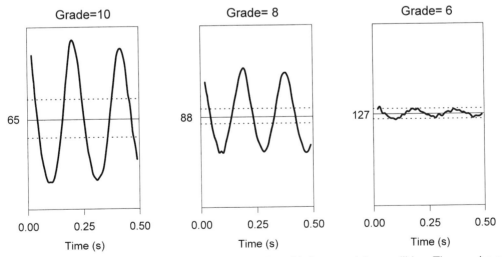

FIG. 9-10. Autocorrelogram grading of tremor cells found in human globus pallidus. The graphs are constructed from a total of 10 seconds of discriminated tremor cell spike trains. The numbers on the y-axis gives the average firing frequency calculated for that neuron. The confidence intervals of 99.5% and 0.5% are shown as dotted lines. Regions of the smoothed autocorrelogram falling above and below represent significant oscillation in the spike train.

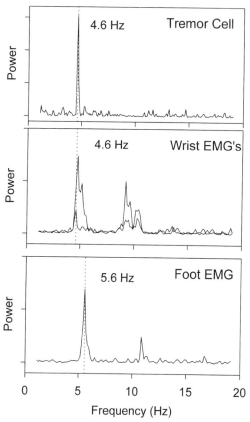

FIG. 9-11. Discrete fast Fourier transform analysis of a tremor cell and EMG records from a patient with a parkinsonian rest tremor in the hand and foot at discordant frequencies. The frequency of the tremor cell matches the forearm EMG traces (superimposed) but not the foot tremor measured in dorsiflexors. Harmonics in EMG traces are related to properties of the EMG signal.

subthalamic portions of the corticobasal ganglia loops, and not in the indirect pathway. Further observation of tremor cells and their distribution in basal ganglia structures is needed before any conclusions can be drawn regarding the neural substrate for rest tremor.

CONCLUSIONS

Techniques and principles of microelectrode recording and microstimulation in the basal ganglia have been outlined and demonstrate the ac-

curacy afforded by these methods in the determination of stereotactic targets. Identification of single units and their characteristics can provide confirmation of the location of structures during procedures and aid in the selection of appropriate trajectories. In addition, single-unit analysis of populations of neurons and their aggregate properties can shed light on the pathophysiology of the basal ganglia in parkinsonism and other movement disorders.

Acknowledgments. I thank Drs. J. Dostrovsky, A. Lozano, and R. Tasker for training in stereotactic recording techniques and collaboration on ongoing projects, and A. Blatz and R. Lobdill of Axon Instruments for helpful discussions on electronics.

REFERENCES

1. Albe-Fessard D, Hardy J, Vourch G, Hertzog E, Aleonard P, Derome P. Dérivations d'activités spontanées et évoquées dans les structures cérébrales profondes de l'homme. *Rev Neurol (Paris)* 1962; 106:89–105.
2. Albin RL. The pathophysiology of chorea/ballism and parkinsonism. *Parkinson Relat Disord* 1995;1:3–11.
3. Albin RL, Young AB, Penney JB. The functional anatomy of basal ganglia disorders. *Trends Neurosci* 1989;12:366–375.
4. Aosaki T, Kimura M, Graybiel AM. Temporal and spatial characteristics of tonically active neurons of the primate striatum. *J Neurophysiol* 1995;73:1234–1252.
5. Bergman H, Wichmann T, Karmon B, DeLong MR. Parkinsonian tremor is associated with low frequency neuronal oscillations in selective loops of the basal ganglia. In: Percheron G, McKenzie JS, Féger J, eds. *The basal ganglia. IV. New ideas and data on structure and function.* New York: Plenum Press, 1994.
6. Bergman H, Wichmann T, Karmon B, DeLong MR. The primate subthalamic nucleus. II. Neuronal activity in the MPTP model of parkinsonism. *J Neurophysiol* 1994;72:507–520.
7. Carpenter MB. Corpus striatum and related nuclei. In: Satterfield TS, ed. *Core text of neuroanatomy,* 4th ed. Baltimore: Williams & Wilkins, 1991;325–360.
8. Chesselet MF, Delfs JM. Basal ganglia and movement disorders. *Trends Neurosci* 1996;19:417–422.
9. Cordeau JP. Further studies on patterns of central unit activity in relation with tremor. *J Neurosurg* 1966;25 [suppl II]:213–218.
10. Crutcher MD, DeLong MR. Single cell studies of the primate putamen. I. Functional organization. *Exp Brain Res* 1984;53:233–243.
11. Dawnay NAH, Glees P. Somatotopic analysis of fibre and terminal distribution in the primate corticospinal pathway. *Dev Brain Res* 1986;26:115–123.
12. DeLong MR. Activity of pallidal neurons during movement. *J Neurophysiol* 1971;34:414–427.

13. DeLong MR. Primate models of movement disorders of basal ganglia origin. *Trends Neurosci* 1990;13: 281–285.

14. Dostrovsky JO, Davis KD, Lee L, Sher GD, Tasker RR. Electrical stimulation-induced effects in the human thalamus. In: Devinsky O, Beric A, Dogali M, eds. *Electrical and magnetic stimulation of the brain and spinal cord.* New York: Raven Press, 1993; 219–229.

15. Filion M, Tremblay L. Abnormal spontaneous activity of globus pallidus neurons in monkeys with MPTP-induced parkinsonism. *Brain Res* 1991;547:142–151.

16. Filion M, Tremblay L, Bédard PJ. Abnormal influences of passive limb movement on the activity of globus pallidus neurons in parkinsonian monkeys. *Brain Res* 1995;444:165–176.

17. Filion M, Tremblay L, Bédard PJ. Effects of dopamine agonists on the spontaneous activity of globus pallidus neurons in monkeys with MPTP-induced parkinsonism. *Brain Res* 1991;547:152–161.

18. Filion M, Tremblay L, Matsumura M, Richard H. Focalisation dynamique de la convergence informationelle dans les noyaux gris centraux. *Rev Neurol (Paris)* 1994;150:627–633.

19. Geddes LA. *Electrodes and the measurement of bioelectric events.* New York: Wiley Interscience, 1972.

20. Guiot G, Hardy J, Albe-Fessard D. Délimitation précise des structures sous-corticales et identification de noyaux thalamiques chez l'homme par l'électrophysiologie stéréotaxique. *Neurochirurgia (Stuttg)* 1962; 51:1–18.

21. Gybels JM. Microelectrode studies of unit discharges in the sensorimotor cortex of monkeys with tremor. In: *The neural mechanism of parkinsonian tremor.* Brussels: Editions Arsia, 1963;83–122.

22. Hallett M. Physiology of basal ganglia disorders: an overview. *Can J Neurol Sci* 1993;20:177–183.

23. Hassler R, Mundinger F, Riechert T. *Stereotaxis in Parkinson syndrome.* Berlin: Springer-Verlag, 1979.

24. Hubel DH. Tungsten microelectrodes for recording from single units. *Science* 1957;125:549–550.

25. Hutchison WD, Levy R, Dostrovsky JO, Lozano AM, Lang AE. Effects of apomorphine on globus pallidus neurons in parkinsonian patients. *Ann Neurol* 1997; 42:767–775.

26. Hutchison WD, Lozano AM, Kiss ZHT, et al. Tremor-related activity (TRA) in globus pallidus of Parkinson's disease (PD) patients. *Soc Neurosci Abstr* 1994;20:783.

27. Hutchison WD, Lozano AM, Tasker RR, Lang AE, Dostrovsky JO. Identification and characterisation of neurons with tremor-frequency activity in human globus pallidus. *Exp Brain Res* 1997;113:557–563.

28. Hutchison WD, Lozano CA, Davis KD, Saint-Cyr JA, Lang AE, Dostrovsky JO. Differential neuronal activity in segments of globus pallidus in Parkinson's disease patients. *Neuroreport* 1994;5:1533–1537.

29. Hutchison WD, Seigneuret E, Lozano AM, Kiss ZHT, Lang AE, Dostrovsky JO. Single unit analysis of movement-related activity during a visually-cued reaching task in globus pallidus (GP) of patients with Parkinson's disease. *Mov Disord* 1996;11 [suppl 1]:11.

30. Jasper HH, Bertrand G. Thalamic units involved in somatic sensation and voluntary and involuntary movements in man. In: Purpura DP, Yahr MD, eds. *The*

31. thalamus. New York: Columbia University Press, 1966;365–390.

31. Kimura M. Behaviorally contingent property of movement-related activity of the primate putamen. *J Neurophysiol* 1990;63:1277–1296.

32. Kimura M. Behavioral modulation of sensory responses of primate putamen neurons. *Brain Res* 1992; 578:204–214.

33. Kimura M, Aosaki T, Hu Y, Ishida A, Watanabe K. Activity of primate putamen neurons is selective to the mode of voluntary movement: visually guided, self-initiated or memory guided. *Exp Brain Res* 1992;89:473–477.

34. Lenz FA, Dostrovsky JO, Kwan HC, Tasker RR, Yamashiro K, Murphy JT. Methods for microstimulation and recording of single neurons and evoked potentials in the human central nervous system. *J Neurosurg* 1988; 68:630–634.

35. Lenz FA, Kwan HC, Martin RL, Tasker RR, Dostrovsky JO, Lenz YE. Single unit analysis of the human ventral thalamic nuclear group: tremor-related activity in functionally identified cells. *Brain* 1994;117:531–543.

36. Lenz FA, Tasker RR, Kwan HC, et al. Single unit analysis of the human ventral thalamic nuclear group: correlation of thalamic "tremor cells" with the 3–6 Hz component of parkinsonian tremor. *J Neurosci* 1988; 8:754–764.

37. Llinás R, Paré D. Role of intrinsic neuronal oscillations and network ensembles in the genesis of normal and pathological tremors. In: Findley LJ, Koller WC, eds. *Handbook of tremor disorders.* New York: Marcel Dekker, 1995;7–36.

38. Loeb GE, Bak MJ, Salcman M, Schmidt EM. Parylene as a chronically stable, reproducible microelectrode insulator. *IEEE Trans Biomed Eng* 1977;24:121–128.

39. Lozano AM, Hutchison WD, Kiss ZHT, Davis KD, Dostrovsky JO. Methods for microelectrode-guided posteroventral pallidotomy. *J Neurosurg* 1996;84:194–202.

40. Matsumura M, Tremblay L, Richard H, Filion M. Activity of pallidal neurons in the monkey during dyskinesia induced by injection of bicuculline in the external pallidum. *Neuroscience* 1995;65:59–70.

41. Millar J. Extracellular single and multiple unit recording with microelectrodes. In: Stamford JA, ed. *Monitoring neuronal activity: a practical approach.* New York: IRL Press, 1992:1–27.

42. Morrison R. *Grounding and shielding techniques in instrumentation,* 3rd ed. New York: John Wiley & Sons, 1986.

43. Nini A, Feingold A, Slovin H, Bergman H. Neurons in the globus pallidus do not show correlated activity in the normal monkey, but phase-locked oscillations appear in the MPTP model of parkinsonism. *J Neurophysiol* 1995;74:1800–1805.

44. Paré D, Curro'Dossi R, Steriade M. Neuronal basis of the parkinsonian resting tremor: a hypothesis and its implications for treatment. *Neuroscience* 1990;35:217–226.

45. Romo R, Scarnati E, Schultz W. Role of primate basal ganglia and frontal cortex in the internal generation of movements. II. Movement-related activity in the anterior striatum. *Exp Brain Res* 1991;91:385–395.

46. Schultz W, Romo R. Role of primate basal ganglia and frontal cortex in the internal generation of movements. I. Preparatory activity in the anterior striatum. *Exp Brain Res* 1992;91:363–384.

47. Schwartzman RJ, Alexander GM, Ferraro TN, Grothusen JR, Stahl SM. Cerebral metabolism of parkinsonian primate 21 days after MPTP. *Exp Neurol* 1988;102:307–313.

48. Tredici G, Pizzini G, Bogliun G, Tagliabue M. The site of motor corticospinal fibres in the internal capsule of man: a computerized tomographic study of restricted lesions. *J Anat* 1982;134:199–208.

49. Turner RS, Andersen ME. Palldial discharge related to the kinematics of reaching movements in two dimensions. *J Neurophysiol* 1997;77:1051–1074.

50. Umbach W, Ehrhardt KJ. Ableitungen mit Mikroelektroden in den Stammganglien des Menschen. *Eur Arch Psychiatry Neurol Sci* 1965;207:106–113.

51. Volkmann J, Joliot M, Mogilner A, et al. Central motor loop oscillations in parkinsonian resting tremor revealed by magnetoencephalography. *Neurology* 1996; 46:1359–1370.

52. Wichmann T, DeLong MR. Functional and pathophysiological models of the basal ganglia. *Curr Opin Neurobiol* 1996;6:751–758.

Pallidal Surgery for the Treatment of Parkinson's Disease and Movement Disorders, edited by J. K. Krauss, R. G. Grossman, and J. Jankovic. Lippincott-Raven Publishers, Philadelphia © 1998.

10

Results of Unilateral Pallidotomy for Parkinson's Disease: Two-Year Experience and Review of the Literature

Anthony E. Lang, *Erwin B. Montgomery, Jr., Janice L. Duff, †Ronald Tasker, †William D. Hutchison, and †Andres M. Lozano

*Division of Neurology, The Toronto Hospital, Toronto, Ontario, Canada M5T 258; *Department of Neurology, Cleveland Clinic Foundation, Cleveland, Ohio 44106, USA; †Division of Neurosurgery, The Toronto Hospital, Toronto, Ontario, Canada M5T 258*

The introduction of levodopa resulted in a striking decline in the use of stereotactic neurosurgical procedures for Parkinson's disease. In recent years, however, there has been a major resurgence in interest in the use of functional neurosurgery that has been encouraged by the high proportion of patients who experience disabling late-stage complications of dopaminergic therapy, including motor fluctuations and dyskinesias. Advances in imaging and intraoperative electrophysiological monitoring have improved the safety and accuracy of stereotactic neurosurgery. Finally, advances in the understanding of the physiological disturbances of basal ganglia function that accompany Parkinson's disease support the current interest in altering the activity of the outflow of the sensorimotor region of the internal segment of the globus pallidus (GPi). Strong evidence exists for the presence of excessive neuronal activity in the GPi, which to a significant extent is driven by overactivity of the subthalamic nucleus (3).

Until recently thalamotomy had largely replaced earlier surgical approaches to the globus pallidus and the pallidofugal fibers, given its apparent superior long-term beneficial effects on tremor versus the perceived inconsistent or short-term benefit obtained with pallidal operations. Thalamotomy may also have a pronounced ame-liorative effect on levodopa-induced dyskinesia (37), although such disabling features of parkinsonism as bradykinesia and ambulatory disturbances (including freezing of gait and postural instability) generally fail to respond and may even worsen (41).

Lesioning the posteroventral portion of the GPi, Leksell and colleagues obtained a pronounced long-lasting response that included alleviation of bradykinesia and other features unresponsive to thalamotomy (41). More recently, Laitinen et al. reported prolonged alleviation of most parkinsonian signs, including levodopa-induced dyskinesias, in 38 patients with advanced Parkinson's disease using a modification of Leksell's target in the medial pallidum (28). Since then there has been widespread interest in and enthusiasm about the procedure. The few studies supporting the beneficial effects of this technique that have been reported to date have generally involved small numbers of patients, and follow-up has been limited to a few months. One-year follow-up data have been provided by two groups, but again in only a small number of cases (1,4). More recently a 2- to 4-year follow-up has been reported in a subgroup of one of these studies (7). In this chapter previous reported series are reviewed and analyzed.

Over the past 3 years our group has performed approximately 150 posteroventral medial pallidotomies (PVMPs). The first 40 of these patients have had detailed evaluations involving clinical assessments in a "practically defined worst-off" state after overnight drug withdrawal and again in the "best on" state in response to their first morning dose of antiparkinsonian medication. Previously we reported results of blinded evaluation of videotapes performed before and 6 months after surgery for the first 14 of these patients (35). Here we describe the results of open clinical evaluations in all 40 patients at 6 months with evaluations of longer-term results in two groups: those followed for 1 and 2 years after pallidotomy. Our group represents the largest cohort with the longest follow-up of patients prospectively evaluated with validated rating scales of parkinsonism in both on and off states and levodopa-induced dyskinesias.

MATERIAL AND METHODS

Patients

Forty patients with a diagnosis of idiopathic Parkinson's disease underwent PVMP. All patients had initially obtained a good response from levodopa but subsequently developed significant disability due to off-period immobility, disabling levodopa-induced dyskinesias, and increasing disability during the on period primarily related to ambulatory disturbances despite optimization of available antiparkinsonian drugs. During this time, four other patients underwent the procedure (see below) but were not lesioned; therefore they were not included in the analysis of efficacy. One patient sustained an intracerebral hemorrhage that required surgical evacuation. She was left with persistent hemiplegia and dysphasia. One patient had unsuccessful microelectrode mapping of the GPi due to technical difficulties. Another also had unsuccessful microelectrode mapping probably due to anatomical disturbances of the GPi. This patient had long-standing Parkinson's disease with severe fluctuations and dyskinesias. Two years before his surgery he sustained a subarachnoid hemorrhage (SAH) with no source of it dis-

covered on subsequent investigations. During the immediate post-SAH period he was comatose briefly and then gradually recovered to his previous functional level with the exception of persistent memory deficits. Magnetic resonance imaging (MRI) demonstrated bilateral symmetrical lesions (? infarcts due to vasospasm) in the GPi. At the time of surgery, multiple recording tracks through the region of the globus pallidus failed to define the usual recognizable patterns of neuronal activity (17,34). Because of inadequate localization data it was decided not to perform a lesion in this patient. A final patient with previous paranoia became agitated during the microrecording studies, and the procedure was abandoned before a lesion could be made.

The 40 patients undergoing PVMP (26 men, 14 women) had a mean age of 58.8 ± 8.2 years (range 44–72 years). The mean duration of their illness was 12.9 ± 4.8 years (range 4–25 years). All patients continued to have a substantial response to dopaminergic therapy as evidenced by the difference between their mean Schwab and England on and off scores (78% versus 39%). Mean Hoehn and Yahr on and off scores were 2.7 and 3.6, respectively. All patients were otherwise medically fit and had a reasonable expectation of surgery. The study was approved by the Human Studies Investigations Committee of The Toronto Hospital, and all patients signed informed consents.

All patients were receiving levodopa preparations. The mean dose of levodopa plus a decarboxylase inhibitor was 1,096 mg (300–2,600). Ten patients took a mean of 23.1 mg bromocriptine (5.0–47.5 mg), and 19 patients took a mean of 3.2 mg pergolide (0.20–11.25 mg). Where possible, postoperative doses of antiparkinsonian medications were maintained at the preoperative levels. Many patients, however, did change their medication doses in response to reduced needs, particularly during the immediate postoperative period. Total "dopa equivalents" were calculated as follows: absolute dosage of regular levodopa (given with peripheral decarboxylase inhibitor) + $0.75 \times$ mg dosage of levodopa in the form of controlled-release (CR) Sinemet + $10 \times$ mg dosage of bromocriptine + $100 \times$ mg dosage of pergolide.

Evaluations

Patients were evaluated clinically as previously reported (34). In brief, this protocol followed a revised form of the Core Assessment Program for Intracerebral Transplantation [CAPIT (32)], which incorporated the Unified Parkinson's Disease Rating Scale (UPDRS) (30) and a simple timed manual task (time to tap the index finger between 2 points 30 cm apart for 10 successive cycles). Other timed tests from the CAPIT protocol were excluded for reasons outlined elsewhere (29). Dyskinesias were evaluated using the modified Obeso scale developed and validated by Goetz et al. (12). Separate scores for dyskinesias of the right and left limbs were obtained, as was a total score that incorporated axial and facial involvement. Clinical assessments were carried out after an overnight drug-free period (minimum 12 hours) in a "practically defined worst off" state and in the typical "best on" state approximately 1 hour after the usual morning dose of medication. In the first 16 patients, two preoperative evaluations were performed at least 1 week apart and two evaluations were obtained at least 1 day apart late during the first week immediately following surgery. In these patients the mean of the two evaluations was used for analysis. One-week postoperative evaluations were obtained for the first 27 patients and then discontinued. Follow-up evaluations were obtained at 3, 6, 12, and 24 months in 39, 39, 27, and 11 patients, respectively. During the follow-up period nine patients underwent further surgical procedures. In one, a second ipsilateral lesion was performed shortly after the 3-month evaluation; this lesion was necessary because the first had resulted in inadequate benefit due to improper placement of the lesion as a consequence of intraoperative patient cooperation problems. Two patients had contralateral pallidotomies at 6 and 18 months following the first surgery, respectively; and six patients underwent contralateral deep brain stimu-lation (four GPi and two Vim 9–18 months following the first surgery). In each of these patients efficacy data are included to the last follow-up point before the second surgical procedure. All patients had detailed neuropsychological evaluations. The preliminary results of these studies have been pre-sented (38), and a formal report has been submitted for publication. All patients underwent video-taping in the off and on states using the CAPIT protocol. These videotapes will be randomized and evaluated blindly when all patients have reached a minimum of 1 year of follow-up.

Surgical Procedure

The methods used by our group for micro-electrode-guided posteroventral pallidotomy have been outlined in detail elsewhere (34) and in Chapter 9 of this volume. A General Electric 1.5-tesla MRI scan was used to display the globus pallidus and allow calculation of target coordinates. Under local anesthesia a single 3-mm twist drill hole was made in the skull 2 cm from the midline at the coronal suture on the side opposite the most disabling symptoms. A right pallidotomy was performed in 26 patients and a left pallidotomy in 14. The initial target was approached at 20–40 degrees anterior to the patient's vertical axis. Microelectrode recording started 15 mm above the proposed target, which was 3 mm anterior to the midcommissural point, 3–6 mm below the intercommissural line, and 21 mm lateral to the midline, as proposed by Laitinen et al. (28). Two to eight electrode tracks were explored in each patient, with neuronal activity recorded using parylene-insulated tungsten or platinum-iridium electrodes with an impedance of 1 to 5 MΩ and 20- to 30-μm exposed tips. When units were identified, testing of the modulation of their activity by passive and active mouth and limb movements was carried out. The optic tract and internal capsule were carefully defined by responses to microstimulation. The optic tract with visual responses to a strobe light was also tested. Lesions were not made until the ventral and posterior borders of the GPi were identified by the characteristic recording and stimulation responses for optic tract and internal capsule. Lesions were made in areas containing neurons whose activity was modulated by movements at least 3 mm away from any point where microelectrode stimulation up to 100 μA (300 Hz) evoked visual or motor responses. Lesions were made with a 1 mm diameter probe, the last 3 mm of which was not insulated. A "test" lesion at 60°C for 60 seconds was followed by permanent lesioning for 60 seconds at 70°C, 80°C, and finally 90°C. Throughout the period of lesioning the patient's speech, motor function, and visual fields were regularly tested.

Statistical Analysis

The data derived from evaluations of patients on a variety of measures obtained prior to pallidotomy and postoperatively at 1 week (the first 27 patients), 3 months, 6 months, 1 year, and 2 years. Evaluation of *early efficacy* (3 and 6 months) was obtained in 39 patients each. At 3 months one patient was unavailable for evaluation. At 6 months one patient had been removed because she had undergone a repeat ipsilateral pallidotomy (see Evaluations, above). The 6-month evaluation was chosen for assessment of "short-term" effects in the hope of reducing the influence of the placebo response, which should have been larger at 3 months than at 6 months. For *long-term efficacy analysis* patients were divided into two groups. The first group comprised patients followed to 1 year ($n = 27$), and the second group (which was included in the first) were those followed for 2 years ($n = 11$). The first group was chosen to have a sufficient number of subjects to draw firm conclusions. However, the long-term effect of pallidotomy is a major concern, and so the second group was also analyzed.

The primary measure of pallidotomy efficacy was the "total" UPDRS score [only Parts II and III: Activities of Daily Living (ADL) and Motor Scores] in the off and on conditions. Secondary measures were of individual subsets of the UPDRS, including tremor, rigidity, and bradykinesia and the dyskinesia rating scale. Tremor scores comprised the sum of rest tremor in the upper and lower limbs plus action tremor in the arm (scores of nos. $20 + 21$); rigidity scores were the sum of rigidity in the arm and leg (no. 20), and bradykinesia scores summed the performance of three manual and one foot rapid movement task (scores of nos. $23 + 24 + 25 + 26$). In addition, a composite score was developed for postural instability and gait disorder (PIGD) composed of the sum of scores (from both the ADL and Motor sections of the UPDRS) for falling, freezing, walking, gait, and postural instability (scores of nos. $13 + 14 + 15 + 29 + 30$). This subsection analysis was performed because significant changes in some subtests could be reversed following pallidotomy, which would tend to be obscured when summed for total UPDRS scores. In addition, the pallidotomy effect may be greatest for only some symptom groups, which would not be observable when considering only the total UPDRS scores. However, the UPDRS is composed of 27 subtests (13 ADL and 14 Motor), and it is not feasible to analyze each subtest owing to the increased risk of type I error (finding a significant change when none truly exists) due to multiple comparisons.

Three questions were addressed by the analysis: (a) Is there an improvement in primary and secondary measures following pallidotomy? (b) When did the improvement occur? (c) Was that improvement sustained? To answer the first and second questions, pairwise comparisons were made between the baseline evaluation and each of the follow-up evaluations. Parametric statistical methods were used where the data met appropriate assumptions (e.g., normal distribution). Either a paired t-test or a Wilcoxon sign rank test were used to compare baseline scores to each of the postoperative evaluations. In view of the number of repeated analyses, a p value of 0.005 was chosen to avoid a type I error.

To answer the third question, two separate analyses were performed. First, an analysis of variance with repeated measures (ANOVA-R) was performed on the difference scores between baseline and each of the follow-up evaluations (degree of improvement). If the data distribution failed tests for normalcy, a Friedman's ANOVA by ranks was performed. Thus the time of evaluation was a factor in the ANOVA-R. If the ANOVA-R showed no statistical difference over time, a sustained benefit over the follow-up period was supported. To be sure that this result was not a type II error (failure to find a change when a change truly exists), a power analysis was performed. The power analysis was based on the sample size and variance calculated for each group, and an estimate of effects size was given to be 10%. Thus the ability to detect a decline in the benefit (i.e., the magnitude of different scores) by as little as 10% with better than 80% chance was determined.

The ANOVA-R may not detect trends over time in an ordered sense. For example, the ANOVA-R determines only if there is a significant difference at any time period. There could be a slight but insignificant decline between week 1 and month 3 or between month 3 and month 6, for example, that would not be detected by an ANOVA-R. The second analysis to evaluate the change in response to pallidotomy over time employed a linear regression of the measures at each evaluation for each patient. Then the mean slope of the regression was determined for all patients. A mean slope greater than zero indicates a change (worsening) in the patients' responses over time. A mean slope of zero indicates no change in response, suggesting sustained benefit.

A secondary hypothesis of the study was that pallidotomy would result in *clinically* significant improvement. This hypothesis was tested by examining the effects of pallidotomy on specific test items of the ADL section of the UPDRS that represent important day-to-day self-care functions (feeding, dressing, personal hygiene), two components of the Motor section of the UPDRS

that relate to ambulatory disability (gait and postural stability), and finally the severity of contralateral dyskinesias as scored on the dyskinesia rating scale. In each of these subsections a score of 2 or more generally indicates some degree of dependence on others for care or a major interference with function. With the exception of dyskinesias, this evaluation was applied only to the practically defined worst off period because there were insufficient numbers of patients who were dependent in the on condition to permit conclusions. Evaluations were assessed at 25 and 52 weeks in the 1-year group and at 52 and 104 weeks in the 2-year group.

RESULTS

Early Response

All 40 patients have been followed for at least 3 months, and data are available at 6 months for 39 of them. Tables 10-1 and 10-2 provide the means and standard deviations for off and on scores, respectively, and the percent improvements of the

TABLE 10-1. *"Off" period scores before and 6 months after unilateral pallidotomy*

Parameter	Before	6 months	p	% Improvement[a]
UPDRS (Parts II and III)	68.8 ± 13.3	47.9 ± 17.0	0.0005	30.4
ADL	24.6 ± 5.1	17.2 ± 7.0	0.000004	30.1
Motor	44.4 ± 11.2	30.7 ± 11.5	0.0000014	30.9
S&E	39.0 ± 17.5	65.1 ± 15.8	< 0.000001	62.8
Total				
Bradykinesia	16.7 ± 4.7	11.4 ± 5.4	0.0000022	31.7
Tremor	6.0 ± 5.3	3.5 ± 3.7	0.00058	41.7
Rigidity	8.6 ± 4.5	5.6 ± 3.2	0.00005	31.4
PIGD	10.3 ± 3.9	7.1 ± 4.1	0.0000019	30.1
Gait	2.3 ± 0.9	1.8 ± 1.1	0.0057	(23.9)
Post. stability	2.1 ± 0.9	1.4 ± 1.0	0.00013	33.3
Freezing	2.3 ± 1.0	1.4 ± 1.1	0.00009	39.1
Ipsilateral				
Bradykinesia	7.3 ± 2.9	5.9 ± 3.1	0.0014	19.2
Tremor	2.0 ± 2.1	1.6 ± 2.1	0.34	
Rigidity	3.0 ± 1.8	2.8 ± 1.5	0.70	
Tapping	13.5 ± 6.0	11.1 ± 2.8	0.0033	17.8
Contralateral				
Bradykinesia	9.4 ± 2.7	5.5 ± 3.1	0.0000013	41.5
Tremor	2.9 ± 2.7	1.3 ± 1.8	0.00014	55.2
Rigidity	3.7 ± 2.2	1.7 ± 1.4	0.0000032	54.1
Tapping	17.8 ± 14.3	12.1 ± 8.5	0.0029	32.0

Results are means ± SD. See text for details of the scores. Ipsilateral and Contralateral indicate the side of the body relative to the pallidotomy.

UPDRS, Unified Parkinson's Disease Rating Scale; ADL, Activities of Daily Living; PIGD, postural instability/gait disorder; S & E, Schwab and England.

[a] Percent improvement of the means given for scores with significant changes.

TABLE 10-2. *"On" period scores before and 6 months after unilateral pallidotomy*

Parameter	Before	6 Months	p	% Improvement
UPDRS (parts II and III)	27.7 ± 11.7	23.6 ± 13.5	0.043	
ADL	10.3 ± 5.0	7.2 ± 5.3	0.0038	30.1
Motor	17.4 ± 8.7	16.5 ± 9.3	0.6	
S&E	78.2 ± 14.3	85.2 ± 9.3	0.007	
Total				
Bradykinesia	7.2 ± 4.0	7.4 ± 4.6	0.86	
Tremor	0.9 ± 1.9	0.5 ± 0.9	0.5	
Rigidity	3.4 ± 2.7	3.3 ± 3.1	0.86	
PIGD	4.7 ± 3.6	3.7 ± 3.6	0.024	
Dyskinesia	5.7 ± 2.3	2.1 ± 1.4	< 0.000001	63.2
Gait	1.0 ± 0.7	0.9 ± 0.9	0.61	
Post. stability	1.2 ± 0.9	1.0 ± 1.0	0.1	
Freezing	0.7 ± 0.8	0.5 ± 0.8	0.098	
Ipsilateral				
Bradykinesia	3.2 ± 2.1	3.4 ± 2.6	0.74	
Tremor	0.2 ± 0.8	0.3 ± 0.5	0.37	
Rigidity	1.1 ± 1.4	1.4 ± 1.5	0.29	
Tapping	10.1 ± 2.5	9.1 ± 2.5	0.0057	(9.9)
Dyskinesia	2.0 ± 1.0	1.1 ± 0.7	0.0000081	50
Contralateral				
Bradykinesia	3.9 ± 2.4	4.1 ± 2.7	0.67	
Tremor	0.4 ± 0.9	0.2 ± 0.6	0.47	
Rigidity	1.4 ± 1.3	1.0 ± 1.3	0.098	
Tapping	11.0 ± 5.8	9.4 ± 3.8	0.0023	14.5
Dyskinesia	2.3 ± 0.9	0.4 ± 0.6	< 0.000001	82.6

Results are means ± SD. See text for details of score.
See Table 10-1 for abbreviations.
Ipsi/Contra = side of body Ipsilateral and Contralateral indicate the side of the body relative to the pallidotomy.

mean scores for the subcomponents that reached statistical significance ($p < 0.005$ given multiple comparisons). The predominant improvements in parkinsonian scores were obtained during the off period. Improvements in off-period UPDRS total Motor and ADL scores averaged 30%. Changes in contralateral parkinsonism accounted for much of this improvement. At 6 months after pallidotomy ipsilateral bradykinesia had also been significantly alleviated (19.2%). All off-period features of parkinsonism demonstrated significant alleviation (i.e., ipsilateral bradykinesia, contralateral bradykinesia, tremor, and rigidity), and the axial features (e.g., gait, postural stability, and freezing) had improved. During the on period there was a significant improvement only in the total ADL score, and improvement in Schwab and England on-period scores showed only a trend toward improvement ($p = 0.007$). In contrast, none of the motor components of the UPDRS changed significantly in the on state. Tapping scores, a measure of bradykinesia, did improve significantly on both the contralateral and ipsilateral sides in the off state and to a lesser but still significant extent dur-

ing the on period. Dyskinesia scores improved markedly on both the contralateral (82.6%) and the ipsilateral (50%) sides.

The effect of age at the time of surgery on outcome was evaluated by dividing the patients into two groups: those age 60 or younger ($n = 22$, mean age 53.2 ± 4.5 years) and those 65 or older ($n = 11$, mean age 68.5 ± 2.5 years). Baseline total UPDRS off scores were not significantly different between the two groups (≤ 60 years 66.7 ± 13.2; ≥ 65 years 69.5 ± 14.4). The total UPDRS off scores at 6 months compared to baseline scores improved by 36% in the younger group but only 16% in the older group ($p = 0.024$). Dyskinesias responded to the same extent in both age groups.

Long-Term Results

Primary Measure: Total UPDRS

Off Condition

Paired comparisons showed a statistically significant difference between baseline scores and each of the follow-up evaluations. Furthermore, the ANOVA-R showed no difference in the degree of improvement (difference scores between baseline and each evaluation) over time, suggesting sustained improvement. Power analysis showed that there was at least an 80% probability of detecting, to an alpha of 0.05, a change in the UPDRS off score of as little as 10%. Regression analysis to detect a change in the pallidotomy benefit over time resulted in a mean slope close to zero, and a zero slope was within the 95% confidence limit, suggesting no change in the patients' benefit during the follow-up period. These findings were true for both the 1-year and 2-year follow-up groups (mean regression slopes and 95% confidence intervals: "off" 1 year = 0.065 (−0.047 to 0.117), "off" 2 years 0.018 (−0.055 to 0.074) (Fig. 10-1). Three patients in the 1-year group did have slopes significantly higher than 0 (0.506, 0.702, and 0.451, respectively), which implies that 3 of the 27 patients may have had some worsening of symptoms over time after the pallidotomy. Only 1 of the 11 patients followed for 2 years had a positive slope outside the 95% confidence limit, indicating significant worsening of symptoms.

In summary, there was a 29% improvement in UPDRS off scores as a result of pallidotomy. This benefit was sustained for at least 24 of the 27 patients over the first year and for 10 of 11 patients for 2 years.

"On" Condition

The data for the 1-year group at the 1-week postoperative evaluation were not normally distributed. Consequently, a Wilcoxon sign rank test was performed. Each postoperative evaluation was significantly different from the baseline with the exception of the 6-month evaluation (Fig. 10-1). Results of the ANOVA-R showed no differences in the improvement (as measured by the differences between baseline evaluations and those at each follow-up time). Power analysis showed a better than 80% chance of detecting as little as a 10% decline in the UPDRS on scores if a decline existed. The mean regression slope (with 95% confidence interval) was 0.009 (−0.075 to 0.151),

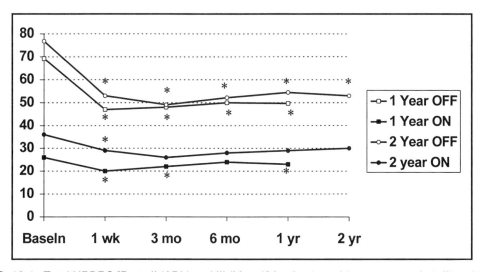

FIG. 10-1. Total UPDRS [Parts II (ADL) and III (Motor)] for the 1- and 2-year groups in "off" and "on" states. Analysis of variance with repeated measures (ANOVA-R) design for the difference scores showed no significant differences from week 1 to 1 year and 2 years in each of the groups for both measures. For all four lines the mean regression slope was not different from zero (see text), indicating that the initial effect is sustained. Statistical significance of the follow-up data from baseline (*Baseln*): *$p < 0.005$.

indicating no change over time and a stable improvement in the UPDRS on scores. None of the patients had an individual regression slope significantly different from zero.

In summary, the patients had a 19% improvement in the UPDRS on scores following pallidotomy that was sustained for the first year. As demonstrated in Fig. 10-1, a sustained improvement in the UPDRS on scores was not seen in the group of 11 patients followed for 2 years.

Secondary Measures

The results of the secondary measures that showed the greatest response are demonstrated in Fig. 10-2A (1-year group) and Fig. 10-2B (2-year group). Tables 10-3 and 10-4 list the parameters that were statistically significant from baseline ($p < 0.005$) along with the results of the ANOVA-R and mean regression slope [with 95% confidence intervals (CI)].

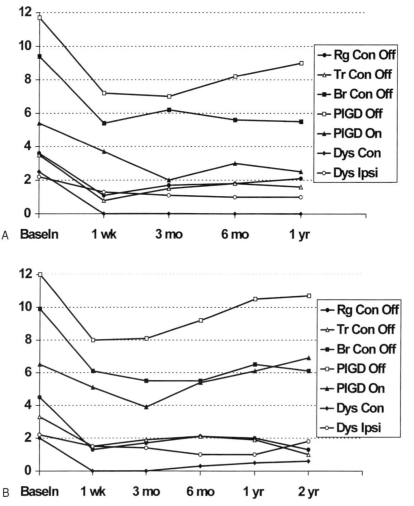

FIG. 10-2A and B. Secondary measures in the 1- and 2-year groups that showed the most significant responses. *Rg Con Off,* rigidity in the contralateral limbs in the off state; *Tr Con Off,* tremor in contralateral limbs in the off state; *Br Con Off,* bradykinesia in contralateral limbs in off state; *PIGD,* postural instability/gait disorder composite score; *Dys Con,* contralateral dyskinesias; *Dys Ipsi,* ipsilateral dyskinesias. See Tables 10-3 and 10-4 for the significance of these changes from baseline.

TABLE 10-3. *One-year group (n = 27)*

1 Week	3 Months	6 Months	12 Months	ANOVA-R	Mean regression slope (95% CI)
Contra brady off	Contra brady off	Contra brady off	Contra brady off	NSD	0.006 (– 0.016 to 0.028
—	Ipsi brady off	—	—	NSD	– 0.014 (– 0.32 to 0.004)
—	Ipsi brady on	—	—	NSD*	– 0.014 (– 0.028 to 0)
Contra rigidity off	Contra rigidity off	Contra rigidity off	Contra rigidity off	NSD*	0.012 (– 0.003 to 0.027)
Contra tremor off	Contra tremor off	Contra tremor off	Contra tremor off	NSD (Friedman's)	0.005 (10.015 to 0.025)
PIGD off	PIGD off	PIGD off	—	Different	0.047 (0.02 to 0.074)
PIGD on	PIGD on (Wilcoxon)	—	—	NSD (Friedman's)	0.013 (0.007 to 0.003)
Ipsilateral dyskinesias	Ipsilateral dyskinesias	Ipsilateral dyskinesias	Ipsilateral dyskinesias	NSD (Friedman's)	0.002 (– 0.006 to 0.010)
Contralateral dyskinesias (Wilcoxon)	Contralateral dyskinesias (Wilcoxon)	Contralateral dyskinesias (Wilcoxon)	Contralateral dyskinesias (Wilcoxon)	NSD (Friedman's)	0.007 (0.000 to 0.009)

Parameters are statistically significant from baseline ($p < 0.005$). Figures 2A and B provide the data for these tables.

NSD, ANOVA-R demonstrated no significant differences over the follow-up time; Different, ANOVA-R demonstrated differences indicating that the benefit was not sustained; brady, bradykinesia; PIGD, postural instability/gait disorder.

*Statistical power less than desirable.

Tremor

Contralateral tremor at rest during the off condition was improved in the 1-year group (53%; this and subsequent percentages are the means of the individual percent improvements) (Fig. 10-2A). The improvement was sustained in this group but tended to fall off in the 2-year group (Fig. 10-2B). There was a tendency for sustained improvement in the 2-year group, but the scores did not reach statistical significance owing to the correction for multiple comparisons and the small number of patients with tremor in this group (only those with tremor at baseline were used for this analysis; $n = 10$). Contralateral tremor during the on condition was unchanged; however, persistent on-period tremor was not a feature in these patients, most of whom continued to have an excellent response to levodopa with respect to this symptom.

Ipsilateral tremor did not improve in the off or the on condition in either the 1- or 2-year group. However, this finding must be interpreted with caution because of the small sample size. Power analysis on the ANOVA-R demonstrated insufficient power.

Bradykinesia

Contralateral bradykinesia in the off condition was improved by 36% in the 1-year group. This improvement was sustained in both the 1- and 2-year groups (Figs. 10-2A and B). Contralateral on-period bradykinesia was unchanged. Ipsilateral bradykinesia in the off condition was improved at 3 months, but this change was not sustained beyond that time.

Rigidity

Contralateral off-period rigidity was reduced by 51% in the 1-year group, and this improvement was sustained in both the 1- and 2-year groups (Figs. 10-2A and B). Changes in contralateral rigidity in the on state were significant only at 1 week for the 2-year group, but the sample size was too small to provide statis-

TABLE 10-4. *Two-year group (n = 11)*

1 Week	3 Months	6 Months	12 Months	24 Months	ANOVA-R	Mean regression slope (95% CI)
Contra brady off	Contra brady off	Contra brady off	Contra brady off	Contra brady off	NSD	0.006 (−0.008 to 0.020)
—	Ipsi brady off	—	—	—	NSD	−0.001 (−0.010 to 0.012)
Contra rigidity off	Contra rigidity off	Contra rigidity off	Contra rigidity off	Contra rigidity off	NSD	0.0 (−0.007 to 0.007)
Contra rigidity on	—	—	—	—	NSD	−0.001 (−0.006 to 0.004)
PIGD off	—	—	—	—	Different ($p < 0.035$)	0.028 (0.005 to 0.051)
PIGD on	PIGD on	—	—	—	Different (Friedman's)	0.024 (0.007 to 0.41)
—	Ipsilateral dyskinesias	Ipsilateral dyskinesias	Ipsilateral dyskinesias	—	NSD (Friedman's)	0.005 (0.001 to 0.009)
Contralateral dyskinesias (Wilcoxon)	Contralateral dyskinesias (Wilcoxon)	Contralateral dyskinesias (Wilcoxon)	Contralateral dyskinesias (Wilcoxon)	Contralateral dyskinesias (Wilcoxon)	NSD (Friedman's)	0.006 (0.001 to 0.011)

Parameters are statistically significant from baseline ($p < 0.005$).

Figures 2A and B provide the data for these tables.

NSD, ANOVA-R demonstrated no significant differences over the follow-up time (i.e., sustained benefit); Different, ANOVA-R demonstrated differences indicating that the benefit was not sustained; Contra, Contralateral; Ipsi, ipsilateral; brady, bradykinesia; PIGD, postural instability/gait disorder.

tical power. Ipsilateral rigidity did not improve in the off or on condition in either the 1- or 2-year group.

Postural Instability/Gait Disorder

The 1-year and 2-year groups had significant improvements in PIGD off scores during the first week following pallidotomy. In the 1-year group the improvement was sustained for 6 months and was lost by 1 year (Fig. 10-2A). In the 2-year group the improvement at 3 months approached statistical significance (Fig. 10-2B) but was not significant thereafter. Both the ANOVA-R and the mean slope of the regression (more than zero) also support the finding that the improvement in PIGD was not sustained. The greatest improvement was 32% at the first week.

Similar to the off condition, the PIGD on scores improved significantly (31% in the 1-year group and 22% in the 2-year group) 1 week after pallidotomy, but this change was lost by 6 months in the 2-year group (Fig. 10-2B) and by the third month in the 1-year group (Fig. 10-2A). Again, the PIGD scores approached but did not reach statistical significance at 3 months. Mean regression slope analysis showed slopes larger than zero for both groups, suggesting that the benefit was not sustained. The ANOVA-R supported this finding in the 2-year group but not in the 1-year group.

Dyskinesia

There was an approximately 40% improvement in ipsilateral dyskinesia scores (evaluated in the drug on condition) in the 1- and 2-year groups. The improvement was sustained in both groups at 1 year (Fig. 10-2A), but in the 2-year group the benefit was lost by the second year (Fig. 10-2B).

There was marked, sustained alleviation of contralateral dyskinesia for the 1- and 2-year (Fig. 10-2B) follow-up groups. Trend analysis did show a worsening of the contralateral dyskinesia in the 2-year group and a tendency to worsen in the 1-year group. However, both groups had statistically significant improvement at the end of the follow-up over the baseline preoperative evaluations.

Changes in Level of Dependence

Figure 10-3 shows the changes from dependence to independence (i.e., reduction of a score of ≥ 2 to < 2) and from independence to dependence (change of the score from < 2 to ≥ 2) evaluated at 6 months and 1 year after pallidotomy in the 1-year group and at 1 year and 2 years in the 2-year group. It can be seen that 44% to 54% of patients dependent, according to measures of ADL function (feeding, dressing, hygiene), in the off state preoperatively were independent at the 6-month follow-up; this level of improvement was maintained at 2 years for feeding and dressing and was reduced to approximately 20% for hygiene at 1 and 2 years. Improvement from dependence to independence with respect to gait and postural stability occurred in a smaller proportion of patients. Reduction in contralateral dyskinesias from a level of intense interference with function to no interference occurred in approximately 75% of cases.

Medications

In the entire group reaching the 6-month follow-up there were no statistically significant changes in levodopa, bromocriptine, or pergolide doses. The total dopa equivalents dosage was reduced from 1155.8 mg to 1006.3 mg, a change that did not reach statistical significance ($p = 0.006$).

In the 1-year group there was a statistically significant reduction in the total daily levodopa level at 1 week and at 3 months. There was no difference at 6 months or 1 year. During the follow-up there was a suggestion of increasing levodopa use, but it was not statistically significant. In the 2-year group there was no significant change in the total levodopa dose. There were no significant changes in the total daily doses of pergolide or bromocriptine. Changes in total dopa-equivalents for the 1- and 2-year groups were not significant.

Complications

Four patients experienced acute confusion and somnolence during the immediate postoperative period that lasted from less than 24 hours to up to 3 to 4 days. One of these patients experienced

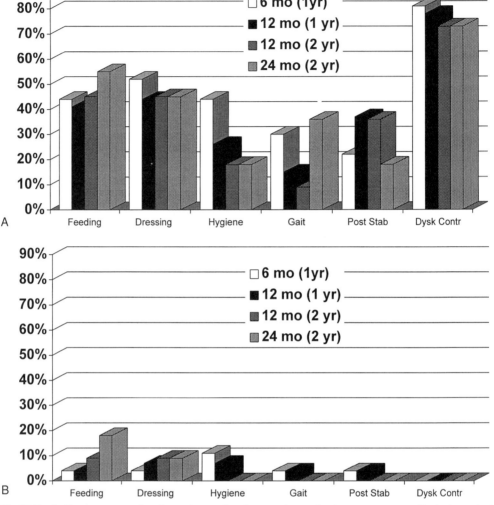

FIG. 10-3. A. Percentages of patients improving from a dependent score preoperatively to an independent score postoperatively (reduction in score from ≥ 2 to < 2) for off-period feeding, dressing, hygiene, gait, and postural stability or from an on-period state of contralateral dyskinesias causing intense interference with function preoperatively to no interference postoperatively (evaluated at 6 and 12 months in the 1-year group and at 12 and 24 months in the 2-year group). **B.** Percentages of patients worsening from an independent state to a dependent state during the off period or experiencing worsening of on-period dyskinesias, changing from noninterfering to interfering with function.

associated acute, transient (< 12 hours) contralateral limb hypotonia. In one patient, shown to have a frontal venous infarct on MRI, postoperative confusion lasted 2 to 3 weeks and was followed by persistent but mild contralateral facial weakness, dysarthria, dysphagia, and changes in concentration, which the patient and the family believed were all outweighed by the benefits obtained from surgery. One patient with mild preoperative dementia had acute confusion and hallucinations during the immediate postoperative period. As this situation resolved it became evident that his persistent level of cognitive dysfunction had increased, and disability from this outweighed the mild motoric benefit that he obtained from the surgery. One patient experienced a brief period of visual hallucinosis during the 2 days following surgery with no subsequent sequelae.

A number of other complications involving limb and bulbar function were usually transient, typically resolving over the first 6 postoperative weeks. They included contralateral facial weakness in 14 (persistent in 2), dysarthria in 10 (persistent in 3), dysphagia in 7 (persistent in 2), mild transient contralateral limb weakness in 3, and contralateral neglect in 1. It was thought that many of these adverse effects were probably related to edema surrounding the lesion, which sometimes coursed along the internal capsule as seen on postoperative MRI scans. Two patients noted persistent worsening of their balance.

One person who had been depressed prior to the surgery experienced an increase in depression 3 to 6 months after surgery. In three cases spouses pointed out changes in personality and behavior (persistent in two), in five cases there were complaints regarding reduced memory, concentration, and judgment (persistent in three), and one noted persistent word-finding difficulty. In these patients the clinical benefit obtained from pallidotomy far outweighed the interference caused by these behavioral complaints. The results of formal neuropsychological evaluations are currently under analysis and have been presented in preliminary fashion (38).

Of the 15 patients who underwent a dominant hemisphere procedure, 4 complained of persistent worsening of handwriting. In all cases it was in striking contrast to the substantial improvements obtained in all other manual activities. Fourteen patients noted weight gain of 8 to 82 pounds over a 6- to 12-month period. After direct questioning it was thought that this gain related to a greater ease of feeding and access to food in nine, reduced dyskinesias in six (weight gain occurred in three patients who had little or no dyskinesia), increased appetite in five, behavioral changes in two (e.g., "foraging" behavior), and better control of diabetes in one. Two or more of the above explanations were present in nine patients experiencing weight gain. None of the patients demonstrated a visual field defect postoperatively.

Excluding weight gain, 25 of the 40 patients experienced one or more complications, and 15 had two or more. Fourteen experienced persistent adverse events; but as stated above, in all but the one patient with worsening dementia, these events were generally mild and considered by patients and families as worth tolerating for the benefit obtained.

DISCUSSION

In 1960 Svennilson et al. (41) provided a retrospective review of 81 patients operated on by Leksell between 1953 and 1957. Three of these patients underwent staged bilateral operations. Rigidity decreased significantly in 79%, and a lasting remission from tremor was seen in 82%. Features of bradykinesia were not directly measured, but it was noted that mobility, range, precision, and speed of movement improved, as did gait and mobility of the trunk.

In 1992 Laitinen et al. reported their 5-year experience with 38 patients undergoing Leksell's pallidotomy (34 unilateral, 4 bilateral) (28). They reported that all aspects of parkinsonism were improved with complete or almost complete relief of rigidity and bradykinesia in 92% and tremor in 81%. Gait and speech dysfunction also consistently improved. Levodopa-induced dyskinesias and "painful muscular spasms" were resolved in almost all patients. In 1995 Laitinen updated his experience with a report of 259 patients (220 unilateral, 12 bilateral, 18 combining PVMP and thalamotomy, and 9 unilateral repeats) (27). Ninety-six percent of patients obtained either a "good" (n = 212) or "fair" (n = 36) response, the former indicating more or less complete relief of all symptoms contralaterally and the latter indicating a substantial improvement.

In that same year Sutton et al. reported poor results of unilateral pallidotomy in three patients (two undergoing a repeat procedure 8 weeks after the first) and in two patients with staged bilateral pallidotomy (40). Although levodopa-induced dyskinesias and dystonia were reduced contralateral to the procedure, little change was obtained in parkinsonism, and postoperative morbidity was common. Some concern should be raised regarding the choice of patients in this study. Two of the five patients had disease durations of only 4 and 5 years and were rated as Hoehn and Yahr stage 5 in both on and off states. These rather "malignant" forms of parkinsonism are suggestive of an alternative diagnosis, such as multiple system atrophy, rather than idiopathic Parkinson's disease (43).

In a series of papers Iacono et al. reported the results after PVMP in 126 patients (58 unilateral and 68 bilateral procedures) (19, 20, 26). They described striking improvements in all motor subscores of the UPDRS and elimination of dyskinesia and profound off periods. Careful evaluation of these papers reveals serious inconsistencies and contradictions. Although it is clear that some patients have benefited considerably from the procedure, overall the data provided are uninterpretable. For example, the details of how scores were obtained and what comprises each score item is confusing, and the data provided are inconsistent with knowledge of the rating scale. It is impossible to discern the relation between clinical signs and the side or sides of surgery, and results of unilateral and bilateral lesions are lumped together. (In fact, one report does not even mention bilateral procedures, and the second indicates that more than half of the patients were treated in this way.)

In 1995 Dogali et al. from New York University reported 1-year results in 18 patients treated with unilateral pallidotomy compared to a non-operated control group of 7 patients who desired surgery but were awaiting initial surgical outcome results (4). Off-condition UPDRS scores improved by 65%, and CAPIT timed subtest scores improved 38.2% in the contralateral limb and 24.2% in the ipsilateral limb. Walk scores improved a mean 45%. Contralateral levodopa-induced dyskinesias were said to have resolved, and on-period scores improved; but no data were provided to support these observations.

More recently this group reported 2- to 4-year follow-up data for 11 of these patients (2 years for all 11 patients, 3 years for 10, and 4 years for 5) (7). In addition to the total UPDRS, they emphasized results of timed maneuvers in the CAPIT protocol, which we have previously criticized with the exception of the tapping task (29). They found that initial responses in the ADL and Motor components of the UPDRS and the timed maneuvers in both the contralateral and ipsilateral limb did not decline over the 3-year post-

operative period and that dyskinesias did not return on the operated side (although, once again, supportive data were not provided). No mention was made of on-period scores in this report.

Baron et al. (1) reported a 1-year follow-up study of 15 patients treated with PVMP. Open evaluations demonstrated a 34.1% reduction in ADL off scores, which remained significant for 1 year, and a 28.5% improvement in ADL on scores at 3 months, which returned to baseline by the 6-month follow-up. The total motor UPDRS scores improved by 24.9% in the off condition at 3 months, and these results remained significant at the 1-year follow-up. Motor on scores improved by 13.3% at 3 to 6 months but returned to baseline by 1 year. Contralateral limb off-period tremor, rigidity, and bradykinesia scores improved significantly as did the off-period gait dysfunction score. Freezing and falling in the on state, however, did not change. Many patients noted a reduction in the amount of off time with less recognizable motor fluctuations. As in other series, levodopa-induced dyskinesias were markedly alleviated and contralateral dyskinesias were evident in only one patient with preexisting dyskinesias at the 1-year follow-up. Patient age was inversely correlated with a better postoperative result with respect to the total UPDRS score at 3 months.

Johansson et al. (21) reported 12-month follow-up data for 22 patients undergoing PVMP performed using electrical macrostimulation to localize the site to be lesioned. Unfortunately, they only assessed patients in the on state using nonvalidated rating scales, which failed to evaluate certain cardinal signs of parkinsonism, such as rigidity. Only 13 of their patients had limb dyskinesias preoperatively, and their severity scores were surprisingly low compared to expected values of patients reported in other studies. They found that PVMP had a pronounced effect on dyskinesias, a moderate effect on tremor, and no effect on bradykinesia, gait, or frequency of off periods.

Kishore et al. reported results for 24 patients undergoing unilateral pallidotomy using computed tomography (CT) scanning and macrostimulation only to localize the site for lesioning (23). All features of off-period parkinsonism improved, mainly on the contralateral side, and dyskinesias were alleviated bilaterally. Changes were stable for at least 6 months. In contrast to our results and those of Baron et al. (1), these authors found that older patients tended to show greater improvement.

Kopyov et al. (24) have also reported 3-month results of microelectrode-guided unilateral pallidotomy in 29 patients. Scoring was said to use blinded videotapes, but much of the data reported, by its nature, had to have come from open evaluations. They reported significant improvements in the off and on contralateral, ipsilateral, and axial parkinsonism, CAPIT dexterity tasks, and dyskinesias. They especially emphasized the ameliorative effects on tremor, which for uncertain reasons improved with time after surgery. They proposed that this response is due to the fact that they made two lesions: one in the anterior aspect and the other in the posterior aspect of the GPi. They claim that, taken individually, the former alleviates dyskinesias but not tremor, and the latter alleviates tremor but not dyskinesias.

In 1995 we reported preliminary 6-month follow-up results in our first 14 patients treated with unilateral pallidotomy (35). This study is the only one reported to date that exclusively provides results of blinded assessments of UPDRS motor scores and dyskinesias rated from videotapes obtained before and 6 months after pallidotomy. The results of this assessment were similar to the open evaluation scores reported here for a much larger group of patients. The present study reports 6-month results for our first 39 patients and long-term follow-up for two overlapping groups: 27 patients followed for 1 year and 11 for 2 years. It represents the largest series with longest follow-up reported to date using validated rating methods of off- and on-period examinations and dyskinesias. We have demonstrated a pronounced reduction in contralateral levodopa-induced dyskinesias (82.6% in the 6-month group) that was sustained through 2 years of follow-up, although there was mild worsening between the 1- and 2-year evaluations. Ipsilateral dyskinesias improved by 40% to 50%, and this change was sustained for 1 year but was lost by the second year of follow-up. Off-period UPDRS scores improved by approximately 30%, and this

improvement remained stable for 2 years of follow-up. The changes in off-period ADL and Motor subcomponents were similar, both improving by approximately 30%. A lesser reduction in on-period total UPDRS scores (approximately 20%) was sustained for 1 year but not 2 years of follow-up. The off-period subscores of the UPDRS for tremor, rigidity, and bradykinesia improved significantly, and this benefit was sustained for 2 years of follow-up. These changes were almost exclusively related to improvement in the contralateral limbs, although some short-term improvement in ipsilateral bradykinesia was also seen. On-period subscores showed little change (all patients were levodopa responders, and preoperatively most continued to obtain good on-period responses with respect to these features). The composite score for postural instability and gait disorder and subscores for gait, postural stability, and freezing in the off condition were all significantly improved in the 39 patients followed for 6 months. In the 1- and 2-year groups the improvements in PIGD scores were evident for the first 3 to 6 months, but changes were not significant thereafter. Milder on-period improvement was also seen initially in the 1- and 2-year follow-up groups but was lost by 3 to 6 months. In the entire 39-patient 6-month follow-up group none of the changes in these parameters of ambulatory disability improved significantly in the on condition. One method for evaluating how clinically significant these improvements were involved the comparison of specific items (feeding, dressing, hygiene, gait and postural stability, and contralateral dyskinesias) before and after surgery with respect to how frequently scores indicated a change from dependence on others for care or major interference of function to a state of independence or little interference. The disability caused by dyskinesias improved markedly, and benefit persisted to 2 years. With respect to measures of ADL function, approximately 50% of patients dependent before surgery were independent 6 months after surgery. This change was sustained for 2 years for feeding and dressing; it partially declined at 1 year for dressing but remained stable between 1 and 2 years. Improvement in gait and postural stability were less substantial but still evident in one-third or more of patients. These observations are particularly striking when one remembers that patients were selected for pallidotomy on the basis that no further clinical improvement could be obtained with adjustments in available medication. Age at the time of surgery clearly affected outcome; those 60 years and under improved by 36% overall, whereas those 65 or older improved by only 16%.

Comparing our experience to previous reports raises a number of important issues that must be addressed in future studies. Laitinen claimed that pallidotomy allowed the dosage of levodopa to be reduced in most patients by 50% to 75%. However, most other studies, including our own, demonstrate that although many patients can reduce their total dosage of dopaminergic medication during the first few months they return to requiring the same doses as before surgery when followed for 1 year or longer. Preliminary evidence that pallidotomy alters the levodoparesponse profile (42) requires further study.

It is still uncertain which parkinsonian signs respond best to the most effective pallidal lesions. Given discrete pallidal output channels (15), it is possible that distinct pallidal areas are responsible for different clinical features; hence there may not be a single "most effective lesion site" applicable to all patients supported by the report of Kopyov et al. (24). In general, it seems that the greatest benefit is obtained regarding the signs and symptoms most responsive to levodopa. Thus off-period symptomatology is most strikingly affected, and the persistent on-period disability, unrelated to dyskinesias, demonstrates much less improvement. It is critical that future studies claiming benefit with respect to late-stage treatment-resistant symptoms clearly distinguish between those symptoms that occur only in the off condition and those that persist at times of optimal benefit (e.g., on-period freezing, postural instability, and falls). It is our impression that the latter features remain relatively resistant to pallidotomy; moreover, whereas other features show persistent benefit over the 2 years following pallidotomy, these symptoms are often worse. Levodopa-induced dyskinesias appear to respond almost universally, and a recent survey of 28 centers performing pallidotomy listed this

as the "best" indication for the procedure (6). However, it does not seem that this effect correlates with the degree of benefit obtained in other spheres. We found that ipsilateral dyskinesias are alleviated initially, but that this effect is lost between 1 and 2 years of follow-up. Contralateral dyskinesias remain markedly improved beyond 2 years postoperatively. Although Fazzini et al. reported that the dyskinesias did not return up to 4 years postoperatively (7), we saw a slight trend toward mild recurrence even at the 2-year mark.

The available series do not allow direct comparison of results obtained using microelectrode-guided surgery to those from operations performed with only macrostimulation. The latter allows localization and avoidance of nearby critical structures during the process of lesioning, whereas microrecording provides the additional ability to define accurately the sensorimotor region of the GPi. Although the large experiences of Svennilson et al. (41) and Laitinen et al. (28) and the more recent report from Kishore et al. (23) suggest that striking benefit can be obtained without microelectrode guidance, proper clinical evaluations using standardized rating scales and assessments of patients in both the on and off conditions were not performed. Although Iacono et al. have not routinely used microelectrode techniques, they too report striking improvements (19, 20). Careful evaluation of these papers raises a number of questions regarding the validity of these data. Sutton et al. (40) obtained poor results with macrorecording and stimulation, but their series was small, and at least two patients may have had atypical clinical features. Johansson et al. (21) used only macrostimulation. Dyskinesias were markedly alleviated, but the effect on the primary signs of parkinsonism were minimal. Evaluations were somewhat idiosyncratic and performed predominantly in the on state. Kishore et al. (23) emphasized that their procedure using CT scanning and macrostimulation only makes pallidotomy more widely accessible (less technically demanding and requiring a much shorter time). Although they suggested that this approach provides results that are comparable to those from studies using microelectrode recording with no greater complication rate (hemiparesis resolving by 3 weeks, 2 patients;

asymptomatic scotomas, 3; persistent facial paresis, 1), we believe that larger series with longer follow-up are required, preferably randomizing patients to microrecording or macrostimulation only. The remaining reports (1,4,7,24,34,35) have used microelectrode guidance techniques. In general, the results of these series are comparable. Finally, although gamma knife surgery has been proposed as a safer alternative to physiology-based functional surgery, aside from improvement in dyskinesias Friedman et al. reported generally poor and complicated results in four patients undergoing gamma knife pallidotomy (8). This emphasizes the poor correlation between the responses obtained for dyskinesias and those for other parkinsonian features as well as the need for at least some form of physiological guidance for the procedure.

The potential cognitive effects of pallidotomy are controversial. Svenillson et al.'s initial report (41) described significant disturbances of cognition especially in patients with "some degree of cerebral atrophy." This was particularly the case in two of the three patients undergoing bilateral procedures, and all three became "mildly demented" following the second procedure. Cognitive changes have been inconsistently documented in subsequent series. Laitinen et al. reported no cognitive or neuropsychological consequences (28), and only one patient reported by Dogali et al. experienced transient sexual disinhibition 24 hours after surgery (4). Acute transient confusion and more delayed psychosis occurred in two patients respectively in the series of Johansson et al. (21). Although Baron et al. (1) described transient postoperative confusion in "several elderly patients," they found no persistent neuropsychological changes that reached statistical significance in the ten patients who lacked postoperative complications. Studying a larger cohort in which we classified patients for analysis according to the side of lesion and evaluated them more often through the postoperative period, we have found discrete neuropsychological and behavioral changes as a consequence of pallidotomy (38). These have included measures of attention and encoding efficiency that were hemisphere-specific. In a small proportion, behavioral changes accounted for weight gain, which was substantial in 35% of our total group. Ten of our patients gained more than 10 kg, and many required dietary counseling. This potential consequence of pallidotomy, which was mentioned in the early literature (16), should be discussed with patients before surgery, and weight should be consistently evaluated during the postoperative period. Although our lesions were directed to the sensorimotor region of the internal segment of the globus pallidus, we cannot exclude the possibility that they impinged on adjacent nonmotor territories of the GPi or globus pallidus externus (GPe). We have found that some neurons in the portion of the GPi populated by movement-responsive cells can modulate their discharge activities in response to cognitive tasks (18). Additional research that carefully evaluates intraoperative neurophysiological responses and pre- and postoperative neuropsychological and behavioral parameters, as well as caloric intake and demand, may provide better understanding of these important potential consequences of pallidotomy.

The mechanisms whereby a lesion in the GPi alleviates parkinsonism are uncertain. It is assumed that the lesion reduces the excessive inhibitory effects of the pallidum on the motor thalamus, thereby allowing more normal activation of the premotor and supplementary motor cortices. Regional cerebral blood flow and metabolic studies using positron emission tomography have demonstrated increased activation of these cortical areas following pallidotomy (5, 13). Our group has demonstrated similar acute changes in response to the presumed inactivation of the GPi that occurs with high-frequency electrical stimulation (2). On the other hand, the current popular model of basal ganglia function might have predicted that pallidotomy would worsen dyskinesias as well as alleviate parkinsonism, as thalamic activation of the cortex might be excessively enhanced by the pronounced reduction in inhibitory input to the thalamus that results from a PVMP lesion. The improvement in both features suggests that elimination of abnormal patterns of pallidal activity may be more important to the clinical effects than changing the discharge rate of the pallidal neurons.

The "optimal" patient for pallidotomy remains to be defined. Our results and those of Baron et al. (1) have shown that younger patients respond better. Patients with greater disability in the on condition unrelated to dyskinesias (usually due to persistent speech disturbances and ambulatory disability) respond less well. Obviously, patients severely disabled by asymmetrical dyskinesias are excellent candidates for the procedure. Our group and others have obtained uniformly poor preliminary results in patients with other parkinsonian syndromes not responding to levodopa [e.g., striatonigral degeneration (31), progressive supranuclear palsy, corticobasal ganglionic degeneration (E. Fazzini, personal communication)]. Thus we do not offer this procedure to patients who have obtained little or no benefit from levodopa, except the rare patient with classic signs of Parkinson's disease who has been completely unable to tolerate dopaminergic medication. Patients with preexisting significant cognitive dysfunction seem to respond less well than others (1) and may be at considerable risk of further cognitive decline secondary to the procedure. Given the neuropsychological and behavioral changes that we have documented following pallidotomy, we regularly decide not to proceed to surgery in patients with impaired baseline neuropsychological function where we believe there is a substantial risk of further decline to a state of disabling cognitive dysfunction. We have also used the premorbid neuropsychological profile and our finding of hemisphere specific postoperative changes (38) to assist the decision of which side to operate on in cases with relatively symmetrical parkinsonian disability. We have also been reluctant to perform bilateral pallidotomy given our concerns about potential cognitive sequelae. This has been reinforced by experience with our first two patients who underwent staged bilateral procedures, both of whom developed disabling degrees of cognitive deterioration following a second procedure (10). We have performed one more staged bilateral pallidotomy in a patient whose neuropsychological function was entirely normal following her first surgery. A cautious, smaller, second lesion performed exclusively to relieve disabling painful off-period dystonia as well as on-period dyskinesias was successful without resulting in further cognitive decline. In five others who were continuing to experience significant disability due to persistent ipsilateral symptoms, we have implanted high-frequency deep brain stimulation (DBS) electrodes into the opposite GPi or Vim thalamus (where tremor was the greatest source of disability). Preliminary evaluation of these patients suggests that clinically important additional benefit can be obtained with this technique (9). However, these results are preliminary, and considerably more data on larger numbers of patients are required before this approach can be recommended more routinely. Iacono et al. have reported on a large number of bilateral contemporaneous pallidotomies (19,20,26); but as mentioned earlier, it is difficult to interpret the data presented in these papers and compare them to the data from other series. The New York University group reported preliminary results of staged bilateral pallidotomy in 11 patients. They concluded that bilateral pallidotomy has a narrow therapeutic window and that chronic pallidal stimulation should be considered for patients who require bilateral procedures (22). The topic of bilateral pallidotomy is dealt with in greater detail elsewhere in this book.

Finally, it is unknown how long the effects of pallidotomy persist and what the long-term outcome is for patients who have previously undergone these procedures. We found that benefit to off-period total ADL and Motor UPDRS scores (approximately 30% improvements) did not decline significantly over 2 years of follow-up. These responses were sustained predominantly for contralateral major features of parkinsonism (bradykinesia, rigidity, tremor). Ipsilateral benefit and axial (postural stability, gait, freezing) responses were modest and short-lived. Ipsilateral dyskinesias were substantially alleviated but returned to baseline between 1 and 2 years of follow-up, but contralateral dyskinesias continued to show pronounced alleviation at 2 years. These results are somewhat divergent from those of Fazzini et al. (7), who obtained more pronounced clinical responses (UPDRS scores

12 hours off medication were as low as 0–2 in some patients postoperatively even after 4 years of follow-up). They also found that ipsilateral parkinsonism declined little during the follow-up period, whereas our results show loss of original benefit. The Atlanta group have also noted progressive changes on the unoperated side (M. DeLong and J. Vitek, personal communication). Additional long-term follow-up data in larger numbers of patients from more centers are required before these differences can be understood and reconciled.

In addition to questions of persistence of benefit, it is also unclear whether patients who have previously had a pallidotomy will respond to new therapeutic strategies, for example, glutamate antagonists (14), fetal mesencephalic implantation (25), or regenerative therapies such as glial derived neurotrophic factor (11). If high-frequency stimulation of the globus pallidus (39) or subthalamic nucleus (33) is shown to be at least as safe and as effective as pallidotomy, it makes sense to offer this nondestructive approach preferentially, especially to younger patients, retaining the potential for future response to as yet undiscovered treatment modalities as they become available. However, practical issues such as cost and the amount of time required to optimize DBS parameters will strongly influence the final surgical decision.

Acknowledgments. Special thanks to Drs. J. Miyasaki and N. Galvez-Jimenez for providing valuable assistance in evaluating and caring for the patients; Dr. J. Dostrovsky for electrophysiological guidance; Dr. A. Harsin for assistance in data analysis; and Ms. S. Malton for assistance in preparing the manuscript. This work was partially supported by the Parkinson Foundation of Canada (A.L.) and a Centre of Excellence grant from the National Parkinson's Foundation (A.E.L.). Dr. Lozano is a Medical Research Council of Canada Clinician-Scientist.

REFERENCES

1. Baron MS, Vitek JL, Bakay RAE, et al. Treatment of advanced Parkinson's disease by posterior GPi pallidotomy: 1-year results of a pilot study. *Ann Neurol* 1996; 40:355–366.

2. Davis KD, Taub E, Housër D, et al. Globus pallidus stimulation activates the cortical motor system during alleviation of parkinsonian symptoms. *Nat Med* 1997;3: 671–674.

3. DeLong MR. Primate models of movement disorders of basal ganglia origin. *TINS* 1990;13:281–285.

4. Dogali M, Fazzini E, Kolodny E, et al. Stereotactic ventral pallidotomy for Parkinson's disease. *Neurology* 1995;45:753–761.

5. Eidelberg D, Moeller JR, Ishikawa T, et al. Regional metabolic correlates of surgical outcome following unilateral pallidotomy for Parkinson's disease. *Ann Neurol* 1996;39:450–459.

6. Favre J, Taha JM, Nguyen TT, Gildenberg PL, Burchiel KJ. Pallidotomy: a survey of current practice in North America. *Neurosurgery* 1996;39:883–892.

7. Fazzini E, Dogali M, Sterio D, Eidelberg D, Beric A. Stereotactic pallidotomy for Parkinson's disease: a long-term follow-up of unilateral pallidotomy. *Neurology* 1997;48:1273–1277.

8. Friedman JH, Epstein M, Sanes JN, et al. Gamma knife pallidotomy in advanced Parkinson's disease. *Ann Neurol* 1996;39:535–538.

9. Galvez-Jimenez N, Lang AK, Lozano A, et al. Deep brain stimulation in Parkinson's disease: new methods of tailoring functional surgery to patient needs and response. *Neurology* 1996;46:A402.

10. Galvez-Jimenez N, Lozano AM, Duff J, Trepanier L, Saint-Cyr JA, Lang AK. Bilateral pallidotomy pronounced amelioration of incapacitating levodopa-induced dyskinesias but accompanying cognitive decline. *Mov Disord* 1996;11:242.

11. Gash DM, Zhang ZM, Ovadia A, et al. Functional recovery in parkinsonian monkeys treated with GDNF. *Nature* 1996;380:252–255.

12. Goetz C, Stebbins GT, Shale HM, et al. Utility of an objective dyskinesia rating scale for Parkinson's disease: inter- and intrarater reliability assessment. *Mov Disord* 1994;9:390–394.

13. Grafton ST, Waters C, Sutton J, Lew MF, Couldwell W. Pallidotomy increases activity of motor association cortex in Parkinson's disease: a positron emission tomographic study. *Ann Neurol* 1995;37:776–783.

14. Greenamyre JT, O'Brien F. *N*-Methyl-D-aspartate antagonists in the treatment of Parkinson's disease. *Arch Neurol* 1991;48:977–981.

15. Hoover JE, Strick PL. Multiple output channels in the basal ganglia. *Science* 1993;259:819–821.

16. Houdart R, Mamo H. Resultats lointains de la coagulation pallidale dans les syndromes parkinsoniens. *Neurochirurgie* 1964;10:455–462.

17. Hutchison WD, Lozano AM, Davis KD, Saint-Cyr JA, Lang AK, Dostrovsky JO. Differential neuronal activity in segments of globus pallidus in Parkinson's disease patients. *Neuroreport* 1994;5:1533–1537.

18. Hutchison WD, Lozano AM, Taub E, et al. Cognitive modulation of human globus pallidus (GP) neurons. *Soc Neurosci* 1996;22:118.

19. Iacono RP, Lonser RR, Ulloth JE, Shima F. Posteroventral pallidotomy in Parkinson's disease. *J Clin Neurosci* 1995;2:140–145.

20. Iacono RP, Shima F, Lonser RR, Kuniyoshi S, Maeda G, Yamada S. The results, indications, and physiology of

posteroventral pallidotomy for patients with Parkinson's disease. *Neurosurgery* 1995;36:1118–1127.

21. Johansson F, Malm J, Nordh E, Hariz M. Usefulness of pallidotomy in advanced Parkinson's disease. *J Neurol Neurosurg Psychiatry* 1997; 62:125–132.

22. Kim R, Alterman R, Kelly P, et al. Efficacy of bilateral pallidotomy. Presented at the 46th Annual Congress of Neurological Surgeons, Sept 28–Oct 3, 1996.

23. Kishore A, Turnbull IM, Snow BJ, et al. Effcacy, stability and predictors of outcome of pallidotomy for Parkinson's disease: six-month follow-up with additional 1-year observations. *Brain* 1997;120:729–737.

24. Kopyov O, Jacques D, Duma C, et al. Microelectrode-guided posteroventral medial radiofrequency pallidotomy for Parkinson's disease. *J Neurosurg* 1997;87:52–59.

25. Kordower JH, Freeman TB, Snow BJ, et al. Neuropathological evidence of graft survival and striatal reinnervation after the transplantation of fetal mesencephalic tissue in a patient with Parkinson's disease. *N Engl J Med* 1995;332:1118–1124.

26. Krayenbuhl H, Wyss O, Yasargil M. Bilateral thalamotomy and pallidotomy as treatment for bilateral parkinsonism. *J Neurosurg* 1961;18:429–444.

27. Laitinen LV. Pallidotomy for Parkinson's disease. *Neurosurg Clin North Am* 1995;6:105–112.

28. Laitinen LV, Bergenheim AT, Hariz MI. Leksell's posteroventral pallidotomy in the treatment of Parkinson's disease. *J Neurosurg* 1992;76:53–61.

29. Lang AK, Benabid A-L, Koller WC, et al. The Core Assessment Program for Intracerebral Transplantation. *Mov Disord* 1995;10:527–528.

30. Lang AK, Fahn S. Assessment of Parkinson's disease. In: Munsat TL, ed. *Quantification of neurological deficit.* Stoneham: Butterworths, 1989:285–309.

31. Lang AK, Lozano A, Duff J, et al. Medial pallidotomy in late-stage parkinson's disease and striatonigral degeneration. In: Marsden CD, Obeso JA, Delong M, Ohye C, eds. *Advances in understanding the basal ganglia and new surgical approaches for Parkinson's disease.* New York: Lippincott-Raven, 1997:199–211.

32. Langston J, Widner H, Goetz C, et al. Core Assessment Program for Intracerebral Transplantations (CAPIT). *Mov Disord* 1992; 7:2–13.

33. Limousin P, Pollak P, Benazzouz A, et al. Effect on parkinsonian signs and symptoms of bilateral subthalamic nucleus stimulation. *Lancet* 1995;345:91–95.

34. Lozano A, Hutchison W, Kiss Z, Tasker R, Davis K, Dostrovsky J. Methods for microelectrode-guided posteroventral pallidotomy. *J Neurosurg* 1996;84:194–202.

35. Lozano AM, Lang AK, Galvez-Jimenez N, et al. Effect of GPi pallidotomy on motor function in Parkinson's disease. *Lancet* 1995;346:1383–1387.

36. Marsden CD, Obeso JA. The functions of the basal ganglia and the paradox of stereotaxic surgery in Parkinson's disease. *Brain* 1994;117:877–897.

37. Narabayashi H, Yokochi F, Nakajima Y. Levodopa-induced dyskinesia and thalamotomy. *J Neurol Neurosurg Psychiatry* 1984;47:831–839.

38. Saint-Cyr JA, Trepanier LL, Lang AK, Lozano AM. Neuropsychological outcome of posteroventral pallidotomy in parkinsonian patients. *Mov Disord* 1996;11:161 (abst).

39. Siegfried J, Lippitz B. Bilateral chronic electrostimulation of ventroposterolateral pallidum: a new therapeutic approach for alleviating all parkinsonian symptoms. *Neurosurgery* 1994;35:1126–1130.

40. Sutton JP, Couldwell W, Lew MF, et al. Ventroposterior medial pallidotomy in patients with advanced Parkinson's disease. *Neurosurgery* 1995;36: 1112–1117.

41. Svennilson E, Torvik A, Lowe R, Leksell L. Treatment of parkinsonism by stereotactic thermo lesions in the pallidal region: a clinical evaluation of 81 cases. *Acta Psychiatr Neurol Scand* 1960;35:358–377.

42. Verhagen L, Mouradian MM, Chase TN. Altered levodopa dose-response profile following pallidotomy. *Neurology* 1996;46:416–417.

43. Wenning GK, Ben Shlomo Y, Magalhaes M, Daniel SE, Quinn NP. Clinical features and natural history of multiple system atrophy: an analysis of 100 cases. *Brain* 1994;117:835–845.

Pallidal Surgery for the Treatment of Parkinson's Disease and Movement Disorders, edited by J. K. Krauss, R. G. Grossman, and J. Jankovic. Lippincott–Raven Publishers , Philadelphia © 1998.

11

Bilateral Pallidotomy for the Treatment of Parkinson's Disease

Jamal M. Taha, *Jacques Favre, and †Kim J. Burchiel

*Division of Functional Neurosurgery, Mayfield Clinic and Department of Neurosurgery, University of Cincinnati Medical Center and Veterans Affairs Medical Center, Cincinnati, Ohio 45219, USA; *Department of Neurosurgery, Centre Hospitalier Universitaire Vaudois, Lousanne, Switzerland; and †Department of Neurosurgery, Oregon Health Sciences University, Portland, Oregon 97201-3098,USA*

Pallidotomy is a safe and effective treatment for Parkinson's disease (1,10,12,13,24). After unilateral pallidotomy, the therapeutic window of dopaminergic medications usually widens secondary to improvements in both "off" symptoms (i.e., bradykinesia, rigidity, tremor) and "on" symptoms (i.e., dyskinesia). In addition, the abrupt fluctuations between off and on cycles diminish, and patients usually spend more time in the on than in the off cycle (25).

After unilateral pallidotomy, appendicular symptoms (e.g., limb rigidity, bradykinesia, tremor, dystonia, dyskinesia, muscle spasms) mostly improve on the side contralateral to the pallidotomy. Some improvement of dyskinesia of the ipsilateral limbs can also occur, but it is rarely spectacular. Other symptoms that can improve after unilateral pallidotomy include some axial symptoms (e.g., walking, balance, speech) and other general symptoms (e.g., freezing, night sleep).

Many patients with Parkinson's disease suffer from severe bilateral appendicular off (i.e., bradykinesia, rigidity, tremor) and on (dyskinesia, dystonia) symptoms. After unilateral pallidotomy several of these patients still suffer from severe rigidity, tremor, or dyskinesia of the ipsilateral side, in which case a contralateral pallidotomy is considered. In addition, many patients with Parkinson's disease suffer from severe axial and general symptoms, such as walking difficulty, freezing, and trunk, neck, or facial dyskinesia, which may not be significantly alleviated after unilateral pallidotomy. In such patients one can argue for consideration of bilateral pallidotomy performed simultaneously or on separate occasions (i.e., staged). There is a sense in the literature of the hazard of creating simultaneous symmetrical deep brain lesions (14). This fear was confirmed by the relatively high complication rates associated with bilateral thalamotomy or bilateral lesions of the mesial temporal structures.

In this chapter we review the results of bilateral pallidotomy in the recent literature as well as our personal experience. We compare the benefits and risks of bilateral pallidotomy with unilateral pallidotomy and of simultaneous pallidotomy with staged pallidotomy. Based on this review, we discuss the indications for bilateral pallidotomy and its role in the overall surgical treatment of Parkinson's disease.

LITERATURE REVIEW

Series reported on the results of bilateral pallidotomy have been rare in the recent literature. In one survey of the practice of pallidotomy in North America in 1996 (4), 20% of 1,015 patients who underwent pallidotomy had bilateral procedures, either staged (7%) or simultaneous (13%), but the clinical results were not reported. There have been mixed "feelings" about the results of bilateral pallidotomy in peer review journals and at international meetings.

Laitinen et al. in 1992 (12) reported the results of four patients who underwent bilateral pallidotomy 6 to 14 months apart. All four patients showed "considerable improvement although one patient had unilateral recurrence of the symptoms 8 weeks after the second operation." He added that "one patient who had been bedridden for 3 years began to walk with assistance after her second pallidotomy. Her condition remained stable for 4 years." In 1995 Laitinen (11) expanded the series to a total of 12 patients who underwent bilateral pallidotomy. Of these 12 patients, 10 had good results and 2 had fair results; none suffered from side effects during a short-term follow-up, the length of which was not specified. One of these patients had been operated in 1960 by Leksell and 33 years later was still in a "fairly good neurological condition." Despite the reports of favorable results with staged pallidotomy, Laitinen advised against simultaneous bilateral pallidotomy to reduce complications such as postoperative walking and balance difficulties (personal communication, March 1995).

The largest experience with bilateral pallidotomy has been reported by Iacono et al. (8). In 1995 this group reported the results of 126 patients who underwent pallidotomy and were followed for 1 week to 12 months (mean 4.5 months). Of these patients, 68 had bilateral pallidotomy: 49 simultaneous and 19 staged 4 to 14 months (mean 7 months) apart. Compared to unilateral pallidotomy, bilateral pallidotomy was not associated with an increased risk of complications. In addition, staged and simultaneous pallidotomies had similar complication rates. In 1996 Iacono et al. (7) expanded their series to 242 patients: 91 patients had unilateral pallidotomy, 128 patients had simultaneous bilateral pallidotomy, and 23 patients had bilateral staged pallidotomies. Of 171 patients who were followed for 6 to 30 months (mean 19 months), 97% who underwent bilateral pallidotomy had excellent or good results compared to 70% who underwent unilateral pallidotomy. Outcomes of cognitive function were analyzed on 10 consecutive patients who underwent simultaneous bilateral pallidotomy. These patients were tested using the Wechsler Memory Scale (WMS) before and 1 week after surgery, during on states. All 10 patients had preoperative impairment of spatial recognition memory. Postoperatively, four of five normative age-weighted indexes for delayed recall, verbal, visual, and general memory improved significantly. In addition, significant improvement occurred in Logical Memory I and II, Visual Reproduction II, and Verbal Paired Associated II, which tested the temporal delay and frontostriatal cognitive functions (6). Based on their experience, Iacono et al. concluded the following: First, after unilateral pallidotomy there was improvement in the contralateral appendicular symptoms and in the axial symptoms, which involved gait, posture, and body bradykinesia; however, patients with severe bilateral appendicular symptoms usually requested another operation for the ipsilateral side. Second, compared to patients who had unilateral pallidotomy, patients with bilateral pallidotomies were able to sustain a more stabilized level of improvement over a longer period. Third, simultaneous bilateral pallidotomy was superior to staged pallidotomy for reasons that included reduced cost, less surgery, and simpler surgery: Data obtained for calculating the pallidotomy target on one side can be immediately used to target the opposite side. Fourth, after simultaneous bilateral pallidotomy, a higher level of motor performance was obtained compared to the preoperative performance. Iacono et al. attributed this improvement to improved sequential programming abilities and processing of information input, especially those related to learned conditional associations, temporal ordering of events, assessment of relative frequency, and recency of stimuli. They attributed this result to postoperative disinhibition of tegmental pedunculopontine pathways and the release of brainstem reticular functioning.

Other investigators also reported briefly on their experiences with bilateral pallidotomy. Patil and Wong (15) reported the results of 80 patients who underwent pallidotomy: 36 patients had unilateral pallidotomy, 22 patients had staged pallidotomies, and 20 patients had simultaneous bilateral pallidotomy. Although they did not specifically analyze the results of each patient group, 74 patients were satisfied with the outcome of surgery. Scott and colleagues (21) studied the intellectual, psychological, and functional outcomes of 20 patients before and 3 months after unilateral (n = 12) and simultaneous bilateral (n = 8) pallidotomy. Postoperatively Unified Parkinson's Disease Rating Scale (UPDRS) scores improved more with bilateral pallidotomy (53%) than with unilateral pallidotomy (27%). A fall in diadochokinetic rates and subjective reports of worsened preexisting dysarthria, hypophonia, and hypersalivation followed bilateral pallidotomy, but these changes did not have functional consequences. One of the eight patients who underwent bilateral pallidotomy had some generalized cognitive impairment postoperatively.

Despite the above-mentioned preliminary favorable results of bilateral pallidotomy, this procedure has not been widely accepted in the neurosurgical and neurological communities. As a matter of fact, many stereotactic surgeons and expert neurologists warn against bilateral pallidotomy at international meetings. This fear stems mainly from unreported complications related mainly to postoperative speech and cognitive impairments following bilateral pallidotomy. In early studies, large bilateral lesions in the globus pallidus caused akinesia (3,16,17), but these lesions may have been placed too medially. Some investigators have now reported increased deficits after bilateral pallidotomy including cognition, speech, and drooling (20). Roberts and Heilbrun (19) reported that 6 of 58 patients who underwent pallidotomy had staged surgery. Although dyskinesia was further improved after the second surgery, 4 patients suffered from increased hypophonia and drooling. Ghika et al. (5) reported significant motoric benefit in four patients after simultaneous bilateral pallidotomy; however, these patients had increased cognitive impairment on detailed postoperative neuropsychological examination. Rabey et al. (18) found no cognitive dysfunction after staged bilateral pallidotomy but achieved no motoric improvement, a finding shared by Kim et al. (9). Vitek and Bakay (25) summarized the experience of the Atlanta group on seven patients who under-

went bilateral pallidotomy. Motor function improved, and salivation problems were mild and intermittent. Hypophonia of varying degrees was a consistent observation, with some experiencing significant hypophonia and others very little. Formal neuropsychological evaluations of two patients revealed no evidence of cognitive decline. Five other patients were not formally evaluated but demonstrated no clinical evidence of cognitive decline.

PERSONAL EXPERIENCE

To clarify the outcome of patients who undergo bilateral pallidotomy, we reviewed our experiences with unilateral (n = 25), staged bilateral (n = 9), and simultaneous bilateral (n = 25) posteroventral pallidotomy on 59 patients with Parkinson's disease. Most of these patients were operated on at Oregon Health Sciences University between 1995 and 1996 using the Leksell stereotactic system, guided by magnetic resonance imaging (MRI). The pallidal target was measured 2 mm anterior to the midcommissure, 3 to 6 mm below the intercommissural line, and 19 to 22 mm lateral to the midline, just lateral to the optic tract. The final target was determined by intraoperative microrecording of pallidal discharges, pallidal base, and optic tract evoked responses, and by macrostimulation techniques (2,22,23). For simultaneous pallidotomy, the location of the final target on one side was translated to the opposite side and confirmed by macrostimulation techniques. The pallidotomy lesion consisted of three thermal lesions on each side, linearly spaced 2 mm apart along the same trajectory. Each lesion was created by heating a 1.16×2.00 mm electrode tip (Radionics, Burlington, MA) to 84°C for 60 seconds. Patients were evaluated using a Visual Analogue Scale that ranged from 0 to 100 mm (0 = no symptom, 100 = worst symptom) before and 6 months after operation.

We analyzed the percentage of patients who improved or worsened after surgery (Table 11-1). It is noteworthy that in several patients postoperative worsening reflected symptoms that had been rapidly becoming more pronounced preoperatively. In addition, many patients were undermedicated after surgery. Compared to unilateral

TABLE 11-1. *Results of unilateral (n=25) and simultaneous bilateral (n=25) pallidotomy*

Symptom	Unilateral pallidotomy (%)			Bilateral pallidotomy (%)		
	Better	Same	Worse	Better	Same	Worse
Bradykinesia	57	7	36	62	17	21
Rigidity	69	2	29	77	16	7
Tremor	54	7	43	70	9	21
Dyskinesia	67	29	14	92	8	0
Walking	50	21	29	67	4	29
Balance	43	21	36	50	14	36
Freezing	43	21	36	64	21	14
Muscle pain	50	43	7	57	36	7
Voice volume	21	29	43	7	22	71
Speech	39	11	50	19	31	50
Swallowing	29	29	43	29	29	43
Drooling	7	64	29	7	22	71
Writing	21	50	29	29	29	43
Memory	36	14	50	0	86	14
Concentration	36	29	36	36	36	29
Depression	36	21	43	18	71	11
Night sleep	64	14	21	43	29	29
Overall "on"	57	7	36	71	29	0
Overall "off"	57	7	36	64	7	29
Duration "off"	57	29	14	71	21	7
Global	50	21	29	50	29	21

pallidotomy, more patients after simultaneous bilateral pallidotomy achieved alleviation of overall dyskinesias, tremor, rigidity, freezing, walking, overall function in the on state, and overall function in the off state. In addition, more patients who underwent simultaneous bilateral pallidotomy spent less time in the off state (Table 11-1). More patients had increased drooling and hypophonia after bilateral pallidotomy than after unilateral pallidotomy. Although formal neuropsychological examination was not performed, patients and their families did not report a difference in postoperative memory, concentration, or overall cognitive function between unilateral and bilateral pallidotomy.

We also analyzed the degree of postoperative change after unilateral and simultaneous bilateral pallidotomy (Fig. 11-1). Compared to unilateral pallidotomy, bilateral pallidotomy achieved better median improvement in bradykinesia, rigidity, tremor, dyskinesia, balance, and walking. Bilateral pallidotomy had a slight higher median worsening of speech; but in only a few patients did speech worsening affect the overall function of the patient. There was no difference in the median postoperative change in memory and depression after unilateral and simultaneous bilateral pallidotomy. Staged and simultaneous bilateral pallidotomy produced similar overall improvement.

TABLE 11-2. *Patient rating of outcome of unilateral and simultaneous bilateral pallidotomy*

Result	Unilateral pallidotomy (*n* = 25)	Bilateral pallidotomy (*n* = 25)
Outcome		
Excellent	43	36
Good	21	36
Fair	7	7
Poor	29	21
Repeat procedure		
Yes	79	79
No	21	21

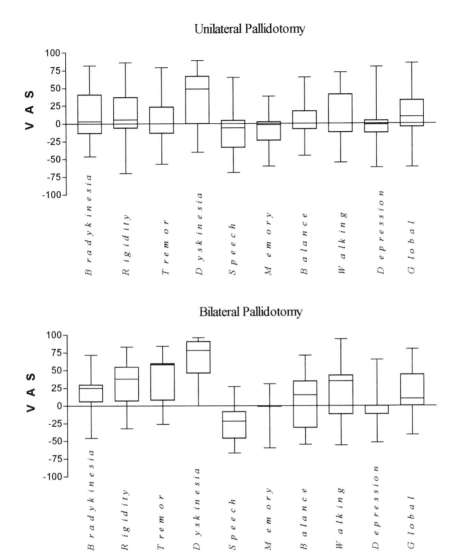

FIG. 11-1. Visual analogue scale (*VAS*) for unilateral and bilateral pallidotomy.

We analyzed the patients' satisfaction of outcome for unilateral and simultaneous bilateral pallidotomy (Table 11-2). Excellent or good results were reported by 64% of patients who had unilateral pallidotomy and by 72% of patients who had bilateral pallidotomy; 79% of those who had unilateral or simultaneous bilateral pallidotomy said they would undergo the procedure again, knowing the final outcome, and would recommend it for other patients.

Based on our results, we conclude that bilateral pallidotomy achieves superior alleviation of nega-

tive and positive symptoms of Parkinson's disease compared to unilateral pallidotomy. There does not appear to be an appreciable, clinically important increased risk of cognitive impairment after bilateral pallidotomy, but there is an increased risk of hypophonia and drooling. These risks do not appear to diminish by staging the procedure.

CONCLUSIONS

Controversy exists about the benefits and risks of bilateral pallidotomy. Several investigators report better improvement in motor function after bilateral pallidotomy than after unilateral pallidotomy but with an increased risk of hypophonia. We can report the same experience, although most of the patients who developed hypophonia did not consider their speech to be severely affected. Some investigators report increased cognitive deficit after bilateral pallidotomy, but others do not share their view. In our experience, patients who had bilateral pallidotomy did not suffer from gross cognitive deficit. We conclude that, compared to unilateral pallidotomy, bilateral pallidotomy achieves better "good outcome" and worse "bad outcome." Staging the procedure does not appear to decrease the risks associated with simultaneous surgery.

REFERENCES

1. Baron MS, Vitek JL, Bakay RAE, et al. Treatment of advanced Parkinson's disease with microelectrode-guided pallidotomy: 1 year pilot-study results. *Ann Neurol* 1996;40:355–366.
2. Burchiel KJ, Taha JM, Favre J. Pallidotomy for Parkinson's disease. In: Rengachary S, Wilkins R, eds. *Neurosurgical operative atlas*, vol 6. Park Ridge, Illinois:AANS Publications, 1997;13–26.
3. Carey JH. Certain anatomical and functional interrelations between the tegmentum of the midbrain and the basal ganglia. *J Comp Neurol* 1957;108:57–62.
4. Favre J, Taha JM, Nguyen TT, Gildenberg PL, Burchiel KJ. Pallidotomy: a survey of current practice in North America. *Neurosurgery* 1996;39:883–892.
5. Ghika J, Favre J, Fankhauser H, Regli F. Neurological and neuropsychological complications of bilateral contemporaneous pallidotomy in Parkinson's disease. *Proceedings of the American Association of Neurology* 1996;46[suppl]:A417.
6. Iacono RP, Mohamed AS, Kraus CE. Motor and cognitive improvement following contemporaneous bilateral posteroventral pallidoansotomy in idiopathic Parkinson's disease. *Presented at the AANS Annual Meeting,* Minneapolis, 1996 (poster).
7. Iacono RP, Mohamed AS, Kuniyoshi S. Complication and avoidance techniques for 242 consecutive Parkinson's patients following pallidoansotomy. Presented at the AANS Annual Meeting, Minneapolis, 1996 (poster).
8. Iacono RP, Shima F, Lonser RR, Kuniyoshi S, Maeda G, Yamada S. The results, indications, and physiology of posteroventral pallidotomy for patients with Parkinson's disease. *Neurosurgery* 1995;36:1118–1125.
9. Kim R, Alterman R, Kelly P, Fazzini E, Beric A, Eidelberg D. Efficacy of bilateral pallidotomy. In: Proceedings of the Congress of Neurologic Surgeons 46th Annual Meeting 1996:269 (abst).
10. Krauss JK, Desaloms M, Lai E, King D, Jankovic J, Grossman RG. Microelectrode-guided posteroventral pallidotomy for treatment of Parkinson's disease: postoperative magnetic resonance imaging analysis. *J Neurosurg* 1997;87:358–367.
11. Laitinen LV. Pallidotomy for Parkinson's disease. *Neurosurg Clin North Am* 1995;6:105–112.
12. Laitinen LV, Bregenheim T, Hariz M. Leksell's posteroventral pallidotomy in the treatment of Parkinson's disease. *J Neurosurg* 1992;76:53–61
13. Lozano AM, Lang AE, Galvez-Jimenez N, et al.: Effect of GPi pallidotomy on motor function in Parkinson's disease. *Lancet* 1995;346:1383–1387.
14. Narabayashi H. Surgical treatment in the levodopa era. In: Stern G, ed. *Parkinson's disease.* London: Chapman & Hall, 1990:597–646.
15. Patil A, Wong S. Bipolar macroelectrode for pallidotomy. *Presented at the AANS Annual Meeting,* Minneapolis (abst).
16. Poirier LJ: Experimental and histological study of midbrain dyskinesias. *J Neurophysiol* 1960;23:534–359.
17. Poirier LJ. Physiopathology of akinesia. In: Siegfried J, ed. *Parkinson's disease,* vol 1. Berlin: Hans Huber, 1973:115–126
18. Rabey JM, Orlov E, Spiegelman R. Levodopa-induced dyskinesias are the main features improved by contralateral pallidotomy in Parkinson's disease: 2-year follow-up. Presented at the AANS 121st Annual Meeting 1996:71 (abst).
19. Roberts JW, Heilbrun PM. Prospective assessment of patients receiving ventroposterolateral pallidotomy in Parkinson's disease. *Stereotact Funct Neurosurg* 1996-1997;67(1):152 (abst).
20. Saint-Cyr J, Trepanier L, Lang A, Lozano A. Neuropsychological outcome of posteroventral pallidotomy in Parkinsonian patients. *Mov Disord* 1996;11[Suppl 1]:161 (P597).
21. Scott R, Gregory R, Carroll C, et al. Neuropsychological, neurological, and functional outcome following pallidotomy for Parkinson's disease: a consecutive series of 8 simultaneous bilateral and 12 unilateral procedures. *Brain* (in press).
22. Taha JM, Favre J, Baumann TK, Burchiel KJ. Characteristics and somatotopic organization of kinesthetic cells in the globus pallidus of patients with Parkinson's disease. *J Neurosurg* 1996;85:1005–1012.
23. Taha JM, Favre J, Baumann TK, Burchiel KJ. Functional anatomy of the pallidal base in Parkinson's disease. *Neurosurgery* 1996;39:1164–1168.
24. Taha JM, Favre J, Baumann TK, Burchiel KJ. Tremor control after pallidotomy for Parkinson's disease: correlation with microrecording findings. *J Neurosurg* 1997;86:642–647.
25. Vitek JL, Bakay RA. The role of pallidotomy in Parkinson's disease and dystonia. *Curr Opin Neurol* 1997;10:332–339.

Pallidal Surgery for the Treatment of Parkinson's Disease and Movement Disorders, edited by
J. K. Krauss, R. G. Grossman, and J. Jankovic.
Lippincott-Raven Publishers, Philadelphia © 1998.

12

Pallidotomy: A Treatment for Parkinsonian Tremor?

Monique L. Giroux and Jerrold L. Vitek

Department of Neurology, Emory University School of Medicine, Atlanta, Georgia 30322, USA

The 1992 report of Laitinen et al. (34) describing complete or near-complete relief of rigidity, hypokinesia, and tremor in patients with Parkinson's disease (PD) undergoing posteroventral pallidotomy revived interest in surgical approaches to the treatment of PD. Subsequently, numerous studies have reported total or partial alleviation of dyskinesia, motor fluctuations, rigidity, and bradykinesia following pallidotomy (4,8,9,26,29,32,41,56, 63,74). The effect of pallidotomy on parkinsonian tremor has been more controversial. This point is of particular importance, as tremor, independent of other parkinsonian symptoms, is often refractory to medical management (28). Therefore for PD patients with functionally disabling tremor, stereotactic surgery may offer the only hope for improvement.

Lesions in both the thalamus (ventralis intermedius, Vim) and the pallidum (internal segment of the globus pallidus, GPi) have been reported to be effective treatment for parkinsonian tremor. The earlier literature generally considered tremor poorly responsive to pallidotomy (15,16,19,20, 30,44). Although pallidotomy was able to improve tremor in some cases, most reports considered it more effective for rigidity. Other sites were explored, and thalamotomy soon became the surgical procedure of choice for the treatment of parkinsonian tremor, with pallidotomy being performed infrequently. Thalamotomy may also alleviate rigidity and drug-induced dyskinesia, but it has little effect on bradykinesia and may be associated with a worsening of gait and speech

(46,66). Thus thalamotomy may provide a less than optimal surgical alternative for PD patients with medically intractable tremor in whom other parkinsonian symptoms coexist.

During the 1950s and 1960s little was known about the underlying functional organization of the basal ganglia and the target for pallidotomy, in general, was more anterior and dorsal in the GPi. Thus lesions were targeted to nonmotor portions of the GPi and likely account for the poor effect of pallidotomy on parkinsonian tremor reported in the past.

At present there are a variety of opinions concerning the effectiveness of pallidotomy for tremor. A survey examining the current practice of pallidotomy in North America has been completed by 28 centers (12). Indications for pallidotomy were rated from 1 (poor indication) to 4 (excellent indication). Tremor was considered a marginal indication for pallidotomy, with a median score of 2. Additional editorial comments concerning the effectiveness of pallidotomy for tremor ranged from "less or no effect on tremor" (17) to "tremor is variably responsive" (49) to "fair to very good" (33). With one exception (33), these editorials did not reference published data or refer to outcome studies to support their conclusions. Thus the basis for these conclusions is unclear and appears to result from personal experience, word of mouth, or dogma taken from the early literature.

This chapter reviews the contemporary literature on pallidotomy and its effect on parkinsonian tremor. In addition, the rationale for pallidotomy for tremor alleviation is discussed in light of current concepts regarding the pathophysiology of parkinsonian tremor. Finally, a variety of factors that may play a critical role in determining the effect of pallidotomy on tremor are examined.

HISTORICAL PERSPECTIVE

James Parkinson's original monograph, *An Essay on the Shaking Palsy,* described a patient whose tremor abated after hemiplegic stroke (52). This observation led to surgical lesioning of the motor and premotor cortex and represents one of the earliest descriptions of surgical intervention for parkinsonian symptoms (6). Although tremor was alleviated, the resultant spastic hemiplegia limited the effectiveness of this procedure; and interest soon turned to other sites (19,42,58,62).

Multiple centers now perform pallidotomy for Parkinson's disease (PD). Despite current reports documenting tremor alleviation following pallidotomy (4,8,9,26,29,32,41,56), previous impressions (15,16,19,20,30,44) of the ineffectiveness of pallidotomy on tremor have persisted. One reason for this impression may lie in the intermittent reappearance of parkinsonian tremor during periods of stress and its often slow disappearance after pallidotomy. This is in stark contrast to the abrupt and complete amelioration of tremor immediately following thalamotomy and may contribute to the belief that pallidotomy is not as effective as thalamotomy for parkinsonian tremor. The basis for these observations and their implication regarding the choice of target sites for the surgical treatment of parkinsonian tremor, however, requires a better understanding of the pathophysiological basis underlying its development.

PATHOPHYSIOLOGY OF PARKINSONIAN TREMOR

The role of the basal ganglia, or more specifically the GPi, in the development of parkinsonian tremor must be interpreted within the framework of two basic hypotheses proposed to describe the pathophysiological basis of tremor: the peripheral feedback and central oscillator hypotheses.

The peripheral feedback hypothesis describes the role of stretch reflex loops and limb mechanics on tremor production, whereas the central oscillator hypothesis implicates bursting activity in a group or groups of neurons in the central nervous system as the cause of tremor. As pointed out by Elble, the expression of tremor follows nonlinear properties; that is, expression of tremor is the property of system variables. Hence a perturbation at one site may interact in a complex manner with a distant site to produce tremor (10). In the case of parkinsonian rest tremor, it is conceivable, even likely, that the peripheral feedback and central oscillator theories are not mutually exclusive. Thus the theoretical basis for the effect of pallidotomy on tremor must be examined within the context of both models and the interaction between them.

Peripheral Feedback Hypothesis

According to the peripheral feedback model, parkinsonian tremor results from the instability of long-latency reflex loops (55,67). Support for this theory comes from the observation that mechanical loads placed on the tremulous limb may alter the amplitude, frequency and phase of tremor (25,54,61,67). Consistent with this theory, PD patients have an increased M2 component of their long loop reflexes (67). The increased magnitude of neuronal responses in the GPi to torque perturbations in the parkinsonian monkey and the altered receptive field properties of neurons in the GPi reported to occur in both parkinsonian monkeys (14,43) and patients with idiopathic PD (a larger percentage of pallidal neurons respond to passive manipulation of the limbs) (60, 64,70) are also consistent with this hypothesis. In these high-gain circuits, it is not difficult to understand how internal oscillations may develop and contribute to the development of parkinsonian tremor.

In the simplified case, where peripheral mechanisms are the sole cause for tremor, tremor frequency would be expected to be proportional to the length of the reflex arc; and interruption of the reflex arc by ablation or electrical stimulation should abolish the tremor. Deafferentation of the upper limb in a patient with postencephalitic parkinsonism by dorsal rhizotomy, however, did not abolish tremor, although its amplitude was reduced (53). These observations suggest that peripheral factors may contribute to, but cannot by themselves account for, the development of parkinsonian tremor and have therefore led to the consideration of other mechanisms.

Central Oscillator Hypothesis

The development of central oscillators may also provide a mechanism for the genesis of parkinsonian tremor (27,36,40,45,47). According to this hypothesis, tremor occurs as the result of unregulated rhythmic activity that occurs in groups of neurons in the central nervous system whose intrinsic membrane properties may promote such patterns of neuronal activity. Support for this concept is provided by in vitro slice recordings from neurons in the guinea pig thalamus (27,40). In this preparation, membrane hyperpolarization of thalamic neurons promotes rhythmically bursting activity by deinactivating low-threshold calcium channels, which induce a rebound excitation. Thus excessive inhibitory output from the GPi to the thalamus could hyperpolarize thalamic neurons and induce a burst-promoting state (14,27, 40).

Additional support for the thalamus as a central oscillator and the central oscillator hypothesis is derived from experiments in monkeys with tremor induced by ventromedial tegmental midbrain lesions (35). In this model of parkinsonian tremor, bursting activity synchronous with electromyographic (EMG) activity has been recorded in portions of the thalamus just anterior to the lemniscal relay nuclei and is unaltered following deafferentation by dorsal rhizotomy or the removal of peripheral feedback via neuromuscular blockade (36,48). Such tremor-synchronous neuronal activity in the thalamus has been recorded in a variety of tremor types, including parkinsonian, essential, and cerebellar tremor; and thalamotomy has proved effective in alleviating each of these tremors (3,11,22,37,39,68). These data provide further support for the role of the thalamus as a central oscillator involved in the genesis of parkinsonian and other types of tremor.

In addition to the thalamus, other sites within the central nervous system may act as oscillators and contribute to the development of parkinsonian tremor. Cells with bursting activity synchronous with 4- to 5-Hz tremor have been found in both the GPi and the subthalamic nucleus (STN) in N-methyl-4-phenyl-1,2,3,6-tetrahydropyridine (MPTP)-treated parkinsonian monkeys (5,73) and in the GPi of patients with idiopathic PD (7, 63,64). Furthermore, neurons in the GPi, similar to those in the thalamus, have inherent oscillatory properties. In vitro slice recordings from guinea pig GPi demonstrated a propensity toward bursting activity when GPi neurons were hyperpolarized (45). In vivo, GPi neurons in the rhesus monkey have been observed to discharge in a 12- to 15-Hz bursting pattern following treatment with MPTP and the development of parkinsonian motor signs (13,43). Interestingly, this bursting pattern of activity has been observed in animals that did not manifest tremor, although a second bursting pattern at a lower frequency (5–7 Hz) has been observed to occur coincident with the development of tremor (13).

Thus the GPi may serve as a central oscillator or promote oscillatory activity in thalamocortical neurons by putting them into a burst-promoting state. Pare et al. (50) offered evidence to suggest that hyperpolarizing pulses from the GPi may serve to entrain thalamic discharges at a rate consistent with parkinsonian tremor. Thus reduction of excessive tonic or burst-related activity in the GPi by pallidotomy would remove the transmission of tonic and bursting activity from the GPi to the thalamus and reduce the incidence of bursting activity in thalamic neurons. Reorganization of membrane and network properties of thalamic neurons and thalamocortical projections, however, may require time and could account for the delayed alleviation of parkinsonian tremor that has been observed to occur over weeks to months following pallidotomy. In addition, because thalamic neurons are still present, they remain capable of generating or transmitting bursting activity from other sites (i.e., cerebellothalamic or the pedunculopontine nucleus, or both). Residual portions of the GPi may also continue to promote or transmit bursting activity to thalamic neurons. Thus under the appropriate conditions, parkinsonian tremor could reemerge following pallidotomy, but the capability of the system to do so is likely to be significantly compromised by lesions in the sensorimotor portion of the GPi.

In addition to the GPi and the thalamus, neurons in the motor cortex may also discharge in bursts when hyperpolarized. Given the reduced mean discharge rate reported in the motor thalamus in parkinsonian monkeys (72), such activity could develop in the motor cortex as a result of loss of excitatory input from the thalamus to layer 5 pyramidal neurons, leading to hyperpolarization and the development of a burst-promoting state (23,31,57). Thus even the motor cortex may, under the appropriate conditions, serve as a central oscillator.

Functional Network Involved in Tremor

In patients with PD central oscillators have been demonstrated to exist at multiple sites within the pallidothalamocortical circuit, and the responsiveness of neurons to afferent input is increased throughout the circuit. Models of parkinsonian tremor, based on recordings of central oscillatory activity and the effect of peripheral afferent feedback, suggest that both central and peripheral factors contribute to its development (55). The combination of central oscillatory activity and peripheral afferent feedback loops form a neuronal network with an intrinsic tendency to oscillate dependent on local environment and network properties—properties that are themselves in a dynamic state. It is not difficult to understand why some patients with tremor respond to dopaminergic therapy and others to anticholinergic medication, whereas still others do not respond to any pharmacological treatment. Similarly, the various combinations of rest, posture, and action tremor seen in different patients likely results from the complex interaction between different oscillators and their interaction with peripheral afferent systems. Should all parkinsonian tremor respond to pallidotomy, given this scenario of multiple oscillators at multiple sites? One might suggest—no. Yet the multiple oscillators appear to form a central circuit, with each component contributing to the development of tremorgenic activity within the circuit. Therefore based on this hypothesis, lesions at the different

sites, so long as they interrupt the circuit or interfere with the network, would be expected to reduce or alleviate tremor.

EFFECT OF POSTEROVENTRAL PALLIDOTOMY ON PARKINSONIAN TREMOR: CONTEMPORARY LITERATURE

Over the last decade numerous reports have emerged describing the effectiveness of pallidotomy in treating parkinsonian motor signs. This section reviews the contemporary pallidotomy literature with a specific focus on tremor and the clinical variables that contribute to its outcome.

Clinical Studies

Laitinen et al. reported favorable results in regard to tremor in patients undergoing pallidotomy between 1985 and 1990 (34). The lesion target was defined by computed tomography (CT)-guided stereotactic coordinates and electrical stimulation. Of 32 patients with rest tremor examined 2 to 71 months postoperatively (mean 28 months), 26 (81%) had excellent to good control of tremor. Fourteen of these patients had a marked decrease or total alleviation of tremor. The remaining patients had periodic relief and showed more gradual improvement. The time course of improvement and measurement of the "degree of tremor dysfunction," however, was unclear as patients were followed at variable intervals and standard tremor rating scales were not used. The six patients whose tremor was not alleviated reportedly had smaller lesions placed more dorsally because they experienced visual symptoms during intraoperative electrical stimulation and the lesioning probe was moved dorsally, away from the optic tract. Lesion locations were not described postoperatively.

Iacono et al. (26), in a study incorporating 126 patients, reported that tremor was reduced in 85% of patients. They reported a 65% improvement in the UPDRS mean tremor subscore while "on," decreasing from 2.2 at baseline to 0.73 postoperatively ($p < 0.01$). Patients self-reported 60% to 90% alleviation of tremor, which occurred on average 1 to 6 months after surgery and then plateaued. Data collection was unconventional, however, based partly on assessment of video recordings provided by family members or the patients' caretakers. Patients were not assessed "off" medications, and follow-up was performed at variable intervals from 1 to 12 months (mean 4.5 months). In a subsequent study, Shima et al. (56) reported significant alleviation of tremor in 90% of patients during a mean follow-up of 8 months. However, similar to Iacono et al. (26), nonstandardized methods were used for tremor assessment based on analysis of video recordings and physical examination, which did not employ standardized rating scales. Paradoxically, they reported that tremor was acutely facilitated in some patients immediately after surgery. In these patients tremor gradually attenuated over a 2- to 3-month postoperative period.

Dogali et al. (8) reported the effect of pallidotomy on tremor in 18 PD patients. UPDRS scores were obtained 12 hours "off" medications and at 3-month intervals up to 12 months after pallidotomy. Inclusion criteria included predominant bradykinesia, rigidity, and motor fluctuations. Although no mention of baseline tremor or data specific to tremor are given, the authors reached the following conclusion: "although pallidotomy may not be as effective as thalamotomy for tremor alleviation, tremor was reduced in all affected patients." The same group (9) reviewed 33 patients for whom similar inclusion criteria were employed. Patients with tremor-predominant PD were excluded. Although UPDRS subscores for tremor were not included, making interpretation of their results difficult, the authors reported marked alleviation of tremor on long-term follow-up still in progress (up to 3 years).

In the study by Lozano et al. (41), 14 patients underwent blinded evaluations in both the on and off states at 3 and 6 months postoperatively. Although patients whose tremor was the most disabling symptom were excluded, and tremor was therefore not a significant component of these patients' disease, contralateral tremor was reported to be significantly reduced following pallidotomy ($p = 0.03$). The number of patients with tremor in this study and their relative improvement following pallidotomy was not reported.

Baron et al. (4) reported significant tremor alleviation in all eight of their patients with tremor prior to surgery, with seven of the eight tremor-free at the 1-year follow-up. Overall the mean ($\pm$ standard deviation) UPDRS tremor score improved from 1.8 ± 0.7 to 0.1 ± 0.3. In addition to significant contralateral improvement, a trend toward ipsilateral alleviation of tremor was noted in three of four patients at the 3- and 12-month follow-up visits. Three patients with tremor did not improve immediately following pallidotomy but experienced a more gradual improvement over the postoperative period (up to 1 year). Gradual improvement was also noted in patients who had more severe tremor.

Moderate benefit following pallidotomy in patients with tremor was reported by Johansson et al. (29). Independent ratings of video recordings were performed using a visual analogue scale (VAS). The VAS is an ordinal scale that rates tremor from 0 (absent) to 100 (most severe) and relies on the patient's interpretation of tremor severity. Using this scale, no change in contralateral tremor median VAS values were noted in ten patients evaluated at 4 and 12 months postoperatively, although the maximum VAS score decreased from 55 to 30 at 4 months postoperatively ($p = 0.004$) and to 10 at 12 months ($p = 0.008$) postoperatively. Four patients with ipsilateral tremor did not change from a baseline maximum VAS score of 40 at 4 months but showed a reduction from 40 to 20 at their 12-month follow-up.

Patients with tremor-predominant PD were included in a study of 24 patients assessed on and off medication and followed up to 12 months postoperatively by Kishore et al. (32). At 6 months after operation the UPDRS tremor scores in the off state improved from 2.61 to 0.55 ($p = 0.003$) contralaterally and from 2.21 to 0.94 ($p = 0.02$) on the side ipsilateral to the lesion. Although data from the 12-month assessment was not reported, review of the data is consistent with a continued improvement in tremor after the 6-month evaluation.

Taha and colleagues (63) specifically assessed the effect of pallidotomy on tremor in 44 patients who underwent microelectrode-guided pallidotomy. Tremor was rated using a VAS similar to that described by Johansson et al. (29) and was defined as severe if the VAS score was more than 50, moderate if it was between 25 and 50, and mild if it was less than 25. Of the 44 patients, tremor was rated as severe in 55% (24/44), moderate in 16% (7/44), and mild in 30% (13/44). Postoperatively, 11% (5/44) had severe, 23% (10/44) moderate, and 66% (29/44) mild tremor. Nine percent (4/44) had complete tremor relief. Patients with the most severe tremor had the greatest degree of improvement, with 67% improving by a VAS score over 50 and 21% by a VAS score of 25 to 50; 12% showed little or no improvement.

Microelectrode recording in these patients revealed tremor-synchronous cells discharging at 3 to 7 Hz in 23% (10/44) of patients. When necessary, the lesion site was modified to include the region of the GPi in which these cells were recorded. All patients with severe tremor in which tremor-synchronous cells were identified during intraoperative recording and included in the lesion reported significant improvement in their tremor, compared with 53% of the patients in whom tremor-synchronous cells were not recorded. The authors concluded that: (a) two-thirds of patients with severe tremor gained at least 50% improvement following pallidotomy; and (b) the inclusion of tremor-synchronous cells in the lesion was associated with improved tremor outcome. This is in contrast to a report by Wilkinson et al. in which cells firing in synchrony with tremor were recorded in patients, but lesions in this area did not give consistent long-term tremor relief (74).

Clinical Variables

Although differences exist between studies, most suggest that parkinsonian tremor is alleviated by pallidotomy, albeit to varying degrees (Table 12-1). The variable improvement reported across these studies may be due to a variety of factors, one of which is the method used to assess tremor. Tremor outcome was assessed differently, under different conditions, and at variable times following surgery. Some utilized the UPDRS tremor subscale (4,8,9, 41), whereas others used patient examination (56), video recording (26, 56), subjective rating scales (29,63), or patient self-reporting (26). Tremor was assessed in the on condition in one (26) and in both on and off states in four (4,8,9,32,41); in three oth-

ers (56, 74) the medication state was not clearly defined. Follow-up at variable times using nonstandardized methods of assessment, as reported in many of these studies, likely contributes to the variable degree of improvement reported in many of these studies as tremor, unlike other parkinsonian motor signs, may continue to improve over time postoperatively (4,26,29,34,56).

In addition to the method and time of assessment, patient selection also may complicate the interpretation of these studies. Most studies (8,9,41) excluded patients with tremor-predominant symptoms, and only one study specifically addressed the effectiveness of pallidotomy on tremor (63). Even this study excluded patients with medically intractable tremor. Thus it is difficult to know whether the results reported in these studies, in which tremor was not severe and may have been responsive to medical therapy, are applicable to patients with severe parkinsonian tremor refractory to medical therapy.

Given the extreme fluctuations in amplitude that may occur throughout the day due to a variety of factors (including medication effects, external stress, fatigue, and anxiety), a representative measure of tremor can be difficult to devise. Many authors have emphasized the difficulty of measuring tremor (18,59). Thus to compare results across studies, methods of assessment should be as similar as possible, standardized rating scales should be used, and patients should be assessed multiple times under the same conditions, preferably in both medicated and nonmedicated states. Finally, the duration of follow-up should be standardized, incorporating longer follow-up intervals to define the time course of tremor alleviation following pallidotomy.

FUNCTIONAL ORGANIZATION OF THE PALLIDUM: RELATION OF LESION LOCATION TO TREMOR ALLEVIATION FOLLOWING PALLIDOTOMY

In addition to the methods and times of tremor assessment, future studies must take into account the role of lesion location and size to evaluate the effectiveness of pallidotomy for treatment of parkinsonian tremor. The importance of this clinical vari-

TABLE 12-1. Summary of the effect of pallidotomy on tremor reported in current studies

Parameter	Laitinen (34)	Iacono (26)	Shima (56)	Dogali (8,9)	Lozano (41)	Baron (4)	Johansson (29)	Taha (63)	Kishore (32)
No. of Patients[a]	32	126	86 (82)	33	14	15 (8)	22 (10)	44	20
Localization technique	CT	MRI Semimicroelectrode	MRI Semimicroelectrode	MRI Microelectrode	MRI Microelectrode	MRI Microelectrode	MRI	MRI Microelectrode	CT
Assessment	Neurologic exam.	UPDRS Video	Neurological exam. Video	CAPIT	CAPIT	CAPIT	VAS	VAS	CAPIT
Medication state	?	On	?	On/off	On/off	On/off	On	?	On/off
Follow-up (months)	2–71 (mean 28)	1–12 (mean 4.5)	3–30 (mean 8)	12	6	12	12	9	6
Tremor response Contralateral	+	+	+	+	+	+	+	+	+
Reported response	81% Improved[b]	85% Improved[b]	90% Improved[b]	"Marked improvement"	Significant improvement	88% Tremor-free[b]	Maximum amplitude decreased	66% > 50% Improved[b]; 100% TSC[c]	79% Improved[b]
Ipsilateral						+	+		+
Reported response						75% Trend improvement[b]			

CT, computed tomography; MRI, magnetic resonance imaging; VAS, visual analogue scale; CAPIT, Core Assessment Program for Intracerebral Transplantation; TSC, tumor synchronous cells; UPDRS, Unified Parkinson's Disease Rating Scale

[a]Numbers in parentheses are the number of patients reported with tremor.
[b]Percent of patients showing improvement in tremor.
[c]100% TSC refers to the percentage of patients with tremor synchronous cells (defined and included in lesion site) whose tremor improved.

able is evident in the previous literature in which clinical benefits were varied and unpredictable when targeting the anterodorsal portion of the GPi. Movement of the target site to the posteroventral portion of the GPi resulted in consistent improvement in each of the cardinal motor signs of PD, including tremor. Thus the importance of lesion location in determining clinical outcome can be extracted from the early and the contemporary literature and has been emphasized more recently in a number of studies in which clinical outcome following pallidotomy was compared to lesion location within the pallidum (62,69,71).

The rationale for lesioning the posterolateral portion of the GPi is based on advances in our understanding of the organization of the basal ganglia. The basal ganglia project to a wide region of the frontal cortex. Five parallel circuits have been identified that project to different regions of the cortex, including the sensorimotor, dorsolateral prefrontal, lateral orbitofrontal, anterior cingulate, and oculomotor (1,51). The sensorimotor circuit is somatotopically organized and involves the posterolateral portion of the GPi, the region targeted by most surgeons performing pallidotomy today. This region contains neurons related to active and passive movement. The altered activity that occurs in this portion of the pallidum is believed to underlie the development of parkinsonian motor signs. Thus if one is to interrupt the motor circuit, involvement of this region is critical when making ablative lesions of the GPi.

Hoover and Strick (24) demonstrated in the monkey the existence of separate subcircuits within the sensorimotor loop, each involving a particular portion of the GPi. Using a virus-labeling technique, injection of virus into the supplementary motor cortex labeled neurons in the dorsal portion of GPi, whereas injections into the ventral premotor area labeled neurons in the ventrolateral portion of the GPi. GPi cells labeled by primary motor cortex injections were found in a region between the above groups. The authors suggested that different regions of the GPi project via discrete output channels to specific motor cortical regions. They speculated that each subcircuit is preferentially concerned with specific aspects of motor control. As an adjunct to this argument, we propose that each subcircuit could also subserve a specific role in the expression of the various cardinal motor signs of PD. The size and location of lesions in the GPi could therefore potentially have a dramatic impact on the effect of specific parkinsonian motor signs. Thus alleviation of parkinsonian motor signs may be dependent not only on involvement of the motor circuit; if the lesion does not encompass the entire sensorimotor region, interrupting all motor subcircuits, certain motor signs may show little or no reduction.

Another factor to be considered in the treatment of parkinsonian tremor or other parkinsonian motor signs is the somatotopic organization of the pallidum. In the GPi the arm area is predominantly represented lateral and ventral to the leg region (70). Thus if lesions are to alleviate tremor in the upper extremity, we argue that they must include that portion of the pallidum in which the hand and arm representation is found. Microelectrode recording may be useful in this regard in that cells related to tremor can be identified and the relative location of the sensorimotor pallidum defined. This information can then be used to guide lesion placement (70), as suggested earlier by Taha and colleagues (63).

Microelectrode Recording: Role in Target Localization

Only a few studies have systematically evaluated the effect of microelectrode recording in determining the site for lesion placement within the GPi (2,21,65,70). In all cases the authors concluded that this technique improved target localization. In one report microelectrode recording led to a change in final location for lesion placement in 14 of 20 (70%) cases, with an average change of 3.5 mm (21). In another report, 75% of cases were within 3 ± 1 mm and 25% (4/6) were more than 5 mm away from the final lesion site (2). Still a third reported a rate of target change that was considered too high to support pallidotomy without microelectrode recording (65). Our own data support these reports (70). In a recent series of patients we calculated a difference of 2.2 mm between the target location determined by MRI to that physiologically determined by microelectrode mapping. Although the accuracy of targeting without the microelectrode is good in many cases, the high incidence of changes in final lesion location reported in these studies suggests that microelectrode recording provides improved target localization. No study has directly compared clinical outcome using conventional versus microelectrode recording techniques, but as a result of improved target localization one would intuitively predict a corresponding improvement in clinical outcome using microelectrode recording.

Microelectrode recording may also be used to identify specific sites or regions within the pallidum that may be more closely related to the development of particular motor signs. Formal analysis of the physiological characteristics of recorded neurons in sites where lesions lead to tremor alleviation may provide a physiological signature that allows identification of the optimal sites within the GPi for tremor relief. Cells in the GPi that discharge at tremor frequency were identified in parkinsonian patients with tremor (63, 74), and the response of tremor to pallidotomy improved when the lesion included these cells (63). This finding is in agreement with a retrospective evaluation of cell clusters with bursting activity in synchrony with EMG activity in patients undergoing thalamotomy for tremor (38). These cells clustered within a particular area of the motor thalamus, and tremor outcome improved if the lesion was placed within 2 mm of this site. Thus previous experience with thalamotomy and more recent experience with pallidotomy suggest that definition of the somatotopic arrangement and identification of tremor-synchronous cell populations is associated with a better outcome when these regions are included in the lesion. The lack of benefit in patients without the identification of such areas suggests either a different pathophysiological subset of patients or, more likely, a different recording location within the GPi. Subsequent verification of lesion location in these patients is critical for differentiating between these two possibilities and for predicting clinical outcome in these patients.

CONCLUSIONS

Evidence from animal and human studies supports the role of the GPi in the production of parkinsonian tremor and offers a scientific rationale for pallidotomy to treat parkinsonian tremor. This role, however, remains controversial despite the fact that almost all studies in the contemporary literature report alleviation of tremor following pallidotomy. Part of this controversy stems from reports in the early literature in which pallidotomy was generally considered minimally effective for parkinsonian tremor, together with some studies in the present literature in which tremor is reported as variably affected by pallidotomy. The lack of adequate objective measures, use of nonstandardized protocols, differences in procedural technique, and lack of documentation of lesion location in the present literature make interpretation of many of these reports difficult. Our own experience strongly supports a role for pallidotomy in the treatment of tremor; but its alleviation, as with other parkinsonian motor signs, is dependent on multiple clinical variables, one of which is lesion location. Future studies must take these variables into account in order to evaluate the effect of pallidotomy on parkinsonian tremor and other parkinsonian motor signs.

Acknowledgments. Some of the studies reviewed in this paper were supported by grants from the NIH (R29 NS30719, R01 NS 32047).

REFERENCES

1. Alexander GE, DeLong MR, Strick PL. Parallel organization of functionally segregated circuits linking basal ganglia and cortex. *Annu Rev Neurosci* 1986;9:357–381.
2. Azizi A, Goldman W, Moreledge D. Posteroventral pallidotomy: comparison of the accuracy of anatomical targets defined by MR and CT imaging with physiological targets defined by microelectrode recording. *Neurology* 1996;46 [suppl]:A199.
3. Bakay RAE, Vitek JL, DeLong MR. Thalamotomy for tremor. In: Rengachary SS, Wilkins RS, eds. *Neurosurgical Operative Atlas*, vol. 2(4). 1992:299–312.
4. Baron MS, Vitek JL, Bakay RAE, et al. Treatment of advanced Parkinson's disease with microelectrode-guided pallidotomy: 1 year pilot-study results. *Ann Neurol* 1996;40:355–366.
5. Bergman H, Wichmann T, DeLong MR. The primate sub-thalamic nucleus. II. Neural activity in the subthalamic nucleus and pallidum in the MPTP model of parkinsonism. *J Neurophysiol* 1993;72:507–520.
6. Bucy PC. Cortical extirpation in the treatment of involuntary movement. *Assoc Nerv Ment Disord* 1942;21:551–595.
7. Chockkan V, Mewes K, Zhang J, et al. A comparison of discharge pattern of internal segment neurons of the

globus pallidus (GPi) in akinetic and tremor parkinsonian patients (PD). *Soc Neurosci* 1997;23:470.

8. Dogali M, Fazzine E, Kolodny E, et al. Stereotactic ventral pallidotomy for Parkinson's disease. *Neurology* 1995;45:753–761.

9. Dogali M, Sterio D, Fazzini E, Kolodny E, Eidelberg D, Beric A. Effects of posteroventral pallidotomy on Parkinson's disease. *Adv Neurol* 1996;69:585–590.

10. Elble R. Central mechanisms of tremor. *J Clin Neurophysiol* 1996;13:133–144.

11. Elble R, Koller W. Parkinson tremor. In: Elble R, Koller W, eds. *Tremor*. Baltimore: The Johns Hopkins Press, 1990:118–133.

12. Favre J, Taha J, Nguyen T, Gildenberg P, Burchiel K. Pallidotomy: a survey of current practice in North America. *Neurosurgery* 1996;39:883–892.

13. Filion M, Tremblay L. Abnormal spontaneous activity of globus pallidus neurons in monkeys with MPTP-induced parkinsonism. *Brain Res* 1991;547:142–151.

14. Filion M, Tremblay L, Bedard PJ. Abnormal influences of passive limb movement on the activity of globus pallidus neurons in parkinsonian monkeys. *Brain Res* 1988; 444:165–176.

15. Gillingham F. Stereotactic surgery: past, present, and future. *Clin Neurosurg* 1966;13:189–203.

16. Gillingham F, Watson W, Donaldson A, Naughton J. The surgical treatment of parkinsonism. *BMJ* 1960; 2:1395–1402.

17. Goetz C, Diederich N. There is a renaissance of interest in pallidotomy for Parkinson's disease. *Nat Med* 1996; 2:510–514.

18. Gresty M, McCarthy R, Findley L. Assessment of resting tremor in Parkinson's disease. In: Findley L, ed. *Movement disorders: tremor*. New York: Oxford University Press, 1984:321–329.

19. Hassler R, Reichert T. Indikationen und lokalisationsmethode der gezielten hirnoperationen. *Nervenarzt* 1954;25:441–447.

20. Hassler R, Reichert T, Mundinger F, Umbach W, Gangleberger JA. Physiological observations in stereotaxic operations in extrapyramidal motor disturbances. *Brain* 1960;83:337–350.

21. Hiner B, Madden K, Neal J. Effect of microelectrode recording on final lesion placement in pallidotomy. *Neurology* 1997;48[suppl 2]:A251.

22. Hirai T, Miyazaki M, Nakajima H, Shibazaki T, Ohye C. The correlation between tremor characteristics and the predicted volume of effective lesions in stereotaxic nucleus ventralis intermedius thalamotomy. *Brain* 1983; 106:1001–1018.

23. Holsapple JW, Preston JB, Strick PL. Origin of thalamic inputs to the "hand" representation in the primary motor cortex. *J Neurosci* 1991;16:425.

24. Hoover JE, Strick PL. Multiple output channels in the basal ganglia. *Science* 1993;259:819–821.

25. Hufschmidt H. Proprioceptive origin of parkinsonian tremor. *Nature* 1963;200:367–368.

26. Iacono RP, Shima F, Lonser RR, Kuniyoshi S, Maeda G, Yamada S. The results, indications, and physiology of posteroventral pallidotomy for patients with Parkinson's disease. *Neurosurgery* 1995;36:1118–1127.

27. Jahnsen H, Llinas R. Electrophysiological properties of guinea-pig thalamic neurons: an in vitro study. *J Physiol (Lond)* 1984;349:205–226.

28. Jankovic J, Fahn S. Physiologic and pathologic tremors: diagnosis, mechanism, and management. *Ann Intern Med* 1980;93:460–465.

29. Johansson F, Malm J, Nordh E, Hariz M. Usefulness of pallidotomy in advanced Parkinson's disease. *J Neurol Neurosurg Psychiatry* 1997;62:125–132.

30. Kelly P, Gillingham F. The long term results of stereotaxic surgery and L-dopa therapy in patients with Parkinson's disease: a 10-year follow-up study. *J Neurosurg* 1980;53:332–337.

31. Kievit J, Kuypers HGJM. Organization of the thalamocortical connections to the frontal lobe in the rhesus monkey. *Exp Brain Res* 1977;29:299–322.

32. Kishore A, Turnbull I, Snow B, et al. Efficacy, stability, and predictors of outcome of pallidotomy for Parkinson's disease: six month follow-up with additional one year observations. *Brain* 1997;120:729–737.

33. Krauss JK, Jankovic J. Surgical treatment of Parkinson's disease. *Am Fam Physician* 1996;54:1621–1629.

34. Laitinen L, Bergenheim A, Hariz M. Leksell's posteroventral pallidotomy in the treatment of Parkinson's disease. *J Neurosurg* 1992;76:53–61.

35. Lamarre Y. Animal models of physiological, essential, and parkinsonian-like tremors. In: Findley L, Capildes R, eds. *Movement disorders: tremor*. London: Macmillan, 1984:183–194.

36. Lamarre Y, Joffroy AJ. Experimental tremor in monkey: activity of thalamic and precentral cortical neurons in the absence of peripheral feedback. *Adv Neurol* 1979;24: 109–122.

37. Lenz FA, Kwan HC, Martin RL, Tasker RR, Dostrovsky JO, Lenz YE. Single unit analysis of the human ventral thalamic nuclear group: tremor-related activity in functionally identified cells. *Brain* 1994;117:531–543.

38. Lenz FA, Normand SL, Kwan HC, et al. Statistical prediction of the optimal site for thalamotomy in parkinsonian tremor. *Mov Disord* 1995;10:318–328.

39. Lenz FA, Tasker RR, Kwan HC, Dostrovsky JO, Murphy JT. Single unit analysis of the human thalamic ventral nuclear group: correlation of thalamic "tremor cells" with the 3–6 Hz component of parkinsonian tremor. *J Neurosci* 1988;8:754–764.

40. Llinas RR. Rebound excitation as the physiological basis for tremor: a biophysical study of the oscillatory properties of mammalian central neurones in vitro. In: Findley LJ, Capildea R, eds. *Movement Disorders: Tremor*. London: Macmillan, 1984:165–182.

41. Lozano AM, Lang AE, Galvez-Jimenez N, et al. Effect of GPi pallidotomy on motor function in Parkinson's disease. *Lancet* 1995;346:1383–1387.

42. Meyers R. The modification of alternating tremors, rigidity and festination by surgery of the basal ganglia. *Assoc Nerv Ment Disord* 1942;20:602–665.

43. Miller WC, DeLong MR. Altered tonic activity of neurons in the globus pallidus and subthalamic nucleus in the primate MPTP model of parkinsonism. In: Carpenter M, Jayaraman A, eds. *Basal ganglia: structure and function II*. New York: Plenum Publishing, 1987:415–427.

44. Mundinger F. 30 years of stereotactic brain operations in parkinsonism (comparison of results of pallido-thalamo-subthalamic elimination and indications). In: Ganshirt H, eds. *Pathophysiology, clinical aspects, and therapy of parkinsonism*. Basel: Roche, 1985:133–158.

45. Nambu A, Llinas R. Electrophysiology of the globus pallidus neurons: an in vitro study in guinea pig brain slices. *Soc Neurosci Abstr* 1990;180:8.
46. Narabayashi H. Striatal symptoms. In: Gildenberg P, eds. *Stereotactic and functional neurosurgery.* Basel: Karger, 1989:200–204.
47. Narabayashi H. Tremor mechanisms. In: Schaltenbrand G, Walker AE, eds. *Stereotaxy of the human brain.* Stuttgart: Thieme Medical Publishers, 1982:510–514.
48. Ohye C, Bouchard R, LaRochelle L. Effect of dorsal rhizotomy on postural tremor in the monkey. *Exp Brain Res* 1970;10:140.
49. Olanow C. GPi pallidotomy: have we made a dent in Parkinson's disease? *Ann Neurol* 1996;40:341–343.
50. Pare D, Curro'Dossi R, Steriade M. Neuronal basis of the parkinsonian resting tremor: a hypothesis and its implications for treatment. *Neuroscience* 1990;35:217–226.
51. Parent A, Hazrati L. Functional anatomy of the basal ganglia I. The cortico-basal ganglia-thalamic-cortical loop. *Brain Res Rev* 1995;20:91–127.
52. Parkinson J. *An essay on the shaking palsy.* London: Whittingham & Roland, 1817.
53. Pollack LT, Davis L. Muscle tone in parkinsonian states. *Arch Neurol Psychiatry* 1930;23:303–319.
54. Rack PMH, Ross HF. The role of reflexes in the resting tremor of Parkinson's disease. *Brain* 1986;109:115–141.
55. Schnider S, Kwong R, Kwan H, Lenz F. Detection of feedback in the central nervous system of parkinsonian patients. *Trans IEEE Decision Control* 1986;25:291–294.
56. Shima F, Ishido K, Sun S, et al. Surgical control of akinesia in Parkinson's disease. *Eur Neurol* 1996;36:55–61.
57. Silva LR, Amitai Y, Connors BW. Intrinsic oscillations of neocortex generated by layer 5 pyramidal neurons. *Science* 1991;251:432–435.
58. Spiegel E, Wycis H, Baird H. Long range effects of electropallidotomy in extrapyramidal and convulsive disorders. *Neurology* 1958;8:743–783.
59. Spiegel E, Wycis H, Freed H. Stereoencephalotomy: thalamotomy and related procedures. *JAMA* 1952;148:446–451.
60. Sterio D, Beric A, Dogali M, Fazzini E, Alfaro G, Devinsky O. Neurophysiological properties of pallidal neurons in Parkinson's disease. *Ann Neurol* 1994;35:586–591.
61. Struppler A, Lehmann-Horn F, Klein W, Lucking CH, Deuschl G. Effect of stereoencephalotomy on long-latency EMG responses and motor control of arm movements in Parkinson's syndrome. *Adv Neurol* 1984;40: 437–445.
62. Svennilson E, Torvik A, Lowe R, Leksell L. Treatment of parkinsonism by stereotactic thermolesions in the pallidal region: a clinical evaluation of 81 cases. *Acta Psychiat Neurol Scand* 1960;35:358–377.
63. Taha J, Favre J, Baumann T, Burchiel K. Tremor control after pallidotomy in patients with Parkinson's disease: correlation with microrecording findings. *J Neurosurg* 1997;86:642–647.
64. Taha JM, Favre J, Baumann TK, Burchiel KJ. Characteristics and somatotopic organization of kinesthetic cells in the globus pallidus in patients with Parkinson's disease. *J Neurosurg* 1996;85:1005–1012.
65. Taha JM, Favre J, Burchiel KJ. The value of macrostimulation in patients who underwent microrecording during pallidotomy. In: *Congress of Neurologic Surgeons Abstracts,* 46th Annual Meeting, 1996:264–265.
66. Tasker R, Siqueira J, Hawrylyshyn P, Organ L. What happened to Vim thalamotomy for Parkinson's disease? *Appl Neurophysiol* 1983;46:68–83.
67. Tatton WG, Lee RG. Evidence for abnormal long-loop reflexes in rigid parkinsonian patients. *Brain Res Amsterdam* 1975;100:671–676.
68. Velasco F, Molina-Negro P. Electrophysiologic topography of the human diencephalon. *J Neurosci* 1973;38: 204–214.
69. Vitek J, Bakay R, DeLong M. Posteroventral pallidotomy for Parkinson's disease. In: Obeso J, DeLong M, Ohye C, Marsden C, eds. *The basal ganglia and surgical treatment of Parkinson's disease.* New York: Lippincott-Raven, 1997.
70. Vitek JL, Bakay RAE, Hashimoto T, et al. Microelectrode-guided pallidotomy: technical approach and application for treatment of medically intractable Parkinson's disease 1998;88:1027–1043.
71. Vitek JL, Baron M, Bakay RAE, Hashimoto T, Mewes K, DeLong MR. Pallidotomy for medically intractable Parkinson's disease: 2 year follow-up. In: *American Neurological Association Abstracts,* 1996; 121st Annual Meeting, 1996:24.
72. Vitek JL, Kaneoke Y, Hashimoto T, Bakay RAE, DeLong MR. Neuronal activity in the pallidum of a patient with hemiballismus. In: *American Neurological Association Abstracts,* 120th Annual Meeting, 1995: 38–39.
73. Wichmann T, Bergman H, DeLong M. Increased neuronal activity in the subthalamic nucleus of MPTP treated monkeys. *Mov Disord* 1990;5[suppl]:78.
74. Wilkinson SB, Overman J, Koller W, et al. Microelectrode guided GPi pallidotomy: volumetric MR and clinical confirmation of electrical recordings. In: *Congress of Neurologic Surgeons Abstracts,* 46th Annual Meeting, 1996:283–284.

Pallidal Surgery for the Treatment of Parkinson's Disease and Movement Disorders, edited by
J. K. Krauss, R. G. Grossman, and J. Jankovic.
Lippincott-Raven Publishers, Philadelphia © 1998.

13

Changes in Postural Control after Pallidotomy

Averell S. Overby, *Deborah Roberts-Warrior, and †Eugene C. Lai

*School of Physical Therapy, Ohio University, Athens, Ohio 45701, USA; *School of Physical Therapy,
Texas Woman's University, Houston, Texas 77030, USA; and †Department of Neurology,
Baylor College of Medicine, Houston, Texas 77030, USA*

Pallidotomy has become the technique of choice for persons with Parkinson's disease (PD) who are experiencing severe motor fluctuations in their on–off cycle and who have severe dopa-induced dyskinesia while on medication. Although there is little doubt that pallidotomy improves the function of some persons (16,23,28–30,34), particularly when "off" medications, it is not clear how long the effects of the pallidotomy last, nor is it clear who benefits most from the procedure. Also unclear is the mechanism by which improvement in postural control takes place, that is, which of the multiple systems that contribute to postural control are affected by pallidotomy. The goals of this chapter are to: (a) review the multiple systems involved in postural control; (b) review studies dealing with postural dyscontrol in PD; (c) describe the preliminary results of our studies with 35 persons who had a unilateral posteroventral pallidotomy; and (d) review the results of pallidotomy studies published thus far particularly as they relate to postural control and gait.

POSTURAL CONTROL

Balance is a multidimensional event requiring several systems, including the sensory, motor, and cognitive systems, to work in concert. A defect in any of these systems can cause a loss of balance or postural dyscontrol. An individual obtains information about the environment through the sensory systems, which also provide continual feedback about the body's relation in space,

to other objects, and to itself. The sensory systems are composed of the visual, somatosensory, and vestibular systems (1,42). Healthy persons tend to rely on the somatosensory system in a feedback situation, particularly when externally perturbed, as it is the fastest of the systems to respond (42). The visual system is generally relied on more heavily in feed-forward situations, that is, in new or novel situations when one needs to assess the environment, make predictions, and formulate a motor plan concerning how to avoid falling. The vestibular system, although continuously active to support posture, is most important when there is a conflict between the other two systems (42). As persons age, there is a decrease in the function of all three of these systems leading to some dyscontrol in the elderly, which may be responsible for falling (35). Along with these decreases in function with age comes more dependence on vision in all situations (35).

The cognitive system comes into play when one needs to recognize and interpret stimuli presented during interactions with the environment. This is done through accessing long-term memory in which information has been categorized from previous experiences. Comparison of the present situation with past experience allows one to initiate a motor program appropriate for the situation, which for the most part in feedback situations is not under cortical control but is rather a stereotyped, automatic postural response. The motor plan assembles which muscles will be used, in what sequence, and the amount of force and speed necessary for the activity (1). The basal ganglia and cerebellum are important in mediating these responses. In feed-forward situations, because any number of responses can be made in response to the destabilizing force more cortical activity is required. Marsden and Obeso (37) suggested that the basal ganglia have a twofold purpose, depending on the context of the situation. They hypothesized that under usual conditions, in which there is more or less automatic running of motor programs, the basal ganglia act to assist cortically driven movements by altering output to the supplemental motor area; hence desired movements are allowed to occur, and opposing muscular contractions are inhibited. They believed that in novel situations (feed-forward), different striatal signals interrupt the running of the motor program to allow new motor sequences appropriate for the situation, thereby allowing flexibility of responses.

Finally, with regard to sensory systems, attentional demands are placed on the individual to recognize and interpret the incoming stimuli. Research in the elderly has demonstrated that older adults' postural control is more affected than that of young adults when attentional demands of a task are increased (38,52). Being able to attend to multiple stimuli in the environment and determine which ones are the most important to monitor and respond to is an important component of postural control.

The motor plan is transmitted to the musculoskeletal system, which is the third complex system involved in postural control. After selecting a motor plan to counteract a destabilizing force, for the most effective postural adjustments to occur sufficient strength, range of motion, speed, timing, and direction are required. Reciprocal inhibition is required to allow muscles to act on the joints of the lower extremity to prevent the person from swaying too far in any direction during quiet stance and in dynamic motion. How far one is able to sway (lean) in any direction with the feet fixed in place is called the limits of stability (LOS) (1,42). Efficiency of movement while exploring the LOS relies on the person's ability to perform an ankle strategy in which muscles are contracted from distal to proximal to allow the body to move as a single unit over the feet.

Range of motion and ability to generate force in the ankle musculature are necessary to perform the ankle strategy. Of equal importance for fast perturbations is the hip strategy, in which muscles contract from proximal to distal in the lower limb. Fast perturbations also require flexibility in the trunk and upper extremity to counteract the destabilizing force. When a person exceeds his or her LOS, a step must be taken to prevent a fall. More attention is being paid to the stepping response in older persons (36) and in those with PD (48), as well as to compensatory upper extremity movements (21,36). As discussed below, all systems concerned with balance have been investigated with no consensus for the main cause of postural dyscontrol in persons with PD.

TESTS OF BALANCE

Tests of balance have been devised for various purposes. To screen for the propensity of the elderly to fall, tests such as the Physical Performance Test (PPT) (33,46), the Performance Oriented Assessment of Balance (POAB) and Gait (POAG) (33,53), the Berg Balance Scale (7,13), and Functional Reach (FR) (17,33) have been assembled and tested and are now commonly used. These functional tests of balance yield a composite score that takes into account constructs such as strength, flexibility, and speed. The tests assume that balance underlies function, particularly in transitional movements from one posture to another. Therefore they are not "pure" tests of balance, and it is difficult to define specifically the impairment that leads to the dysfunction exhibited during the test. An advantage of these tests (except for FR) is their ability to demonstrate fairly objective changes in function, such as turning while walking, standing up, and sitting down in a chair; picking up an item from the floor; standing with a narrowed base of support; or resisting an external push.

Other tests of balance are designed to identify a specific impairment. These tests include the Sensory Organization Test (SOT), which determines the sensory contributions to balance under six separate conditions, that is, eyes opened and eyes closed on a fixed and sway referenced surface and two visual conflict tests (1,42). Also analyzed during this task is the motor strategy (hip or ankle) the subject uses to prevent falling. The SOT and motor control tests are usually called posturography (42). Motor control tests (MCTs) analyze the automatic response of the lower extremity musculature to perturbations while the subject stands on a platform. Horizontal or angular (toes up) translations of the platform may be applied; and the latency, duration, and integrated electromyographic (EMG) responses are recorded for the short, medium, and long responses. These can be useful for determining whether a lesion is central or peripheral, and there are some identifying characteristics for central nervous system disorders; for example, an enhanced medium latency has been documented in persons with PD (6,8,51).

Additional tests utilizing the same equipment as the SOT and MCT (NeuroCom International, Clackamus, OR, USA) are tests of motor function. One is the limits of stability test, which analyzes volitional movement of the center of gravity while the subject leans toward eight different targets arranged in an ellipse on a computer screen without moving his or her feet. Targets are set at 75% of the LOS according to the individual's height (1). Anticipatory postural adjustments have also been measured while persons attempt to perform a functional movement involving the upper limbs, lower limbs, or whole body (5). Of course, specific impairments that lead to balance dysfunction, such as strength, flexibility, reaction time, and coordination, can be tested by many clinical tools, including dynamometers, electrogoniometers, and electromyography.

In summary, because of the multiple systems affecting an individual's postural control, no one test can measure balance. Rather, a battery of tests, carefully chosen for the patient population of interest, is needed.

POSTURAL DYSCONTROL IN PARKINSON'S DISEASE

Sensory Studies

Many researchers have attempted to determine the cause of postural instability in persons with PD. The studies have been related to the multiple systems that contribute to postural control discussed above. In the past, the sensory systems have been the most studied, probably because of the observation that persons with akinesis can produce movement with visual input. There is not a great deal of consensus in the findings.

Bronstein and associates (11) studied 13 ambulatory persons with PD (mean age 59 years). They reported that all basic sway parameters were normal in the eyes-open and eyes-closed conditions on a stable surface; the sway in response to a moving surround was significantly greater than in a control group, and this response was not adaptable over time. The authors thought it represented overreliance on vision even when it was incorrect but questioned whether it was a primary component of the disease process or a compensation for failure in the other systems. One difficulty with the study was that some persons had additional neurological findings, and two patients were not using antiparkinsonian medications but the others were, and the results were not analyzed separately.

Schieppati and associates (50) found that the anterior/posterior sway area was slightly increased during quiet standing in 18 persons with PD, but it was significant only for persons who had had the disease for a long time. They found no difference between the eyes-open and eyes-closed conditions; however, seven subjects were examined in the "on" phase. It was not clear whether the others were on or off medication.

Trenkwalder and associates (55) studied 10 persons with advanced PD (mean age 64.8 years) who demonstrated step hesitation and difficulty initiating walking. They used an SOT on the Equitest (NeuroCom International) to measure anterior/posterior (A/P) and medial/lateral (M/L) displacement of the center of pressure. In the eyes-open condition for both surfaces, the patients with PD scored in the normal range; however, in the eyes-closed condition the authors noted that the A/P sway was greater than the lateral sway on a fixed surface, and sway was significantly worse than that of the controls on the foam surface. Authors indicated that this was consistent with vision compensating under stressful conditions. Again, in this study, seven of ten patients were tested during the "off" phase because of motor fluctuations with medications.

In contrast, Mitchell and associates (39), who studied 22 subjects while on medication found that subjects with PD had larger maximal displacements than controls in the M/L direction but not in the A/P direction. The radial area generally was significantly larger in subjects with PD, indicating more sway. Kitamura and associates (25) studied nine patients with idiopathic PD (mean age 60.7 years) while on medication during quiet stance with eyes open and eyes closed. They noted that with eyes closed the normal subjects shifted their weight forward, whereas persons with PD shifted their weight backward. They concluded that under normal circumstances persons with PD use vision to maintain a forward position of their body.

Waterston and associates (57), using the SOT, studied 20 persons with PD (11 HY3 and 9 HY2, where HY represents the Hoehn and Yahr stage) with a mean age of 63.8 years off medication. They found that HY3 patients had an overall greater sway in all conditions. In condition 5 (eyes closed on a sway referenced surface), subjects in HY3 lost balance, possibly suggesting vestibular dysfunction, which correlated with the incidence of falls in this group. However, they found that only two of the patients who fell had vestibular dysfunction as measured by calorics. They concluded that the main pathology related to balance was in the motor system, not the sensory system.

Bodis-Wollner (9) noted that one-half of persons with PD whom he evaluated showed delayed visual evoked potentials. He also noted that persons with PD had reduced contrast sensitivity, which is a quantified measure of the contrast needed to detect coarse targets. This information is important if persons with PD rely more heavily on vision for balance.

The threshold for detecting changes in body position may be increased in persons with PD. Cooke and colleagues (14) concluded that during a tracking task involving the upper extremity persons with PD were unable to maintain the proper arm position in the absence of visual cues but stopped short of saying that this was indicative of proprioceptive loss. Richards et al. (47) found no impairment on two visuospatial tasks, but they discovered that persons with PD had difficulty when asked to trace a sawtooth pattern with two consecutive angles of the sawtooth occluded. They interpreted this to mean that "PD patients can't use sensory information to plan and execute complex and/or new movement," or at least they had difficulty with prediction.

Testing for vestibular dysfunction in PD has produced conflicting reports. Reichert and associates (45), using caloric testing and electronystagmography, found that significantly more persons with PD, when compared to controls, had decreased or absent vestibular responses; however, Pastor et al. (43), who measured body sway induced by galvanic vestibular stimulation while the patient stood with feet together and eyes closed on a stable surface, found that there was no difference between subjects with PD and a control group.

In summary, there is some evidence of impairment in sensory systems in persons with PD, but the effect of that impairment on postural control has not been demonstrated consistently. Studies suffer from small sample sizes and excessive heterogeneity of the sample. Indeed, the effect of sensory impairment on the elderly, without pathology, has not been well documented, although early signs of PD are often considered a cause of postural dyscontrol in the elderly.

Motor Tests

Toole and associates (54) tried to identify variables that affect balance in persons with PD. They studied 11 patients (mean age 71.9 years) with PD staged from 1 to 4; their staging was a composite score with the Hoehn and Yahr (HY) and motor subscale of the Unified Parkinson's Disease Rating Scale (UPDRS). Because of the multidimensional nature of balance, they used many tools as testing instruments, including the SOT, motor responses to perturbations, LOS test, and strength and flexibility testing of the knee and ankle. For the regression equation they developed, because of high correlations among variables they used only six variables: medium loop reflex onset time, range of motion of ankle dorsiflexion, percent peak torque of knee flexion relative to knee extension, percent peak torque of inversion at the ankle, the strategy score on the SOT test, and path sway from the LOS test. This model explained 88% of the variance in the scores, but only three variables were significant. Two of the three were the strength variables, the other was strategy. Although this was an excellent attempt to delineate the cause of postural instability, the dependent variable the model predicted was the composite score on the SOT, which is only a portion of the many variables that represent postural control.

Schiepatti et al. (50) found that when subjects were asked to lean forward or backward to their maximal positions, subjects with PD demonstrated contracted limits of stability (displacement of the center of foot pressure was about 30% of foot length with eyes open and 20% with eyes closed) when compared to healthy elderly subjects, and scores were significantly different in subjects who had the disease long term. These authors thought that defective body leaning could not be explained in terms of insufficient muscle force because the clinical examination for strength was normal. They found the restriction in leaning to be related to the degree of bradykinesia and rigidity.

Perhaps this defective leaning could also be related to the study performed by Lee and co-workers (32), who found that preparatory postural adjustments were absent or decreased in persons with PD during a leg-raising task performed as rapidly as possible. PD subjects in early disease stages did have a brief postural adjustment phase but still had difficulty maintaining equilibrium for several seconds during the leg-raising task and stumbled or fell. Bazalgette and associates (5), in a simple reaction time test of the upper extremities, found that in only 10% of the 18 persons with PD they examined were postural adjustments present prior to the task being performed, and the adjustments were not specific to that movement, whereas in the control group the movements were specific and preceded the task. Without the anticipatory postural adjustment, movements must be slower to compensate for the changes in the center of gravity as the movement proceeds.

In summary, the results of studies on motor impairment have been fairly consistent. Generally, strength or motor recruitment have been noted to

contribute to balance deficits, limits of stability have been demonstrated to be contracted, and anticipatory postural responses have been found to be decreased or absent in persons with PD.

RESULTS

Subjects were the first 40 individuals consecutively scheduled for a unilateral posteroventral pallidotomy. Patients were excluded for the following reasons: Two patients did not return for testing after surgery, two patients did not have presurgical data collected due to scheduling, one patient fractured her hip 1 week after surgery, and one patient fell resulting in a subdural hematoma 3 weeks after the surgical procedure, limiting the evaluation of balance and gait. Thirty-five patients remained in the data pool to be assessed; of these 35, two subjects were missing before surgery data (pretest data) for most variables while in the "off" medication phase. Therefore, for the most part, results are reflective of 33 patients tested. One subject fractured her hip in a fall after the 3-month evaluation period, so only 32 patients were available for testing at 6 months. Whenever possible, the testing was scheduled so the "off" cycle testing was done after 12 hours without medication (12 HOM). If scheduling did not permit testing at 12 HOM, the off phase was determined by the subject's report and the examiner's observations. Although "on" testing was done also, it is not reported here.

The average age of the subjects (18 men, 17 women) was 60.0 ± 8.82 years (median 61 years). Mean Activities of Daily Living (ADL) and Motor scores on the (UPDRS) were 31.2 ± 6.2 and 57.2 ± 13.9, respectively (median scores were 32.0 and 57.5, respectively). The mean HY score was 4.1 ± 0.7 (range 3–5); thus all subjects demonstrated advanced stages of the disease, including significant balance deficits. The surgical procedure was performed on the left side in 24 subjects and on the right side in 11. The procedure, in general, was performed contralateral to the more affected side.

Subjects were tested immediately before surgery (within 2–3 days) and at intervals of 2 weeks, 3 months, 6 months, and 1 year after surgery. Data at 2 weeks are not reported except to say that they were consistent with data at 3 and 6 months after pallidotomy. Therefore, positive results can be seen at a relatively short interval after surgery; in general, the results for individuals did not change much from the 2-week period to the 3- and 6-month period with the exception of one subject who had not improved at 2 weeks but showed marked improvement at 3 and 6 months.

Because of the wide variability among the subjects and the potential richness of the data, results are presented in a descriptive manner. To determine overall change the 3- and 6-month periods were averaged together, as there was little difference between the scores and statistical tests revealed no difference between the 3- and 6-month data for most variables. Data were imputed when necessary because of one or two subjects not returning for testing at either 3 or 6 months. The mean of the subject's scores was used to impute the data. For the 6-month period, if 12-month data were not available for that subject, no imputation was performed because it was difficult to identify a trend. In addition, at the time of this writing data have been collected on only 18 persons 1 year after surgery; the remainder have not yet reached the 1-year anniversary or were not available for follow-up.

Several variables were tested in our laboratory to analyze changes in postural control and gait after pallidotomy. For gait, just two of these variables are reported here: the timed walk for 25 feet and the POAG. Because balance is a multidimensional activity, as we have discussed, many measures were taken that reflect the factors contributing to balance in an older population. Strength in the lower extremities was measured by the performance of five chair stands, which the subject was instructed to do as quickly as possible, and five step-ups as quickly as possible onto a surface 8 inches from the floor. Subjects were instructed not to hold on during either test. Functional balance was determined by the subjects' ability to reach as far forward as possible without moving their feet (Functional Reach), the POAB, and the time it took to turn 360 degrees in the right and left directions. Posturography, using eyes open, eyes closed, and control of the center of gravity with visual feedback was performed to analyze the effect of pallidotomy on the sensory components of balance. Finally, an LOS test, examining the time it took for the subjects to lean toward the eight targets and the accuracy of the trajectory, was done.

Gait Assessment

Timed Walk

Subjects were asked to walk 25 feet in a straight line utilizing a purposeful walking speed as "if they were going somewhere," which included getting up from a straight-back chair. The test was performed twice, and times were averaged. The repeatability of this measure has been reported to be 0.88 in persons with PD on peak dose medication (41). The pretest score was recorded as 120 seconds for those who could not initiate gait using any means at their disposal (visual imagery, verbal cues, visual cues) after determining that 103 seconds was the maximum score for those who could complete the test. After surgery, four persons could walk who could not initiate gait prior to surgery. Among 34 subjects, between pretest and 3 and 6 months, 5 persons were worse, although 3 were minimally worse (< 3 seconds); 9 had minimal or no improvement; and 20 persons had moderate or marked improvement (Table 13-1). Mean scores for the timed walk at pretest and at 3 and 6 months were 39.1 ± 37.5, 18.3 ± 21.0, and 18.5 ± 22.0, respectively. The mean change in timed gait between pretest and 3 months was 20.7 ± 41.2 seconds (22% gain) and 18.1 ± 38.8 seconds (16%) between pretest and 6 months. Fourteen persons had more than 50% decrease in the time it took for the timed walk during the 3- and 6-month testing periods. At 1 year after surgery, 5 of 18 subjects (28%) were worse than at pretest due to increased freezing and difficulty initiating gait. Four of them had continually shown no improvement, and one had shown moderate improvement (6.5 seconds) at 3 and 6 months. One person who could walk before surgery was unable to walk at 3 and 6 months due to progressive frailty.

POAG

The POAG score reflects seven items, including hesitancy, step length, step symmetry, and step

TABLE 13-1. *Improvements in functional scores between baseline 3 and 6 months combined*

Test	No.	Marked/moderate	Minimal/no change	Worse[a]
TW	34	20 (59%)	9 (26%)	5 (15%)
POAG	33	16 (49%)	13 (39%)	4 (12%)
Chair stands	31	20 (65%)	3 (9%)	8 (26%)
Step-ups	31	19 (61%)	7 (23%)	5 (16%)
FR	33	23 (70%)	NA	10 (30%)
POAB	33	17 (52%)	10 (30%)	6 (18%)
Turn left	33	21 (64%)	7 (21%)	5 (15%)
Turn right	31	19 (61%)	5 (16%)	7 (22%)

NA, not available.

TW, timed walk: minimal change (< 3 sec); moderate/marked change (≥ 3 sec). POAG/POAB, performance-oriented assessment of gait/balance: minimal (1–2 points), moderate (3–4 points), marked (> 5 points). Chair stands/Step-ups: minimal (1–2 sec); moderate/marked (≥ 3 sec). FR, functional reach: marked/moderate (> 0). Turning: minimal (< 3 sec); marked/moderate (≥ 3 sec).

[a] To be considered worse, at least one negative score was recorded during the 3- or 6-month testing period.

clearance. Interrater reliability has been established to be 85% to 90% (33). Between presurgery and 3 and 6 months after surgery, 4 of 33 persons were worse; 13 persons had minimal or no improvement; and 16 had moderate or marked change (Table 13-1). Of the 13 with minimal or no improvement, 4 already had the maximum score of 12, and 4 others had presurgery scores of 10 or above; therefore they could not demonstrate any greater change. The median score was 6.0 prior to surgery and 11.0 and 10.5 at 3 and 6 months postsurgery, respectively, demonstrating great improvement. The average percent changes between pretest and 3, 6, and 12 months were 63%, 65%, and 41%, respectively.

Generally, the same subjects had minimal or no improvement or were worse in both tests of gait. None of them had had incidents at or following surgery that might explain the lack of improvement. However, as noted, several persons had high or maximum scores prior to surgery, which precluded great changes from occurring. In those who did improve, most improvement appears to have occurred by 6 months and may decline at 1 year based on the limited sample reported here. Of the 18 patients, 5 were worse than they were at baseline at 1 year, and 4 of the 5 had consistently shown no improvement. The improvements in gait appear to be related to the subject's ability to overcome the akinesia and freezing that were prevalent prior to surgery.

Walking speed was increased, as was the quality of the gait. Although freezing was still observed to occur, it appeared that subjects were able to overcome it more easily to initiate and maintain movement.

Many authors have reported improvement in gait and gait velocity following pallidotomy (16,28,30,34). Laitinen et al. (30) reported that gait was improved "similar" to hypokinesia, which was decreased in 92% of patients (n = 46) who had undergone pallidotomy. Although measurement tools were not well defined in that report, the change in akinesia was measured by the Purdue pegboard test 1 day before and after surgery. The authors went on to say that, even in the long term, bradykinesia and rigidity were "more or less abolished" on the side contralateral to the surgery. Lozano and associates (34) indicated that postural instability and gait score (walking, freezing, and falling from the ADL component of the UPDRS) and gait and postural instability as measured by the motor score on the UPDRS, decreased by 23% at 6 months. Dogali and associates (16), who studied patients both "on" and "off" medication, reported that a timed walk for 23 feet, which included turning and a return to the start position, improved by 24% in their sample. They saw no effect of age on their result and noted that the greatest improvement was noted when the patient was in an "off" stage.

Only Johansson et al. (24), who studied patients in the "on" phase, found no changes in gait velocity at 4 and 12 months after pallidotomy. Baron et al. (4) reported the results from 15 subjects at 3, 6, and 12 months after unilateral pallidotomy using the Core Assessment Program for Intracerebral Transplantation (CAPIT) protocol. They reported that patients in the "off" phase demonstrated a reduction in gait disorder, postural instability, falling, and freezing at 3 months, but these improvements had declined at 1 year. Lang and associates (31) reported that they also have observed that functional disability increased over a 2-year period (although still improved from baseline) in 12 patients following unilateral pallidotomy.

Why unilateral pallidotomy results in positive changes in walking performance and how long those changes are maintained is still being investigated. Most authors ascribe to the current theory that akinesia results from overactivity of neurons in the globus pallidus internus (GPi), resulting in excessive inhibition of the ventrolateral thalamus with a resultant decrease in thalamocortical drive. Voluntary movements, or those initiated in the cortex, are inhibited (19). By lesioning the GPi, excessive output is reduced, which then allows movement to occur (3,4,16,19,34). To support this theory, researchers have demonstrated, using positron emission tomography (PET) before and after pallidotomy, increased activity in the supplemental motor area of the cortex (12,20). Iacono and associates (22) believed that reduction in akinesia is a result of the disinhibition of the reticulospinal brainstem areas. Whatever the mechanism, reduction in akinesia can explain the improved velocity seen in gait. To our knowledge, no one has studied extensively the kinematics of gait after pallidotomy, although some authors have studied gait in patients on and off medication, which may provide some insight into why pallidotomy improves gait velocity.

The gait pattern in persons with PD is usually characterized as a "flexed" gait with slowness, shuffling steps, reduced arm swing, reduced stride length, and increased double limb support (10,18,40,56). Bowes and associates (10) described walking speed as 76% that of controls with increased cadence and shorter strides. They found that passive range of hip flexion was im-

portant as a predictor of speed in persons with PD; reduced muscle strength was not significant. Speed of walking was not related to tremor, rigidity, or body sway in this study; however, they tested subjects on medication.

Morris et al. (40) studied 34 patients with idiopathic PD while on medication. They found that gait velocity was slower and attributed it to decreased stride length and increased cadence. Subjects were able voluntarily to increase or decrease stride length, but the response was reduced compared to that in controls. When provided with visual cueing, persons with PD could improve their stride length to that approaching normal. The authors thought that persons with PD have a "fundamental deficit in their ability to automatically regulate stride length" through internal cueing, possibly because they cannot generate the appropriate amplitude of movement necessary. Morris et al. suggested that increased cadence is used as compensation. Bagley and associates (2) found similar increases in stride length and time, but noted that velocity did not improve.

Ferrandez and Blin (18), who studied gait parameters in patients with PD on and off medication, found that L-dopa produced an increase in velocity and stride length and a decrease in double support time. They thought that this improvement was related more to controlling force output than to rhythmicity. Although stride length was not measured in the present study, the mechanism for increasing speed may be similar for pallidotomy.

Our results suggest that there may be two mechanisms for increasing gait velocity. Four persons walked after surgery who could not walk prior to surgery, indicating alleviation of akinesia or an increase in the neural drive. In light of other studies, and combined with results on strength presented below, we can hypothesize that diminished control of force production or lack of sustained activity may also be responsible for many of the difficulties in walking and other functional activities.

Postural Control Variables

Strength

Strength in the lower extremities was measured by the subjects' performance of five chair stands and five step-ups performed as quickly as possible. Tests were performed twice, and the times it took to complete each set of five were averaged. For chair stands, 95 seconds was the highest score recorded among those who could perform the task; therefore 100 seconds was recorded if the subjects were unable to stand up from the chair; 10 seconds was added to the score to indicate greater disability if they needed to use their arms as support to stand up from the chair. For step-ups, 68 seconds was the highest score recorded for those who could perform the task; therefore 70 seconds was recorded if the subjects were unable to step up onto the platform, and 10 seconds was added to their score if they needed minimal assistance from their arms. Two subjects had knee pain, which precluded their being able to perform the tests; therefore the number of subjects for these tasks is 31. Refer to Table 13-1 for the improvements in chair stands and step-ups.

Chair Stands

Four persons could not perform the task before or after surgery. Twenty subjects had a moderate or marked improvement at 3 and 6 months; three had minimal or no change, but these patients also had the best scores (< 18 seconds); and eight took longer than before surgery, although three were minimally slower (< 3 seconds). The mean score was 36.7 ± 27.6 seconds prior to surgery. The mean change in timed score at 3 months was 15.0 ± 24.3 seconds (average change of 21%), and at 6 months it was 5.1 ± 29.9 seconds (average change of 18%). Eight persons improved their time more than 50%, and six persons who needed to use their arms before surgery could do the task without their arms after surgery. Of 16 subjects tested at 1 year, 5 had worse scores than their pretest scores; however, all of them had demonstrated minimal or no improvement at 3 and 6 months after surgery.

Step-ups

Four subjects were unable to perform step-ups before surgery and were able to perform them after surgery; six subjects were able to step-up independently after surgery, whereas they needed as-sistance of their arms before surgery. Nineteen subjects had a moderate or marked change between their pretest scores and at 3 and 6 months; seven had no change or minimal improvement; and five got worse. Of the five who were worse, three were minimally worse (< 2 seconds). Seven persons improved their score by more than 50%. The mean score was 31.7 ± 19.9 seconds prior to surgery. The mean change in score at 3 months was 10.7 ± 16.9 seconds (average change of 35%), and at 6 months it was 9.9 ± 17.9 seconds (average change of 32%). Of 16 persons tested at 1 year, 6 were worse than they were before surgery; however, except for one individual, all of them had demonstrated minimal or no improvement at 3 and 6 months.

These data are somewhat difficult to interpret because they are not a pure measure of strength in the lower extremities. They are a measure of functional strength. In the two patients who were markedly worse, it appeared that the PD continued to be progressive. The improvement in scores could reflect a change in force production, a change in perception of balance (which is necessary to perform the movement smoothly and safely), or a change in bradykinesia/akinesia. The same subjects who got worse on the step test could not stand up from the chair, which appears to be related more to force production. Koller and Kase (26) noted that even in the early stages of the disease patients complained of weakness. Utilizing an isokinetic dynamometer, they demonstrated that persons with PD were weaker than age-matched controls. In hemiparkinsonism greater weakness was observed on the affected side.

Pedersen and Oberg (44) demonstrated that, off medication, isometric, concentric, and eccentric contractions demonstrated decreased peak torque in ankle dorsiflexors; however, there was no decrease in the area under the curve using the surface EMG. No co-contraction was observed in the soleus muscle group. They concluded that the strength reduction "points to a dysfunction in the organization of the control of contraction" by the central nervous system.

Kunesch and associates (27) studied isometric contractions in the upper extremities of subjects who were on medication. They studied the subjects' abilities to hold a constant force, to produce and release a force, reaction time and movement time, and maximal force production. A major finding in the study was that persons with PD had difficulty releasing a force once produced. This finding agrees with the theory that the basal ganglia turn off a postural set to allow movement to occur; and with dysfunction in the basal ganglia, persons are slower to release the previous force and switch to another motor program.

Corcos and associates (15) studied isometric contractions in the biceps and triceps muscles in nine persons with PD on and off medication while simultaneously recording the surface EMG. They found that, off medication, subjects demonstrated a reduction in peak torque that was much greater in extensor muscles (34%) than in the flexors. In addition, time to peak torque was greater off medication than on medication. They speculated that the decrease in extensor torque may be responsible for the difficulty rising from a chair and the flexed posture so characteristic of this group of patients. Bradykinesia was considered responsible for the delay in reaching peak torque, and changes in contraction rate correlated with the change in strength. Therefore the improvement in the subjects' ability to stand up and step up may also be due to two different mechanisms responsible for decreasing bradykinesia and improving modulation of force production so that movement is smoother and maintained.

Functional Tests of Balance

Refer to Table 13-1 for the criteria for improvement and the percentages of those who had improved functional tests of balance.

Functional Reach

Subjects were asked to reach forward with their arm outstretched as far as possible without moving their feet. The distance was measured three times (in inches). The reliability of this measure has been found to be 0.99 with normal subjects in our laboratory. In persons with PD, on medication, the intraclass correlation coefficient was reported as 0.84 (49). Of 33 subjects, 23 (70%) improved the distance they were able to reach before surgery at the 3- and 6-month evaluation pe-

riods. Ten persons were worse, although four had a decrease of less than 1 inch. Seven persons increased their distance by 50% or more. Fourteen subjects reached 6 inches or less before surgery and only 6 persons at 3 months, and five patients at 6 months reached 6 inches or less. In elderly persons it has been found that less than 6 inches forward reach is associated with falling (33). The mean score was 7.4 ± 3.7 inches prior to surgery. The mean change at 3 months was 1.8 ± 3.9 inches (an average gain of 47%), and at 6 months it was 1.4 ± 4.0 inches (average gain of 43%). The mean change in score at 1 year was 1.1 ± 4.6 inches. At 1 year four persons were doing worse after having done better at 3 and 6 months after surgery. Seven of sixteen (44%) were doing worse than before surgery at 1 year. Forward reach appears to peak at 3 months, is maintained at 6 months, and then begins to decline—but not to the presurgery values in all subjects.

POAB

The POAB analyzes nine activities, such as standing up from a chair, initial balance, stance width, eyes closed, a sternal nudge, and turning in a circle. Of 33 subjects, 17 demonstrated moderate or marked change; 10 demonstrated minimal improvement or no change; and 6 persons were worse. Of the 10 subjects with minimal change, 3 had scores of 15/16 or 16/16; hence there was no possibility for improvement. The median score presurgery was 9/16 and at 3 months was 13/16. The mean change score between presurgery and 3 months was 3.8 ± 4.9 (average change of 149%); between presurgery and 6 months the mean change in score was 3.2 ± 4.6 (average change of 144%). At 1 year, with 17 persons tested, the mean change was 1.5 ± 4.9 (average change of 78%). It was interesting to note that the one item on the POAB that showed no improvement while subjects were "off" medication was the sternal nudge, or an external perturbation. Functional tasks improved, but automatic postural responses did not.

Turning Left and Turning Right

Subjects were asked to walk in a small circle to the left and to the right. The time (in seconds) was recorded. The reliability of this measure has been reported to be 0.80 in persons with PD who are moderately impaired when they are on medication (49). The maximum time recorded for those who could perform the task was 53 seconds; therefore 60 seconds was recorded if the subject could not perform the task. When turning to the left, seven persons could not perform the task before surgery but could after pallidotomy. Most of the operations were performed on the left side because the right side was more affected; therefore turning to the left was more difficult. Altogether 21 persons showed moderate to marked improvement after surgery, 7 had minimal or no improvement, and 5 were worse. Eleven persons improved their score more than 50%. The mean score presurgery was 26.0 ± 20.9 seconds. The average change score at 3 months was 9.6 ± 20.9 seconds (average change of 35%) and at 6 months 8.5 ± 21.2 seconds (average change of 30%). Values ranged from a normal score of 2 to 3 seconds to 60 seconds. At 1 year, with 17 subjects evaluated, the change score was 1.1 ± 18.5.

For turning right, two persons could not perform the task prior to surgery and could after surgery; only one could not do it before or after surgery. Nineteen persons showed moderate to marked change at 3 and 6 months after surgery; five persons showed minimal or no change (of these three had scores of ≤ 10 seconds); and seven persons were worse. Eleven persons improved their timed score by 50% or more. The mean score prior to surgery was 23.7 ± 19.6 seconds. The average change scores between 3 and 6 months were 8.8 ± 13.3 (average change of 32%) and 9.1 ± 16.5 seconds (average change of 33%), respectively. At 1 year, with 16 patients evaluated, the change score was 0.49 ± 18.6.

From functional tests of balance, it appears that postural control improves until at least 6 months postsurgery and then begins to decline at 1 year after pallidotomy; however, some persons maintain the improvement or at least do not return to presurgery states. For the POAB and for turning, bradykinesia/akinesia and freezing were observed to reappear as symptoms or were unaffected by the surgery. The forward reach is not as affected by bradykinesia or freezing because it is not timed and does not represent a great deal of force production; therefore functional reach may be more of a pure marker for balance. Forty-four percent of patients tested at 1 year had a score lower than before surgery, and ten persons were worse after surgery. This, coupled with the fact that the sternal nudge did not show significant improvement, may reflect that postural control continues to deteriorate despite the pallidotomy. However, this test is strongly influenced by the patient's perception of ability or fear of falling, not necessarily their capability. To the authors' knowledge, no others have used these precise, quantitative tests in patients after pallidotomy, so it is difficult to compare results. As noted before, many authors have remarked on the improvement in postural stability when measured by the ADL and Motor scores on the UPDRS, although these scores are more subjective.

Correlations With Presurgical Variables

Presurgery Variables

To determine if there was a relationship between the Hoehn and Yahr, the Motor and ADL scores on the UPDRS, and the functional variables that were measured, Spearman correlations were calculated and are presented in Table 13-2. The HY score correlated highly significantly with all measured variables. The Motor score on the UPDRS correlated significantly with all variables except the POAG and turning to the right. The POAG reflects more of the quality of the gait, which may be the reason for the lack of correlation. It is possible that turning while walking was not significantly related to the Motor score because the Motor score reflects the examiner's rating of items such as rigidity, tremor, rapid alternating movements, rising from a chair, and postural stability as well as bradykinesia and gait. The ADL score on the UPDRS correlated significantly with all variables except the turns to the left and to the right. This score reflects freezing, falling, and walking, so this lack of correlation is somewhat surprising; however, only three of the ten items in this score are related to walking, with the others measuring such things as

TABLE 13-2. *Spearman correlations among presurgery functional variables*

Parameter	H & Y	ADL	Motor	TW	POAG	POAB	FR	TRS	TLS	CS	SUps
H & Y		0.63 (n = 34) 0.000*	0.69 (n = 34) 0.000*	0.55 (n = 34) 0.001*	−0.52 (n = 33) 0.002*	−0.79 (n = 33) 0.000*	−0.69 (n = 33) 0.000*	0.61 (n = 31) 0.000*	0.53 (n = 33) 0.001*	0.47 (n = 31) 0.007*	0.61 (n = 31) 0.000*
Motor	0.69 (n = 34) 0.000*	0.58 (n = 34) 0.000*		0.50 (n = 33) 0.003*	−0.29 (n = 32) 0.103	−0.66 (n = 32) 0.000*	−0.51 (n = 32) 0.003*	0.35 (n = 30) 0.056	0.44 (n = 32) 0.011*	0.46 (n = 30) 0.012*	0.66 (n = 30) 0.000*
ADL	0.63 (n = 34) 0.000*		0.58 (n = 34) 0.000*	0.52 (n = 33) 0.002*	−0.41 (n = 32) 0.020*	−0.66 (n = 32) 0.000*	−0.44 (n = 32) 0.011*	0.35 (n = 30) 0.055	0.33 (n = 32) 0.062	0.60 (n = 30) 0.000*	0.62 (n = 30) 0.000*

POAG, performance-oriented assessment of gait; POAB, performance-oriented assessment of balance; TW, timed walk; FR, functional reach; TRS, turning to the right (in seconds); TLS, turning to the left (in seconds); CS, time for five stand-ups from a chair; SUps, time for five step-ups onto an 8-inch platform; H & Y, Hoehn and Yahr score; ADL, freezing, falling, walking, turning in bed, bradykinesia; Motor, tremor, rigidity, coordination, arising from chair, gait, postural stability, bradykinesia.

*Significant at $p \leq 0.05$.

swallowing and drooling. Interesting to note is that age correlated with none of the variables. Of great interest was the moderately high correlations between the HY scores and the UPDRS with the POAB and step-ups, and the HY with the FR. The moderate correlations of the variables indicate that they are measuring a similar construct.

Postsurgery Variables

Change scores on all of the variables measured were correlated with the HY and the ADL and Motor scores of the UPDRS to determine which of them might be used to predict the patients who would have the best results from surgery. These data are presented in Table 13-3. Generally speaking, the more impaired the individual was, the greater were the change scores. The HY score correlated best with changes in the strength measures of the time required for five chair stands and five step-ups, although correlations with the POAB scores at 3 and 6 months were moderately high. The motor score correlated best with the timed variables of turning, standing up, and stepping up. The greater the motor score, the greater was the change score. The motor score had a moderately high correlation with the POAB; the higher the motor score, the greater was the improvement in balance. It was not related to the simple task of reaching forward or to the performance on the POAG. The ADL score related to all change scores except for turning while walking.

Posturography

Static Variables

The Smart Balance Master (NeuroCom International) was used to collect data on the changes in the sensory contributions to postural control. The variables measured were eyes open and eyes closed on a stable platform and center target, which provides visual feedback while demanding that the subject move his or her center of gravity to the most biomechanically correct posture and maintain it there for 20 seconds. Means and standard deviations are presented for these variables

in Table 13-4. To determine how many subjects did not have normal postural control, normal scores are discussed that were obtained from a sample of 45 persons tested in our laboratory. Generally, there was a decrease in the variability in scores after surgery, and all conditions demonstrate improvement; that is, the subjects demonstrated less sway. For the center target, mean scores improved by 50%. Seven persons experienced marked decrease in sway after surgery (> 0.10% of LOS); four subjects increased sway at 3 months and seven persons at 6 months. When compared to the normal values for center target, among those less than 60 years of age 12 were not in the normal range prior to surgery, 7 were still not in the normal range 3 months after surgery, and 6 were still out of the normal range 6 months after surgery. Among those over 60 years of age, 6 were outside the normal range prior to surgery, 3 at 3 months, and 9 at 6 months, indicating that younger persons continued to improve while older persons tend to get better at 3 months but then begin to decline. Maki and McIlroy (35) stated that excessive sway is not likely to result in a loss of balance unless the person's center of mass is already near the limits of stability. Persons with PD may already be at their posterior limits of stability due to their tendency to shift their weight backward during quiet stance. This test was noted to be difficult for persons with advanced PD because it required them to hold a position in which they felt insecure, and it placed a large attentional demand on them. Moreover, if vision is not accurate, this task is all the more difficult. Photographs of subjects (Fig. 13-1) before and after surgery showed marked improvement in the static posture of all subjects after surgery; therefore it is possible that with the improvement in posture it was easier to maintain the center of gravity closer to a more normal position.

We must address the fatigue issue. Almost all of the patients after pallidotomy reported that they had much more energy and were able to accomplish much more during the day, including fairly heavy work, such as gardening and housekeeping. Although this improvement may certainly be a result of the release from tonic inhibition, it could also be related to the decreased attentional demands placed on the patient's sys-

TABLE 13-3. *Significant Spearman correlations among presurgery descriptions of disease severity and change scores in functional strength and balance measures*

Parameter	POAG		POAB		TW		FR		TRS		TLS		CS		SUps	
	3 Mo.	6 Mo.	3 Mo.	6 Mo.	3 Mo.	6 Mo.	3 Mo.	6 Mo.	3 Mo.	6 Mo.	3 Mo.	6 Mo.	3 Mo.	6 Mo.	3 Mo.	6 Mo.
H & Y	NS	NS	0.67 (n = 33) 0.000	0.53 (n = 32) 0.002	NS	NS	NS	0.39 (n = 32) 0.027	NS	0.46 (n = 30) 0.011	NS	NS	0.41 (n = 30) 0.026	0.45 (n = 29) 0.016	0.60 (n = 31) 0.000	0.57 (n = 30) 0.001
ADL	0.36 (n = 32) 0.046	NS	0.65 (n = 32) 0.000	0.63 (n = 31) 0.000	0.40 (n = 32) 0.021	0.42 (n = 32) 0.018	NS	0.43 (n = 31) 0.016	NS	NS	NS	NS	0.59 (n = 29) 0.001	0.48 (n = 28) 0.008	0.55 (n = 30) 0.002	0.49 (n = 29) 0.007
Motor	NS	NS	0.71 (n = 32) 0.000	0.66 (n = 31) 0.000	NS	0.40 (n = 32) 0.022	NS	NS	0.41 (n = 30) 0.025	0.50 (n = 29) 0.006	0.47 (n = 32) 0.006	0.50 (n = 31) 0.004	0.58 (n = 29) 0.001	0.58 (n = 28) 0.001	0.69 (n = 30) 0.000	0.71 (n = 29) 0.000

POAG, performance-oriented assessment of gait; POAB, performance-oriented assessment of balance; TW, timed walk; FR, functional reach; TRS, turning to the right (in seconds); TLS, turning to the left (in seconds); CS, time for five stand-ups from a chair; SUps, time for five step-ups onto an 8-inch platform.

NS, $p > 0.05$.

TABLE 13-4. *Descriptive statistics for static posturography variables*

Variable	Center target $\overline{X} \pm SD$	ChSc	Eyes closed $\overline{X} \pm SD$	ChSc	Eyes open $\overline{X} \pm SD$	ChSc
PCT	0.27 ± 0.72		0.38 ± 0.43		0.21 ± 0.29	
CT$_3$	0.11 ± 0.14	0.17	0.24 ± 0.27	0.13	0.13 ± 0.13	0.08
CT$_6$	0.14 ± 0.17	0.13	0.25 ± 0.24	0.13	0.11 ± 0.11	0.10
CT$_{12}$	0.12 ± 0.09	0.22	0.27 ± 0.31	0.07	0.12 ± 0.16	0.09

PCT, center target sway before surgery; CT$_3$, center target sway 3 months after surgery; CT$_6$, center target sway 6 months after surgery; CT$_{12}$, center target sway 12 months after surgery; ChSc, mean change score from PCT.

tem to hold the body up against gravity, resulting in less fatigue.

For the eyes-open condition, there were ten outside the normal range of scores among those under age 60 years before surgery, eight at 3 months, and eight at 6 months. For those over age 60, there were eight outside the normal range of scores before surgery, four at 3 months, and two at 6 months. In the eyes-closed condition, ten persons in each age group had scores outside the normal range before surgery, eight in each group at 3 months, and eight in each group at 6 months. It was interesting to note that the eyes-closed sway was about twice that of the eyes-open sway, just as it is with normal subjects. The eyes-open condition had about the same change as the eyes-closed condition; therefore it is not likely that the change in the eyes-closed condition is due to increased use of somatosensation but, rather, to a change in overall control or perception of control. Although older persons performed better than the younger group in the eyes-open condition, it should be noted that the range of normal values is much larger for this age group.

Dynamic Variables

For the dynamic variables test, subjects were asked to look at a computer screen while standing upright. Eight targets appeared on the screen in an ellipse representing the subject's theoretical limits of stability. The subject was asked to lean from the ankles so his or her center of gravity was in the center target. When a target was highlighted, the subjects were asked to move their center of gravity to that target without moving the feet. The time required to reach the target was recorded, as was the accuracy of the path taken to get to the target (path sway). If the subject did not reach the target, 8 seconds was recorded as the maximum time. Values for the average time taken for the eight targets and the change scores appears in Table 13-5

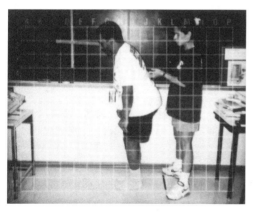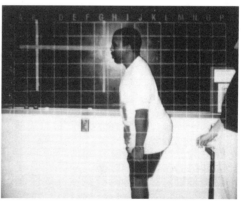

A   B

FIG. 13-1. Standing posture of a patient with PD before **(A)** and after **(B)** posteroventral pallidotomy procedure.

TABLE 13-5. *Descriptive statistics for posturographic dynamic variables*

Time	ATM			APL		
	$\overline{X}$	SD	ChSc	$\overline{X}$	SD	ChSc
Pretest (*n* = 33)	6.65	1.22		217.58	87.18	
3 Months (*n* = 33)	6.01	1.39	0.73	196.25	64.00	20.93
6 Months (*n* = 32)	5.79	1.50	0.91	182.45	42.58	39.25
12 Months (*n* = 19)	5.96	1.50	0.68	186.99	49.71	18.05

ATM, averaged time for eight targets; APL, averaged path deviation for eight targets; ChSc, mean change score from pretest.

and are compared with normal times recorded in our laboratory for a sample of 45 persons. Before surgery, all 12 subjects who were less than 60 years of age had out of normal range averaged time for the eight targets; 19 of 21 subjects more than 60 years of age had out of normal range scores. At 3 months there was only one person in each age category with normal scores; four subjects' scores were worse than their presurgery scores, but only one person was greatly worse. At 6 months, for those less than 60 years of age, still only one subject was in the normal range; for those more than 60 years of age, 5 were close to the normal range and 16 were outside the normal range. Six persons were worse at 6 months, but only one was greatly worse. Subjects in the younger group never improved to a normal score except one at 6 months who declined again at 1 year.

The mean path sway to reach the eight targets appears in Table 13-5. Before surgery six persons

in the less than 60 years age group and eight persons in the more than 60 age group were outside the normal range for the age group. At 3 months, four and five persons were outside the normal range for their age group in the less than and more than 60 year age groups, respectively. At 6 months, four and three persons were outside the normal range for this variable for their age groups in the less than and more than 60 years groups, respectively. Only eight persons were worse than their presurgery scores at 3 months, and only two persons had scores at 6 months worse than their presurgery scores. Generally, it was noted when looking at the raw tracings (Fig. 13-2) that subjects seemed to exert finer control over their movement to the targets, as it was smoother and more organized. Therefore even though time was not improved and many targets were still missed, it is possible that time was sacrificed for the sake of accuracy and control. Whereas subjects were still having difficulty

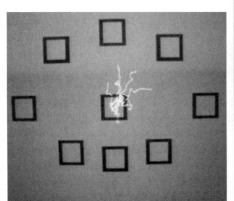
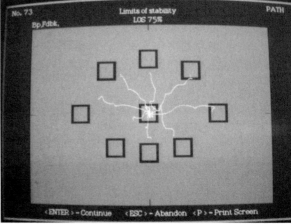

A

FIG. 13-2. Limits of stability (LOS) test results in a patient before **(A)** and 3 months after **(B)** posteroventral pallidotomy demonstrating improved ability to reach targets set at 75% LOS and better organization of the response.

reaching 75% of their limits of stability in a reasonable amount of time, voluntary control over the movements appears to be improved, as evidenced by the straighter path tracings.

Spearman Correlations of Presurgery Variables with Posturography Variables

Presurgery Variables

The HY and Motor and ADL scores on the UPDRS are significantly correlated with sensory scores on posturography, specifically eyes open and eyes closed on a stable surface (Table 13-6). The more involved the subject is, the greater sway he or she exhibits in these stable conditions. The moderately low correlations indicate that the tests may be measuring a similar construct, but they are not the same. The HY and the UPDRS may be measuring more functional performance and the sensory testing measures pure postural control. Although one is needed for the other, they are not the same thing.

TABLE 13-6. *Spearman correlations: among presurgery posturography variables and descriptors of disease severity*

Variable	H & Y	Motor	ADL
Pre-ATM	0.41	0.23	0.22
	(n = 33)	(n = 32)	(n = 32)
	0.017*	0.215	0.244
Pre-APL	0.40	0.20	0.13
	(n = 33)	(n = 32)	(n = 32)
	0.023*	0.277	0.465
Pre-CT	0.27	0.20	0.14
	(n = 33)	(n = 32)	(n = 32)
	0.126	0.264	0.454
Pre-EO	0.44	0.39	0.44
	(n = 34)	(n = 33)	(n = 33)
	0.009*	0.024*	0.011*
Pre-EC	0.36	0.42	0.47
	(n = 34)	(n = 33)	(n = 33)
	0.036*	0.014*	0.006*

H & Y, Hoehn & Yahr score; Motor, motor score on UPDRS; ADL, ADL score on UPDRS; Pre-ATM, pretest score for averaged time for eight targets; Pre-APL, pretest score for averaged path length for eight targets; Pre-CT, pretest score for sway, center target; Pre-EO, pretest score for sway, eyes open, fixed surface; Pre-EC, pretest score for sway, eyes closed, fixed surface.
    * Significant at $p \leq 0.05$.

Only the HY correlates with the averaged time for the eight targets and the averaged length of the path. The more involved the subject is, the longer are the time and path length to reach the targets with visual feedback. One would expect there to be some relation with the Motor and ADL scores on the UPDRS, as bradykinesia/akinesia is the most plausible reason for a slow time and tortuous path. Interestingly, the sway in the center target is not correlated with any of the functional measures.

Postsurgery Variables

Generally speaking, the HY and the Motor and ADL scores are not related to the amount of change in the subjects' scores after pallidotomy. Isolated cases demonstrating a relation are easily seen in Table 13-7. The ADL score does not correlate with any of the posturographic changes; however, the Motor score correlates with the averaged path length of the LOS during the sixth month and with decreased sway in the eyes-closed position at 3 months. The greater the disability, the more change takes place in the sway in the eyes-closed condition and in the averaged path length. The presurgery values for sway in the eyes-open, eyes-closed, and center target are all significantly correlated with the magnitude of the change score in these same conditions. To determine the maximum improvement on these tests, one need only to look at the presurgery scores.

CONCLUSIONS

The greatest changes in all of the variables are noted in persons with the greatest disability; therefore although persons with mild disability can improve with the pallidotomy procedure, their gain is not as great. Positive changes were seen in all of the variables mentioned when the group was taken as a whole, although several patients demonstrated minimal or no improvement or even got worse. This was not related to any event that occurred during surgery. In most cases patients did not improve sufficiently to be in the normal range for tests of balance. Generally, from the limited sample tested at 12 months

TABLE 13-7. *Spearman correlations: change in posturography variables (3 and 6 months) and presurgery variables*

Variable	ATM		APL		CT		EO		EC	
	3 Mo.	6 Mo.	3 Mo.	6 Mo.	3 Mo.	6 Mo.	3 Mo.	6 Mo.	3 Mo.	6 Mo.
H & Y	0.03 (n = 31) 0.856	−0.33 (n = 31) 0.062	0.13 (n = 31) 0.489	0.29 (n = 30) 0.120	0.04 (n = 32) 0.842	0.17 (n = 33) 0.341	0.33 (n = 34) 0.056	0.35 (n = 32) 0.050*	0.29 (n = 33) 0.199	0.12 (n = 33) 0.517
Motor (UPDRS)	0.16 (n = 31) 0.401	−0.25 (n = 30) 0.186	0.14 (n = 31) 0.453	0.42 (n = 29) 0.022*	0.11 (n = 32) 0.557	0.29 (n = 32) 0.106	0.24 (n = 33) 0.187	0.32 (n = 31) 0.081	0.36 (n = 33) 0.040*	0.20 (n = 32) 0.280
ADL (UPDRS)	0.12 (n = 31) 0.531	−0.27 (n = 30) 0.156	0.13 (n = 31) 0.499	0.11 (n = 29) 0.579	−0.08 (n = 32) 0.649	0.16 (n = 32) 0.393	0.05 (n = 33) 0.799	0.34 (n = 31) 0.066	0.21 (n = 33) 0.238	0.20 (n = 32) 0.268
Pre-ATM	0.06 (n = 31) 0.753	−0.16 (n = 31) 0.401	−0.22 (n = 31) 0.226	−0.07 (n = 30) 0.711	−0.22 (n = 32) 0.231	−0.21 (n = 33) 0.247	0.04 (n = 33) 0.835	0.11 (n = 32) 0.534	−0.15 (n = 32) 0.414	−0.08 (n = 33) 0.653
Pre-APL	−0.22 (n = 31) 0.236	−0.31 (n = 31) 0.088	0.43 (n = 31) 0.015*	0.66 (n = 30) 0.000*	0.21 (n = 32) 0.248	0.16 (n = 33) 0.365	0.55 (n = 33) 0.001*	0.23 (n = 32) 0.210	0.20 (n = 32) 0.281	0.26 (n = 33) 0.520
Pre-CT	−0.14 (n = 31) 0.466	−0.12 (n = 31) 0.518	0.27 (n = 31) 0.14	0.46 (n = 30) 0.011*	0.67 (n = 32) 0.000*	0.60 (n = 33) 0.000*	0.71 (n = 33) 0.000*	0.61 (n = 32) 0.000*	0.55 (n = 32) 0.001*	0.56 (n = 33) 0.001*
Pre-EO	−0.13 (n = 31) 0.499	−0.205 (n = 31) 0.268	0.17 (n = 31) 0.358	0.29 (n = 30) 0.123	0.45 (n = 32) 0.011*	0.39 (n = 33) 0.024*	0.68 (n = 34) 0.000*	0.81 (n = 32) 0.000*	0.46 (n = 33) 0.007*	0.47 (n = 33) 0.006*
Pre-EC	0.004 (n = 31) 0.981	−0.14 (n = 31) 0.459	0.18 (n = 31) 0.322	0.36 (n = 30) 0.050*	0.42 (n = 32) 0.016*	0.40 (n = 33) 0.020*	0.41 (n = 34) 0.017*	0.67 (n = 32) 0.000*	0.52 (n = 33) 0.002*	0.63 (n = 33) 0.000*

ATM, averaged time; APL, averaged path length; CT, center target sway; EO, sway with eyes opened, fixed surface; EC, sway with eyes closed, fixed surface; Pre, pretest scores.
* Significant at $p \leq 0.05$.

some decline in function is observed, although the change scores are still in a positive direction. Age is not a factor in the amount of change, as it correlated with none of the postsurgery scores. Two persons, both female, fell after surgery, demonstrating that their balance was still a problem. At least one of those persons had fairly severe postural deformities that were fixed; therefore pallidotomy could not effect any changes in the posture overall. The one person who got progressively worse (also a woman) was extremely frail prior to surgery, and her disease seemed to be progressive, regardless of the surgery.

Although there is a model proposed for how the basal ganglia function to support movement, it does not explain completely why postural control improves or does not improve after pallidotomy. From the work that we have done, it appears that posture and gait improve owing to the release of the thalamocortical pathway from excessive inhibition. Postural dyscontrol in persons with PD appears to be predominantly a dysfunction in the motor system, particularly as it relates to sequencing muscle contractions, releasing a postural set, and generating sufficient force in a timely and controlled manner, rather than in short bursts of activity. Although balance is improved on functional tasks, such as standing up from a chair and stepping up, there is less improvement on pure measures of balance, which may mean that balance is resistant not only to medication effects but also to surgical effects and therefore may require some training postoperatively for the maximum benefit to be realized. More research is needed to determine other ways of influencing the postural control mechanism.

Acknowledgments. This work was supported in part by a grant from the NIDRR (191180043).

REFERENCES

1. Allison L. Balance disorders. In: Umphred DA, ed. *Neurological rehabilitation,* 3rd ed. St. Louis: Mosby, 1995: 802–837.
2. Bagley S, Kelly B, Tunnicliffe N, Turnbull GI, Walker JM. The effect of visual cues on the gait of independently mobile Parkinson's disease patients. *Physiotherapy* 1991;77:415–420.
3. Bakay RA, DeLong MR, Vitek JL. Neurosurgical forum. *J Neurosurg* 1992;77:487–488.
4. Baron MS, Vitek JL, Bakay RAE, et al. Treatment of advanced Parkinson's disease by posterior GPi pallidotomy: 1-year results of a pilot study. *Ann Neurol* 1996;40: 355–366.
5. Bazalgette D, Zattara M, Bathien N, Bouisset S, Rondot P. Postural adjustments associated with rapid voluntary arm movements in patients with Parkinson's disease. *Adv Neurol* 1986;45:371–374.
6. Beckley DJ, Bloem BR, van Dijk JG, Ross RAC, Remler MP. Electrophysiological correlates of postural instability in Parkinson's disease. *Electroencephalogr Clin Neurophysiol* 1991;81:263–268.
7. Berg KO, Wood-Dauphines SL, Williams JI, Gayton D. Measuring balance in the elderly: preliminary development of an instrument. *Physiother Can* 1989;41: 304–311.
8. Bloem BR, Beckley DJ, vanDijk JG, Zwinderman AH, Ross RAC. Are medium and long latency reflexes a screening tool for early Parkinson's disease? *J Neurol Sci* 1992;113:38–42.
9. Bodis-Wollner I. Visual deficits related to dopamine deficiency in experimental animals and Parkinson's disease patients. *TINS* 1990;13:296–302.
10. Bowes SG, Charlett A, Dobbs RJ, Lubel DD, et al. Gait in relation to ageing and idiopathic Parkinsonism. *Scand J Rehabil Med* 1992;24:181–186.
11. Bronstein AM, Hood JD, Gresty MA, Panagi C. Visual control of balance in cerebellar and parkinsonian syndromes. *Brain* 1990;113:767–779.
12. Ceballos-Baumann AO, Obeso JA, Vitek JL, et al. Restoration of thalamic cortical activity after posteroventral pallidotomy in Parkinson's disease. *Lancet* 1994;344:814.
13. Cole B, Finch E, Gowland C, Mayo N. In: Basmajiian J, ed. *Physical rehabilitation outcome measures.* Toronto: Canadian Physiotherapy Association, 1994.
14. Cooke JD, Brown JD, Brooks VB. Increased dependence on visual information for movement control in patients with Parkinson's disease. *Can J Neuro sci* 1978;5: 413–415.
15. Corcos DM, Chen CM, Quinn NP, McAuley J, Rothwell JC. Strength in Parkinson's disease: relationship to rate of force generation and clinical status. *Ann Neurol* 1996;39:79–88.
16. Dogali M, Fazzini E, Kolodny E, et al. Stereotactic ventral pallidotomy for Parkinson's disease. *Neurology* 1995; 45:753–761.
17. Duncan PW, Weiner DK, Chandler JM, Studenski S. Functional reach: a new clinical measure of balance. *J Gerontol* 1990;45:M192–197.
18. Ferrandez AM, Blin O. A comparison between the effect of intentional modulations and the action of L-dopa on gait in Parkinson's disease. *Behav Brain Res* 1991;45: 177–183.
19. Goetz CG, Delong MR, Penn RD, Bakay RAE. Neurosurgical horizons in Parkinson's disease. *Neurology* 1993;43:1–7.
20. Grafton ST, Waters C, Sutton J, Lew MF, Couldwell W. Pallidotomy increases activity of motor association cortex in Parkinson's disease: a positron emission tomographic study. *Ann Neurol* 1995;37:776–783.
21. Hines C, Mercer V. Anticipatory postural adjustments: an update. *Neurol Rep* 1997;21(1):17–22.
22. Iacono RP, Lonser RR, Oh A, Yamada S. New pathophysiology of Parkinson's disease revealed by posteroventral pallidotomy. *Neurol Res* 1995;17:178–180.

23. Iacono RP, Shima F, Lonser RR, Kuniyoshi S, Maeda G, Yamada S. The results, indications, and physiology of posteroventral pallidotomy for patients with Parkinson's disease. *Neurosurgery* 1995;36:1118–1127.

24. Johansson F, Malm J, Nordh E, Hariz M. Usefulness of pallidotomy in advanced Parkinson's disease. *J Neurol Neurosurg Psychiatry* 1997;62:125–132.

25. Kitamura J, Nakagawa H, Iinuma K, et al. Visual influence on center of contact pressure in advanced Parkinson's disease. *Arch Phys Med Rehabil* 1993;74:1107–1112.

26. Koller W, Kase S. Muscle strength testing in Parkinson's disease. *Eur Neurol* 1986;25:130–133.

27. Kunesch E, Schnitzler A, Tyercha C, Knecht S, Stelmach G. Altered force release control in Parkinson's disease. *Behav Brain Res* 1995;67:43–49.

28. Laitinen LV. Ventroposterolateral pallidotomy. *Stereotact Funct Neurosurg* 1994;62:41–52.

29. Laitinen LV, Bergenheim AT, Hariz MI. Ventroposterolateral pallidotomy can abolish all parkinsonian symptoms. *Stereotract Funct Neurosurg* 1992;58:14–21.

30. Laitinen LV, Bergenheim T, Hariz MI. Leksell's posteroventral pallidotomy in the treatment of Parkinson's disease. *J Neurosurg* 1992;76:53–61.

31. Lang AE, Lozano A, Galvez-Jimenez N, et al. Posteroventral-medial pallidotomy for late stage Parkinson's disease: a 2 year follow-up. *Ann Neurol* 1996;40:538 (abst).

32. Lee RG, Tonolli I, Viallet F, Aurenty R, Massion J. Preparatory postural adjustments in parkinsonian patients with postural instability. *Can J Neurol Sci* 1995;22:126–135.

33. Lewis CB, McNerney T. *Clinical measures of functional outcomes: the "functional tool box."* Washington, DC: Learn Publications, 1994.

34. Lozano AM, Lang AE, Galvez-Jimenez N, et al. Effect of GPi pallidotomy on motor function in Parkinson's disease. *Lancet* 1995;346:1383–1387.

35. Maki BE, McIlroy WE. Postural control in the older adult. *Clin Geriatr Med* 1996;12:635–658.

36. Maki BE, McIlroy WE. The role of limb movement in maintaining upright stance: the "change in support" strategy. *Phys Ther* 1997;77:488–507.

37. Marsden CD, Obeso JA. The functions of the basal ganglia and the paradox of stereotaxic surgery in Parkinson's disease. *Brain* 1994;117:877–897.

38. Maylor EA, Wing AM. Age differences in postural stability are increased by additional cognitive demands. *J Gerontol B Psychol Sci Soc Sci* 1996;51b:P143–154.

39. Mitchell SL, Collins JJ, DeLuca CJ, Burrows A, Lipsitz LA. Open-loop and closed-loop postural control mechanisms in Parkinson's disease: increased mediolateral activity during quiet standing. *Neurosci Lett* 1995;197:133–136.

40. Morris ME, Iansek R, Matyas TA, Summers JJ. The pathogenesis of gait hypokinesia in Parkinson's disease. *Brain* 1994;117:1169–1181.

41. Morris ME, Matyas TA, Iansek R, Summers JJ. Temporal stability of gait in Parkinson's disease. *Phys Ther* 1996;76:763–789.

42. Nashner L. Computerized dynamic posturography. In: Jacobsen GP, Newman CW, Kartush JM, eds. *Handbook of balance function testing.* St. Louis: Mosby Year Book, 1993:261–307.

43. Pastor MA, Day BL, Marsden CD. Vestibular induced postural responses in Parkinson's disease. *Brain* 1993;116:1177–1190.

44. Pedersen SW, Oberg B. Dynamic strength in Parkinson's disease. *Eur Neurol* 1993;33:97–102.

45. Reichert WH, Doolittle J, Phil M, McDowell FH. Vestibular dysfunction in Parkinson disease. *Neurology* 1982;32:1133–1138.

46. Reuben D, Siu AL. An objective measure of physical function of elderly outpatients: the physical performance test. *J Am Geriatr Soc* 1990;38:1105–1112.

47. Richards M, Cote LJ, Stern Y. The relationship between visuospatial ability and perceptual motor function in Parkinson's disease. *J Neurol Neurosurg Psychiatry* 1993;56:400–406.

48. Rogers MW. Disorders of posture, balance, and gait in Parkinson's disease. In: Studenski S, ed. *Clin Geriatr Med* 1996;12:825–843.

49. Schenkman M, Cutson TM, Kuchibhatla M, Chandler J, Pieper C. Reliability of impairment and physical performance measures for persons with Parkinson's disease. *Phys Ther* 1997;77:19–27.

50. Schieppati M, Hugon M, Grasso M, Nardone A, Galante M. The limits of equilibrium in young and elderly normal subjects and in parkinsonians. *Electroencephalogr Clin Neurophysiol* 1994;93:286–298.

51. Scholz E, Diener HC, Noth J, Friedman H, Dichgans J, Bacher M. Medium and long latency EMG responses in leg muscles: Parkinson's disease. *J Neurol Neurosurg Psychiatry* 1987;50:66–70.

52. Stelmach GE, Zelaznck HN, Lower D. The influence of aging and attentional demands on recovery from postural instability. Aging 1990;2:155–161.

53. Tinetti M. Performance oriented assessment of mobility problems in elderly patients. *J Am Geriatr Soc* 1986;34:119–126.

54. Toole T, Park S, Hirsch MA, Lelman DA, Maitland CG. The multicomponent nature of equilibrium in persons with parkinsonism: a regression approach. *J Neural Transm* 1996;103:561–580.

55. Trenkwalder C, Paulus W, Krafczyk S, Hawken M, Oertel WH, Brandt T. Postural stability differentiates "lower body" from idiopathic parkinsonism. *Acta Neurol Scand* 1995;91:444–452.

56. Wall JC, Turnbull GI. The kinematics of gait. In: Turnbull GI, ed. *Physical therapy management of Parkinson's Disease.* New York: Churchill Livingstone, 1992:49–67.

57. Waterston JA, Hawken MB, Tanyeri S, Jantti P, Kennard C. Influence of sensory manipulation on postural control in Parkinson's disease. *J Neurol Neurosurg Psychiatry* 1993;56:1276–1281.

Pallidal Surgery for the Treatment of Parkinson's Disease and Movement Disorders, edited by J. K. Krauss, R. G. Grossman, and J. Jankovic. Lippincott-Raven Publishers, Philadelphia © 1998.

14

Neuropsychological Evaluation of Patients with Parkinson's Disease Before and After Pallidal Surgery

Gayle M. Rettig, *Eugene C. Lai, Joachim K. Krauss, Robert G. Grossman, and *Joseph Jankovic

*Departments of Neurosurgery and *Neurology, Baylor College of Medicine, Houston, Texas 77030, USA*

Improvements in stereotactic surgery, neuroradiological imaging, and electrophysiological targeting of the lesion site, combined with a better understanding of the pathophysiology underlying Parkinson's disease (PD), have led to a resurgence in stereotactic surgery for PD. It has been particularly used in patients in whom prolonged use of levodopa has led to a loss of the drug's effectiveness and has induced disabling side effects. For these patients, microelectrode-guided posteroventral pallidotomy (PVP) has proved to be a safe, effective treatment for the motor symptoms of rigidity, bradykinesia, levodopa-induced dyskinesias, and tremor.

The effect of PVP on neuropsychological functioning is less clear, in part because the effect of PD on cognition and other neuropsychological parameters is poorly understood. Previous studies of cognition in patients with advanced PD have shown significant impairments in speed of information processing, visuospatial abilities, executive functioning, and recall memory (16,23,41, 42,44,69). The neuropsychological effects of PVD in patients with PD have been investigated in even fewer studies. Most of these studies have reported on a small number of patients and for brief follow-up periods. The tentative conclusions provided by these studies offer little consensus concerning the probable impact of PVP on cognitive functioning.

The purpose of this chapter is to review the findings of studies done at other institutions and, together with data obtained at our institution, discuss the present state of knowledge concerning the neuropsychological effects of PVD in patients with PD. More specifically, we address (a) the neuropsychological changes that occur following PVP; (b) the patient variables, including the side of surgery, associated with neuropsychological changes following PVP; and (c) the effects of PVP on the patient's mood or emotional adjustment.

NEUROPSYCHOLOGICAL IMPAIRMENT IN PARKINSON'S DISEASE

In the original report by Parkinson in 1817, the symptoms of the disease were described as tremor, rigidity, and motor slowing. The concept of PD as a purely motor disorder persisted until the 1960s owing to the relative absence of obvious language deficits and other deficits associated with cortical dementia. During the 1960s neuroanatomical evidence of large, direct connections between the prefrontal cortex and the basal ganglia led to studies comparing the cognitive and behavioral deficits observed in PD patients with the deficits observed in patients with frontal lobe damage. Results from the evaluation of various higher-order cognitive tasks revealed a number of similarities between the two groups of patients (11,13,24,30,49,70), although later studies have shown that differences also exist (20,27,28,53). In addition, primate studies have demonstrated that when a lesion placed within the dorsolateral cortex or orbital frontal cortex produced a performance deficit on a cognitive task, the same deficit could be replicated by placing a lesion within the specific basal ganglia region to which the cortical area projected (30,38). Subsequent research has shown that the direct connections between the dorsolateral frontal cortex and the basal ganglia (the frontostriatal circuit) represent but one of three nonmotor, parallel, closed feedback circuits involved in cognition and emotion (4). Nevertheless, it is the frontostriatal circuit that figures most prominently in understanding the higher-order cognitive deficits that occur in PD (59).

In PD, important neuropathological changes occur in pigmented cells in the substantia nigra and in dopamine-producing cells in the ventral tegmentum (34). These changes result in (a) depletion of dopamine output to the striatal complex (via the nigrostriatal pathway), which adversely affects portions of the caudal end of the frontostriatal circuit; and (b) depletion of dopamine output from the ventral tegmentum to the prefrontal cortex and limbic system (via the mesocortical and mesolimbic pathways), which adversely affects the rostral end of the frontostriatal circuit and the limbic structures (1,34).

Collectively, the depletion of dopamine in the rostral dorsolateral prefrontal cortical portion of the circuit and dopamine depletion in the caudal portion of the circuit (which includes the dorsolateral head of the caudate, dorsomedial globus pallidus, substantia nigra, and ventroanterior and dorsomedial thalamus) are thought to account for most of the higher-order cognitive impairments observed in PD (26,54,67).

In a larger sense, damage to the dorsolateral, lateral orbital, and anterior cingulate frontal lobe circuits forms the primary neural substrate for the concept of "subcortical dementia" (48). This concept was introduced by Albert and associates in 1974 to describe the changes that occur in supranuclear palsy (3). The term has since been expanded to include the changes in mood and cognition seen in a variety of diseases in which the cellular pathology is most prominent in the striatum, globus pallidus, and substantia nigra and in which there is functional involvement of the frontal lobes (2,18,19). Cummings and Benson, in 1984, were among the first clinicians to describe and popularize the concept of subcortical dementia (17,18) and to defend it against its critics, some of whom pointed to the involvement of the cerebral cortex (73) and some of whom took issue with the level of severity of the cognitive and behavioral deficits needed to meet the criteria for this form of dementia (10).

In patients with PD the cardinal cognitive features of subcortical dementia, which may be present in mild to moderate degrees of severity, include impaired speed of cognitive processing (bradyphrenia), visuospatial disturbances (14), impaired ability to use previously acquired knowledge, impaired fluency, impaired executive functioning, impaired recall memory, abnormalities of procedural memory (70), and prominent mood disorders. When severe dementia is present in PD, it is usually associated with Alzheimer-type pathology (8) or Lewy body dementia. For a more in-depth discussion of frontostriatal cognitive impairments in patients with PD, the reader is referred to review articles by Owens and associates (52), Morris and associates (50), and Gabrieli and associates (29).

EFFECTS OF PVP ON NEUROPSYCHOLOGICAL FUNCTION: REVIEW OF CURRENT LITERATURE

Although the number of articles describing reduction of motor symptoms following pallidotomy has steadily increased over the past several years, few studies have described changes in neuropsychological functioning. Baron and associates studied 12 patients at 3 and 12 months after PVP (5). Of the 25 cognitive variables they analyzed, only four were significantly changed postoperatively. All of the changes were in memory or frontal lobe functioning. If the two patients who sustained small postoperative subdural hematomas were omitted, none of the cognitive variables were significantly changed. These authors did not find the side of surgery to be a significant variable. They acknowledged that their small sample size could have limited the study's ability to detect significant differences.

More recently, a study by Soukup and associates came to a similar conclusion (61). They reported on 14 patients with a relatively short duration of PD symptoms (mean 7 years), none of whom were judged to have dementia. Eight of the patients underwent a right pallidotomy, and six underwent a left pallidotomy. None of the 21 cognitive variables Soukup and associates studied were significantly changed at 3 months after surgery. They did, however, report statistically significant improvements in motor coordination speed (as measured by the Purdue Pegboard test) for both hands regardless of the side of surgery ($p < 0.01$).

In contrast to these two studies, Riordan and associates found that the side of surgery had a significant effect on several outcome variables (58). Patients who underwent a left pallidotomy ($n = 10$), for example, experienced a mild decline in verbal learning, verbal memory, phonemic and semantic verbal fluency, and cognitive flexibility, whereas patients who underwent a right pallidotomy ($n = 8$) experienced a mild decline in verbal learning, cognitive flexibility, and visuospatial constructional abilities but improved on a delayed facial memory test. Riordan and associates also found that patients who underwent a left pallidotomy reported significantly fewer symptoms of depression or anxiety postoperatively than did those who underwent a right pallidotomy.

There is a surprising diversity of outcomes and little consensus about what, if any, cognitive changes occur following pallidotomy (Table 14-1). When changes have been observed, they have generally been related to some aspect of fluency (semantic or phonemic), speed of cognitive processing, verbal memory, or executive functioning. Decreased levels of depression after surgery were frequently reported, particularly when the surgery was performed on the right side.

With respect to the effect of age or dementia on cognitive outcome after PVP, the results of various studies are equivocal. Of the 18 patients studied by Riordan and co-authors, one-third were noted to have moderately to severely impaired cognition prior to surgery. This impairment, however, was not observed to affect the post-PVP outcome on measures of motor functioning or overall ratings of surgical outcome (58). The authors suggest that cognitively impaired patients can benefit from pallidotomy, a concept that challenges using dementia as an exclusionary criterion. However, in Baron and associates' study the two patients with dementia experienced a "poor surgical outcome" and showed a mean improvement of only 12.5% on the Unified Parkinson's Disease Rating Scale (UPDRS) (5). This compared with 32% UPDRS improvement by the patients without dementia. Interestingly, one of the two patients who showed no improvement on the Schwab and England scale 3 months after surgery displayed 27.9% improvement when tested at 12 months. With regard to age at the time of surgery, Baron and associates found that age was inversely related to the total UPDRS score at 3 months after PVP (5). In their study, the mean UPDRS score for the younger patients improved 53%, whereas the mean UPDRS score for the older patients worsened by 13.8%. They did not observe similar changes on the Schwab and England level of independence scale.

The current literature on cognitive changes following PVP is not yet robust enough to allow more than tentative conclusions. Studies with small numbers of patients and short follow-up periods that utilize somewhat broad measures of neuropsychological functioning and univariate analysis may not demonstrate statistically significant cognitive changes. Nevertheless, the current literature points to a number of variables that are likely to be important in subsequent studies of the effects of pallidotomy on cognitive function. These variables include the side of surgery, age at onset of PD symptoms, duration of PD symptoms, age at the time of surgery, and the Mini-Mental Status Examination (MMSE) (26). In addition, specialized tests that place maximal demands on the functional capacity of frontostriatal memory and executive functioning, such as measures of spatial working memory, attentional

TABLE 14-1. *Summary of recent studies analyzing neuropsychological outcome following pallidotomy for Parkinson's disease*

Study	No. of pts.	Postop. interval (mo)	Variables	Results
Bowers (9)	21	NA	Verbal memory	Improved
			Free recall	Unchanged
			Other standard tests	Unchanged
Cahn (12)	16	3	Motor speed	Improved
			Motor coordination	Improved
			Grip strength	Contra declined
			Memory, language	Unchanged
			Working memory	Unchanged
Cullum (15)	19	NA	Verbal learning	Improved
			Nonverbal memory	Improved
			Figural fluency	Improved
			Depression	Improved
Jahanshani (37)	11	3	Executive functions	Unchanged
			Spatial working memory	Unchanged
Manning (43)	10	NA	Motor dexterity (nondom. hand)	Declined
			Verbal fluency	Declined
			Verbal memory	Improved
			Depression	Improved
			Executive functions	Declined
Masterman (45)	24	NA	Category fluency	Mild decline
			Behavioral assessment	Unchanged
Riordan (57)	16	NA	Verbal memory (with left PVP)	Declined
			Fluency (with left PVP)	Declined
			Nonverbal memory (with right PVP)	Improved
Stebbins (64)	9	6	Reading span; listening span	Declined
			Digit ordering	Declined
			Cognitive processing speed	Declined
			Abstract reasoning	Declined
			Non-WM declarative memory	Unchanged
Uitti (71)	20	3	Global cognitive functioning	Unchanged
			Semantic fluency	Declined
			Controlled oral association	Declined

NA, not available; PVP, posteroventral pallidotomy; WM, working memory; Contra, Contralateral side; nondom., nondominant.

set-shifting, and strategic memory (50, 53, 68), are more likely to show statistically significant changes following PVP than are broader measures of memory and executive functioning.

EFFECTS OF UNILATERAL PVP ON NEUROPSYCHOLOGICAL FUNCTION: BAYLOR COLLEGE OF MEDICINE STUDY

Patient Selection

A total of 44 consecutive patients who underwent unilateral PVP between August 1995 and December 1996 are included in the present study. Details of the procedure are described in Chapter 8. All 44 patients underwent a preoperative and a 3-month postoperative examination. Of the 44 patients, 26 also underwent a 12-month post-PVP examination. Each examination consisted of a complete neurological evaluation using the Core Assessment Program for Intracerebral Transplantations (CAPIT) protocol (40) by a neurologist (J.J. or E.C.L.); measures of motor function, balance, and reaction and movement time; a video-assessment protocol; speech testing; and a comprehensive neuropsychological evaluation. It should be noted that the neuropsychological battery was adjusted slightly early in the study, and that not all patients were able to complete all of the neuropsychological tests. Because of these two factors, the number of results analyzed for individual tests may be slightly fewer than the number of patients who underwent post-PVP evaluations at 3 and 12 months. Also, although the initial exclusion criteria included moderate to severe dementia (as measured by an MMSE score of ≤ 25), these guidelines were relaxed later in the study, and 2 of the 44 patients presented here had MMSE scores between 20 and 24.

The demographics of the 44 patients at the time of surgery included (a) mean age of 59.3 years (range 40–75 years); (b) mean age at PD symptom onset of 44.8 years (range 22–61 years); (c) mean symptom duration of 13.8 years (range 4–26 years); and (d) mean education of 13.7 years (range 8–19 years). There were 20 women and 24 men, all of whom were right-handed. The pallidotomy was performed, in general, contralateral to the more affected body side. More patients (68.2%) underwent a left PVP than a right PVP. The mean preoperative Hoehn and Yahr staging score was 2.7 when "on" levodopa and 4.1 while "off" levodopa. Patients were tested during their best "on" periods and typically continued their preoperative antiparkinsonian medication regimen, except for minor adjustments, for at least 12 months after surgery.

Neuropsychological Tests

The neuropsychological test battery was designed to assess the pattern of cognitive and affective difficulties most commonly seen with advanced PD. All tests were administered using standardized instructions and procedures with the exception of the Wisconsin Card Sorting Test (WCST). During the pre-PVP administration of this test, several patients with severe dyskinesia, tremors, or bradykinesia had difficulty finding and pressing the appropriate computer keys. These patients were allowed to make their choices by touching the computer screen and their selections were entered by the examiner. Most of the tests used were selected to measure four aspects of neuropsychological function, as outlined below. For a more detailed

description of the tests used in the study, see the Appendix.

Verbal Learning and Memory

The tests used to measure verbal learning and memory included the California Verbal Learning Test (CVLT) (22), Wechsler Logical Memory I and II tests (72), and Boston Naming Test (a measure of semantic verbal memory) (39).

Executive Abilities

Tests utilized to measure executive function included the WCST (32), Trail Making B test (56), Multilingual Aphasia Examination—Controlled Oral Word Association (MAE-COWA) test (7), and Semantic Cluster versus Serial Cluster scores from the CVLT (22).

Visuospatial Abilities

To test visuospatial abilities we used the Hooper Visual Organization Test (33).

Cognitive Processing Speed

To assess cognitive processing speed, we used the Symbol Digit Modalities Test—Verbal Response (60), Trail Making A test (56), and Stroop Color and Word Naming Test (66).

Statistical Methods

Statistical analyses were performed using SAS software (Cary, NC, USA). First we computed simple t-tests to compare pre-PVP and post-PVP (pre–post PVP) scores and identify any significant changes (Tables 14-2, 14-3). We also examined the possible mediating effects of other variables, including (a) MMSE score, (b) Beck Depression Scale scores, (c) age at baseline testing, (d) age of PD symptom onset, (e) symptom duration, (f) side of surgery, and (g) severity of PD symptoms. Pearson r correlations were performed between each of these control variables and the outcome variables. If a statistically significant correlation was found ($p < 0.01$), an analysis of variance (ANOVA) was performed with the control vari-

TABLE 14-2. *Univariate analysis of change between pre-PVP and 3-month post-PVP neuropsychological scores (n = 44)[a]*

Test[a]	Results; mean (SD)		p
	Preoperative	Postoperative (3 mo)	
Beck Depression Scale	11.45 (7.70)	9.32 (6.50)	0.065
Boston Naming Test	−0.45 (1.39)	−0.26 (1.31)	0.16
CVLT—Total List A	−0.95 (1.24)	−1.50 (1.32)	0.0004
CVLT—Short Delay Free Recall	−0.85 (1.30)	−1.13 (1.49)	0.08
CVLT—Long Delay Free Recall*	−0.68 (1.15)	−0.90 (1.32)	0.04
CVLT—Semantic Cluster Score*	−0.38 (0.82)	−0.79 (0.95)	0.002
CVLT—Serial Cluster Score*	0.09 (0.83)	0.47 (1.17)	0.018
CVLT—Discrimination Memory*	−0.78 (1.60)	−0.40 (0.96)	0.002
Hooper Visual Organization Test*	54.63 (8.62)	52.30 (7.73)	0.003
MAE-COWA*	37.66 (10.29)	34.02 (9.16)	0.002
Mini-Mental State Examination	27.95 (2.19)	28.19 (1.97)	0.42
Stroop Color Naming Test	1.24 (0.90)	1.32 (0.79)	0.34
Stroop Word Naming Test	−0.88 (0.97)	−1.02 (0.85)	0.10
Stroop Color and Word Naming Test	−0.97 (0.99)	−0.95 (0.97)	0.84
Stroop C/W Test—Interference	−0.18 (0.79)	−0.20 (0.75)	0.83
Symbol/Digit—Verbal Response	−1.43 (1.03)	−1.48 (1.04)	0.90
Trail Making A	−1.18 (1.63)	−1.08 (1.45)	0.53
Trail Making B	−1.42 (1.60)	−1.61 (1.49)	0.33
Wechsler Logical Memory I*	45.36 (30.36)	53.95 (32.19)	0.004
Wechsler Logical Memory II*	50.30 (31.80)	55.87 (30.75)	0.023
WCST—Categories Achieved	−1.14 (1.14)	−1.09 (1.37)	0.93
WCST—Perseverative Errors	−0.96 (0.89)	−0.87 (1.24)	0.94

CVLT, California Verbal Learning Test; MAE-COWA, Multilingual Aphasia Examination—Controlled Oral Word Association; PD, Parkinson's disease; PVP, posteroventral pallidotomy; Stroop C/W Test, Stroop Color and Word Naming Test; Symbol/Digit, Symbol Digit Modalities Test; WCST, Wisconsin Card Sorting Test.

[a] See Appendix for a description of the tests. Owing to slight changes in the test battery and scheduling problems, some analyses are based on fewer than 44 patients.

*$p < 0.05$.

ables as the between-subjects factor and time (pre–post PVP assessments) as the within-subjects factor. If this interaction was not statistically significant, the control variable was not contributing to the change observed; and we concluded that the *t*-test was describing the effects of surgery independent of the control variables. Although regression toward the mean may account for a portion of the pre–post differences, the magnitude of these changes suggests that PVP contributed significantly to the changes observed.

When a significant moderating effect was found for one of the control variables, an additional step was taken to simplify the interpretation of the change. In these instances the patients were divided into two groups: those with values above the median and those with values below the median for that control variable. The mean preoperative and postoperative scores were then determined for each group, which al-

lowed a comparison of the pre–post PVP mean scores within subsets of the control variables, for example between the older and younger patients at onset of PD symptoms and between the patients with shorter and longer durations of PD symptoms. We reasoned that these subgroups might affect the outcome variables in ways that could not be determined by analyzing the ungrouped data.

The analyses described above were also used to study the long-term effects of pallidotomy by comparing the changes observed between the 3- and 12-month postoperative evaluations in the 26 patients who were evaluated at both time points.

The significance level was set at $p < 0.05$ for the *t*-test results and at $p < 0.01$ for the Pearson *r* correlations. For the repeated-measures ANOVAs, a significance level of $p < 0.05$ was chosen to avoid making a type II error. The Beck Depression

TABLE 14-3. *Univariate analysis of change between 3- and 12-month neuropsychological scores following PVP for PD (n = 26)[a]*

Test[a]	Postoperative results; mean (SD)		p
	3 Months	12 Months	
Beck Depression Scale	9.32 (6.50)	8.17 (7.34)	0.30
Boston Naming Test*	−0.22 (1.32)	0.40 (1.33)	0.01
CVLT—Total List A	−1.50 (1.30)	−1.04 (0.95)	0.15
CVLT—Short Delay Free Recall	−1.15 (1.47)	−1.10 (1.33)	0.30
CVLT—Long Delay Free Recall	−0.91 (1.31)	−0.80 (1.10)	0.64
CVLT—Semantic Cluster Score	−0.79 (0.94)	−0.60 (0.94)	0.33
CVLT—Serial Cluster Score*	0.46 (1.16)	0.05 (0.89)	0.05
CVLT—Discrimination Memory	−0.42 (0.96)	−0.75 (1.68)	0.23
Hooper Visual Organization Test	52.09 (7.77)	51.52 (8.11)	0.55
MAE-COWA	33.95 (9.06)	36.17 (11.08)	0.23
Mini-Mental State Examination	28.23 (1.96)	28.26 (1.84)	0.07
Stroop Color Naming Test	−1.35 (0.80)	−1.44 (0.81)	0.88
Stroop Word Naming Test	−1.04 (0.84)	−1.29 (0.66)	0.38
Stroop Color and Word Naming Test	−0.97 (0.97)	−0.70 (0.99)	0.10
Stroop C/W Test—Interference*	−0.20 (0.74)	0.38 (0.74)	0.03
Symbol/Digit—Verbal Response	−1.50 (1.03)	−1.52 (1.25)	0.88
Trail Making A	−1.04 (1.45)	−1.50 (1.58)	0.25
Trail Making B	−1.61 (1.47)	−1.98 (2.02)	0.52
Wechsler Logical Memory I*	53.61 (31.86)	68.18 (28.44)	0.003
Wechsler Logical Memory II*	55.74 (30.34)	70.18 (31.14)	0.01
WCST—Categories Achieved*	−1.12 (1.36)	−1.08 (1.26)	0.02
WCST—Perseverative Errors	−0.87 (1.22)	−0.88 (1.69)	0.15

CVLT, California Verbal Learning Test; MAE-COWA, Multilingual Aphasia Examination—Controlled Oral Word Association; PD, Parkinson's disease; PVP, posteroventral pallidotomy; Stroop C/W, Stroop Color and Word Naming Test; Symbol/Digit, Symbol Digit Modalities Test; WCST, Wisconsin Card Sorting Test.

[a]See Appendix for a description of the tests. Owing to slight changes in the test battery and scheduling problems, some analyses are based on fewer than 26 patients.

*$p < 0.05$.

Scale was analyzed using the Kruskal-Wallis nonparametric test because of the skewed nature of some of the scores.

Because the Hooper Visual Organization, Boston Naming, and Wechsler Logical Memory Scales I and II tests have only one version, the same test was repeated at 3 and 12 months for all patients. In addition, approximately 15 of the 44 patients also underwent these tests at 6 and 9 months after surgery, before testing at these intervals was discontinued. Most patients improved as a function of the number of times they took the same test, and so the tests may have been particularly susceptible to practice effects. The tests, however, were retained in the battery to help identify patients who might be undergoing a dementing process. Because of the potential for practice effects to distort any measured change, the results from these tests were generally excluded from consideration when assessing pre–post cognitive change following PVP. The

only exception was when one of the control variables was significantly related to the pre–post change observed and was therefore believed to have potential prognostic value.

Preoperative Patient Status

Motor Status

The mean preoperative Hoehn and Yahr staging (H & Y) score was 2.7 while "on" and 4.1 while "off." The mean UPDRS motor score was 30.0 while "on" and 57.2 while "off"; and the mean UPDRS Activities of Daily Living (ADL) score was 15.9 while "on" and 30.9 while "off."

Neuropsychological Status

Table 14-2 shows the *t*-test results comparing 22 outcome variables pre-PVP and 3 months post-PVP. Consistent with advanced PD, many of the preoperative test scores were mildly impaired. Analysis of the pre-PVP scores revealed a pattern of deficits associated with dysfunction of the frontostriatal circuit, as manifested by mild to moderate deficits in memory, executive functioning, speed of information processing, and verbal fluency. Preoperative performance was within the normal or near-normal range for the following measures: (a) verbal memory for logical prose (Wechsler Logical Memory I and II); (b) semantic memory (Boston Naming Test); (c) portions of the verbal list learning test (CVLT); (d) executive abilities (Stroop C/W Test—Interference); and (e) visuospatial abilities (Hooper Visual Organization Test). The preoperative MMSE scores ranged from 20 to 30, with a mean ± SD of 27.39 ± 2.70; the mean ± SD Beck Depression Scale score for the 44 patients was 11.45 ± 7.70.

Postoperative Outcome at 3 and 12 Months

Motor Status

Significant symptomatic improvements were observed on all of the motor measures of PD. Between the pre-PVP and 3-month post-PVP testing, the mean H & Y score "on" improved by 30% ($p < 0.001$), and the "off" score improved by 29% ($p < 0.001$). Similarly, the UPDRS motor score "on" improved by 45% ($p < 0.001$), and the "off" score improved by 39% ($p < 0.001$). The UPDRS ADL score "on" improved by 50% ($p < 0.001$), and the "off" score improved by 41% ($p < 0.001$).

At 12 months post-PVP, no statistically significant changes from the 3-month scores were observed on any of the measures of motor function or activities of daily living. Nevertheless, there was a tendency to observe additional improvement at 12 months, with more pronounced improvement observed while the patient was "off" levodopa.

Neuropsychological Outcome

The 44 patients performed significantly better on the CVLT—Discrimination Memory subtest and on the Wechsler Logical Memory II test (delayed recall) at 3 months post-PVP (Table 14-2). A worsening was seen on the CVLT measures of immediate recall (Total List A), long delay free recall, and strategic memory (demonstrated by an increased reliance on serial clustering rather than semantic clustering). In addition, a decline was observed on the MAE-COWA test, which measures verbal fluency.

At 12 months post-PVP (Table 14-3), no cognitive measures were statistically worse when compared with the 3-month results, but there was an overall trend toward better performance and three measures were statistically better. All three were measures of executive functioning: the Stroop C/W Test—Interference, the WCST—Categories Achieved, and the CVLT—Semantic versus Serial Cluster Scores. A slight worsening at 12 months post-PVP from the scores at 3 months was seen on four tests (Trail Making A and B and the Stroop Color and Word tests), all of which test speed of information processing.

Cognitive Improvements

The univariate analysis of pre–post changes at 3 months after pallidotomy reflected a statistically better performance on the discrimination portion of the CVLT ($p = 0.002$) (Table 14-2, Fig. 14-1). Multivariate analysis showed that side of surgery contributed to the change. Patients who underwent a right pallidotomy improved significantly, with a pre–post PVP difference score of +0.87, whereas patients who underwent a left-sided procedure were slightly worse postoperatively, with a pre–post PVP difference score of −0.18.

The scores on the Wechsler Logical Memory II Test (20-minute delayed recall) were also significantly better at 3 months after surgery ($p < 0.02$), with the duration of parkinsonian symptoms contributing to the pre–post PVP change (Fig. 14-2). Patients with PD symptoms for more than 14 years performed poorly preoperatively but improved significantly after pallidotomy (from 33.5 to 50.7). Patients with a shorter duration of PD symptoms (14 years or less) performed relatively well preoperatively but exhibited little improvement postoperatively (from 67.3 to 69.5).

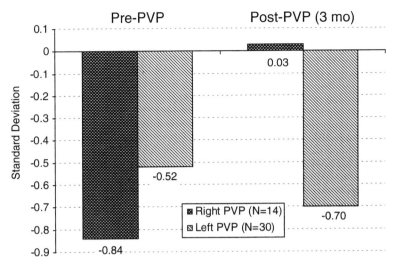

FIG. 14-1. Mean pre–post PVP scores (expressed as standard deviations from 0 where 0 = norm) on the California Verbal Learning Test—Discrimination Memory Scale by side of surgery. *PVP,* posteroventral pallidotomy.

At 12 months after pallidotomy, three measures of cognitive function were significantly improved from the results at 3 months post-PVP (Table 14-3): two measures of executive functioning (Stroop C/W Test—Interference and WCST—Categories Achieved) and one measure of strategic memory (CVLT—Serial Cluster Score). None of these cognitive measures were moderated by the control variables between 3 and 12 months post-PVP, and therefore

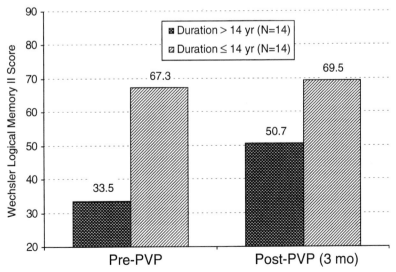

FIG. 14-2. Mean pre–post PVP scores on the Wechsler Logical Memory II Scale (20-min delayed recall), by duration of PD. Higher scores are better. *PD,* Parkinson's disease; *PVP,* posteroventral pallidotomy.

the observed changes are thought to represent the effects of PVP surgery alone. Although the mean CVLT—Total List A score declined significantly at 3 months post-PVP (discussed below under Cognitive Declines), there was a noticeable improvement at 12 months compared with the 3-month scores. Figure 14-3 shows a typical example of change across all three time points. The mean CVLT—Total List A scores, with age at PD symptom onset as a covariate, are shown for the patients who have undergone both 3- and 12-month follow-up evaluations. Although there was an initial worsening at 3 months in both subgroups (with the subgroup that performed best preoperatively declining the most), both groups showed mild to moderate improvement at 12 months post-PVP, such that their scores at 12 months were comparable to their pre-PVP scores.

Cognitive Declines

Univariate t-test pre–post analysis at 3 months after PVP showed a significant worsening on four CVLT measures (Total List A, Long Delay Free Recall, Semantic Cluster Score, and Serial Cluster Score) as well as on the MAE-COWA verbal fluency test (Table 14-2). Multivariate analysis did not show a moderating effect by any of the control variables for the worsening of the CVLT—Semantic Cluster scores. On the other hand, both duration of PD and the age at symptom onset had a significant moderating effect on the pre–post PVP change for CVLT—Total List A ($p = 0.017$). Patients with a shorter duration of PD symptoms (≤ 14 years) declined considerably more after PVP, with a difference score of -1.0, compared with patients with a longer duration of PD (> 14 years) who declined less, with a difference score of -0.32 (Fig. 14-4). Age of PD onset also had a significant effect on the pre–post PVP change for CVLT—Total List A at 3 months. Patients with a later age at onset (> 45 years) performed better before PVP than patients with an earlier age of onset (≤ 45 years). However, later age of onset patients declined significantly more (pre–post PVP difference score of -0.85) than did earlier onset patients (pre–post difference score of -0.40).

The CVLT Long Delay Free Recall results were also significantly worse at 3 months post-PVP ($p < 0.04$), with the Beck Depression Scale score having a moderating effect (Fig. 14-5).

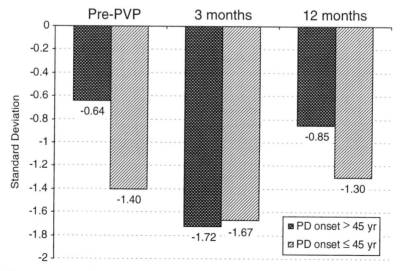

FIG. 14-3. Mean pre–post PVP scores (expressed as standard deviations from 0 where 0 = norm) of patients with 3- and 12-month evaluations on the California Verbal Learning Test—Total List A, by age of PD onset. *PD*, Parkinsons's disease; *PVP*, posteroventral pallidotomy.

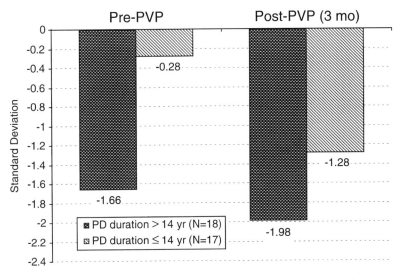

FIG. 14-4. Mean pre–post PVP scores (expressed as standard deviations from 0 where 0 = norm) on the California Verbal Learning Test—Total List A, by duration of PD. *PD,* Parkinson's disease; *PVP,* posteroventral pallidotomy.

Preoperatively, the patient groups with Beck scores above and below the median score of 10 performed almost the same (−0.72 and −0.71, respectively), but following PVP the patients with less depression (a Beck Depression Scale score of 10 or less) performed considerably worse (pre–post PVP mean difference score of −0.47) than did the patients with a Beck Depression Scale score greater than 10 (mean pre–post difference score of −0.17).

The MAE-COWA verbal fluency score was also worse at 3 months post-PVP, with the side of

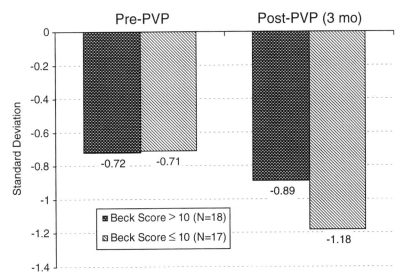

FIG. 14-5. Mean pre–post PVP scores (expressed as standard deviations from 0 where 0 = norm) on the California Verbal Learning Test—Long Delay Free Recall scale, by Beck Depression Scale scores. *PVP,* posteroventral pallidotomy.

PVP surgery having a significant effect ($p < 0.05$) on the pre–post change (Fig. 14-6). Patients who underwent a right PVP declined only slightly (the raw score declining by a mean of −0.54 points), whereas patients who underwent a left PVP performed significantly worse (the raw score declining by a mean of −5.18 points).

At 12 months post-PVP, no cognitive measures were statistically worse when compared to the results at 3 months. Mild but not significant declines were seen on the Trail Making A and B and Stroop Color and Word tests. These tests require attention, concentration, and speed of information processing, which may decline with disease progression.

Changes in Mood

The Beck Depression Scale (BDS) (6) scores for the 44 patients were not significantly changed at 3 months post-PVP, but the mean score declined from 11.45 to 9.32 (Table 14-2), indicating some reduction in overall levels of depression. Interestingly, the preoperative mean scores for patients, by side of surgery, were significantly different ($p < 0.05$), with patients undergoing a right procedure being more depressed. Patients ($n = 44$) who underwent a right PVP scored a mean preoperative BDS score of 11.4, whereas patients who underwent a left procedure scored 9.9 preoperatively. This difference was still significant at 3 months post-PVP (right = 12.6, left = 7.8; $p = 0.02$).

The change in the BDS score between the 3- and 12-month follow-up evaluations was not significant for the pooled scores. However, although the depression scores declined considerably for both left and right PVP patients at 3 months, left PVP patients showed a slight increase in depression at 12 months (+2.59) whereas right PVP patients were relatively unchanged (−0.40) (Fig. 14-7).

DISCUSSION

The Baylor College of Medicine pallidotomy study at the time of this analysis had 44 advanced PD patients who had undergone a unilateral PVP and had completed a 3-month follow-up evaluation. Of these patients, 26 had also completed a 12-month follow-up evaluation. Analysis of the neuropsychological data from these patients provides tentative answers to several of the questions posed at the beginning of the chapter. Our findings, in conjunction with those from other studies, may help to clarify the choice of reason-

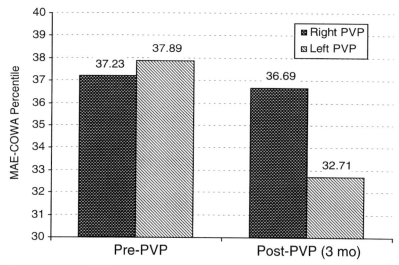

FIG. 14-6. Mean pre–post PVP scores (expressed as percentiles; 50 = norm) on the Multilingual Aphasia Examination—Controlled Oral Word Association test of verbal fluency, by side of surgery. *PVP,* posteroventral pallidotomy.

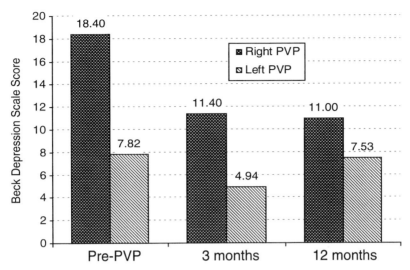

FIG. 14-7. Mean pre–post PVP raw scores on the Beck Depression Scale (higher scores = greater depression), by side of PVP, for patients with 3- and 12-month follow-up evaluations. *PVP,* posteroventral pallidotomy.

able exclusionary criteria for PVP and better define the roles of age of onset and duration of PD symptoms in patient outcome.

In our patients with advanced PD, preoperative analysis of selected cognitive variables revealed a pattern of deficits known to be associated with dysfunction of the frontostriatal circuitry, including mild to moderate deficits in (a) list learning and memory, (b) executive functions, (c) speed of information processing, and (d) verbal fluency. Memory for logical prose material, visual organization, and object naming were within the average range.

At 3 months after PVP, significant improvements were seen in the CVLT—Discrimination Memory scores (Fig. 14-1) and the Wechsler Logical Memory II scores (Fig. 14-2).

The discrimination subtest of the CVLT measures delayed recognition memory corrected for false-positive responses. Side of surgery had a significant effect on these scores. Patients who underwent a right PVP improved (+0.87 standard deviations), whereas those who underwent a left PVP declined (−0.18 standard deviations). The improvement observed was largely the result of fewer false-positive results, suggesting less bias to give "yes" responses in right PVP patients.

Postoperative improvement in attentional abilities may also be a contributing factor. Such improvements have been reported by Baron and associates following unilateral pallidotomy (5) and by Riordan and associates, who also reported improvements in visual recognition memory in their right-sided pallidotomy patients (58). Other studies have shown that patients with PD or Huntington's disease exhibit similar patterns of memory deficits on the CVLT, typified by relatively intact storage but impairment in the utilization of effective retrieval strategies. Discrimination memory tests using a yes/no paradigm minimize the memory retrieval deficits commonly seen in patients with subcortical disease while providing evidence of their relatively intact memory storage (65).

As seen in Fig. 14-2, the Wechsler Logical Memory Scale II scores were significantly improved at 3 months post-PVP. Although test/retest effects may account for some of the improvement, this scale was retained in the analysis because the duration of PD had a significant effect on the post-PVP changes observed. Preoperatively, patients with PD symptoms for longer than 14 years performed significantly worse than did patients with a shorter duration of symptoms (mean scores of 33.5 and 67.3, respectively). However, at 3 months post-PVP the patients in the "longer duration" group had improved significantly (from 33.5 to 50.7), whereas the patients in the "shorter duration" group improved only slightly (from 67.3 to 69.5).

The pattern of change described above is one of the two patterns that were commonly seen when analyzing the CVLT memory subtests with the time-related covariates (age at symptom onset and duration of disease). As shown in Fig. 14-2, when there was an overall significant improvement in function at 3 months post-PVP, the patient group that performed worse preoperatively showed the greatest improvement postoperatively. The second pattern, as demonstrated in Fig. 14-3, was seen when there was overall significant worsening at 3 months post-PVP, in which case the patient group that performed the best preoperatively declined the most postoperatively. These two patterns were not seen when using other control variables, such as severity of motor symptoms, MMSE scores, or age at the time of PVP, as covariates and were most apparent when analyzing the memory variables. It is unclear why age at the time of surgery was inconsistent in showing the direction of change, but it may be that the average age of patients in our study was below that which is necessary for the effect to be demonstrated consistently.

Postoperative declines at 3 months were also seen on various measures of executive functioning, which demonstrated relatively mild declines, and on several CVLT measures of memory, which were significantly worse. The latter included CVLT—Total List A and CVLT—Long Delay Free Recall, as well as the comparison of the Semantic and Serial Cluster Scores, which measures strategic memory.

The CVLT—Total List A is the sum of five free recall trials of the 16-word List A of the CVLT. The univariate pre–post analysis of this test was the most significant ($p = 0.0004$) of any variable analyzed. Multivariate analysis showed that both age at PD symptom onset ($p < 0.03$) and duration of disease ($p < 0.02$) had a significant effect on outcome at 3 months. When the patients were divided into two subgroups by age at onset, the "later onset" group, which had performed better pre-PVP, declined more post-PVP (change −0.85), whereas the "earlier onset" group declined less (change −0.40).

The fact that the "later onset" group performed better preoperatively than the "earlier onset" group was unexpected based on previous studies (25), but this trend was apparent when we performed preliminary analyses of the data from the first 20 patients and has persisted through the present time with increased significance. Two factors in patient selection may have contributed to this finding. First, selections were made from a waiting list of several hundred patients, and there may have been a greater likelihood of selection if a patient was relatively young and had relatively severe motor impairments, especially rigidity and bradykinesia, for which PVP is especially effective. Both of these motor symptoms are associated with increased cognitive dysfunction in PD (47, 51, 55). The second contributing factor may have to do with the fact that the mean MMSE score of the 22 patients who were older than 45 years of age was 28.27, whereas the mean MMSE of the 22 patients who were 45 years of age or younger was 27.63, suggesting a trend toward selecting only cognitively intact older patients. Together these two factors—a younger group of patients who were perhaps more cognitively impaired than expected and an older group of patients selected for less cognitive impairment than expected—could help to explain the present findings.

The postoperative findings on the CVLT—Total List A subtest were also significantly related to duration of PD (Fig. 14-4) ($p = 0.017$). [*Note:* Although duration of disease and age at symptom onset were not found to be significantly correlated (Pearson r coefficient = −0.28) in this study, the two variables may not be independent; and it is likely that they are confounded by each other to some degree.] The subgroup of patients with a shorter duration of disease (≤14 years) performed better preoperatively than did the subgroup of patients with a longer duration of disease (> 14 years) (−0.29 and −1.66, respectively). As expected, the patient group that performed better pre-PVP (i.e., the "shorter duration" group) accounted for the major portion of the decline post-PVP (−0.99 versus −0.31 for the "longer duration" group). Although the significance of this finding is unclear, it may be that PVP accelerates a change in the globus pallidus that occurs in PD patients as a function of the duration of their illness so the patients with the most to lose are the ones who sustain the greatest loss post-PVP.

The CVLT–Long Delay Free Recall subtest is a free recall trial conducted after a 20-minute delay during which time only nonverbal tasks are administered. Preoperatively, the Beck Depression Scale scores were unrelated to performance on this scale, but at 3 months after pallidotomy patients with a score below the median of 10 performed more poorly than did patients with a score above the median ($p = 0.04$). These results are not consistent with what we expected because, in general, studies have shown that nondepressed PD patients perform better cognitively than do depressed PD patients (46,63). However, considering that our patients had been screened for major depression and that the preoperative mean Beck Depression Scale score was only 11.97, even those patients who scored highest on the scale were no more than mildly depressed. Another factor that could have some bearing on this finding is the relatively large number (68%) of patients who underwent a left PVP. Previous studies have shown that patients whose PD symptoms begin on the right side of the body tend to have milder cognitive deficits than patients whose symptoms begin on the left side of their body (62). In addition, our findings and those of Riordan et al. (58) suggest that PD patients who have primary involvement of the left side of their brain and who undergo a left PVP tend to be less depressed than patients who have primary involvement of the right side of their brain and who undergo a right PVP. It is possible that our patient group is less depressed and has milder cognitive deficits than a group of patients balanced for side of PVP surgery, and that this bias offsets the effects of the expected trend for higher depression scores to be related to poorer cognitive performance. The relation between cognitive functions and Beck Depression Scale scores before and after PVP needs further study. We plan to do a follow-up study using a method of analysis, described by Gotham et al. (31) and

Huber et al.(35,36), that analyzes specific features (e.g., mood, self-reproach, and somatic and vegetative symptoms) of the Beck Depression Scale. The latter two symptoms may be of special interest in PD and may also have a higher correlation with cognitive changes than the first two features.

The CVLT Semantic Cluster Scores were significantly worse at 3 months post-PVP. This index measures strategic memory and reflects the degree to which a patient is able to organize conceptually the CVLT's 16-word "shopping list" into four semantically related categories. The decline on the Semantic Cluster Score observed at 3 months after PVP indicated reduced reliance on this effective recall strategy, whereas a higher Serial Cluster Score indicated an increased reliance on recalling the words in the same order as presented, which is an ineffective recall strategy. Because of the executive nature of these functions, it is likely that their decline is related to changes in the functional status of the frontostriatal cognitive circuit.

At 12 months post-PVP, none of the cognitive variables were significantly worse. However, a further slight decline was seen on Trail Making tests (A and B) and on the Stroop Color and Word tests. These results appear to be associated with a further slowing of information-processing speed, which may be related to further progression of the disease process at 12 months post-PVP.

Significant improvements were observed at 12 months post-PVP on tests relating to executive functioning, including the number of categories achieved in the Wisconsin Card Sorting Test, and reduced reliance on the ineffective recall strategy measured by the Serial Cluster Scale. None of the control variables contributed to these improvements, suggesting that the surgery and time were the primary contributors to the favorable changes. In general, memory variables also improved between 3 and 12 months postoperatively, although these improvements were not statistically significant.

Figure 14-3 shows a common pattern of change observed when plotting change over time. In this instance, although the mean scores on the CVLT—Total List A subtest, which measures immediate recall, declined significantly between pre-PVP and 3 months post-PVP, there was a noticeable improvement for both low and high performing groups over the subsequent 9 months.

CONCLUSIONS

As with virtually all previous studies, the Baylor College of Medicine's pallidotomy program has demonstrated a high degree of efficacy in the treatment of the cardinal motor symptoms of advanced PD and the disabling effects of levodopa-induced dyskinesias and on–off fluctuations. The significant improvements in motor function and activities of daily living seen at 3 months post-PVP were essentially unchanged at 12 months post-PVP.

Accompanying these motor improvements was an initial worsening in short and long delay memory, executive functions, and verbal fluency. These cognitive changes persisted for at least 3 months; but at 12 months post-PVP there were measurable trends toward improvement in most cognitive areas, with the exception of speed of mental processing, which tended to be slightly worse.

Based on our findings, certain patient variables (including age at onset of PD symptoms, duration of disease, and side of surgery) appear to be useful predictors of cognitive outcome at 3 months post-PVP and may be useful for predicting several patterns of change. These patterns are dependent on whether the cognitive variable being studied declined or improved postoperatively and on whether a patient scores above or below the median of the covariate being studied. In general, for those neuropsychological tests that decline significantly at 3 months post-PVP, it is the patients who perform the best preoperatively who decline the most postoperatively. Conversely, for those tests that improve significantly at 3 months post-PVP, it is the patients who perform poorest preoperatively who improve the most postoperatively. Our results also suggest that, for patients with young-onset PD, prolonged duration of disease and greater cognitive dysfunction, learning, and memory do not further worsen post-PVP as initially feared.

The present data further suggest that for patients with similar demographics the age at the time of PVP, MMSE scores, and the severity of motor symptoms do not play a significant part in determining cognitive outcome at 12 months post-PVP. As at many other centers performing PVP, we are gradually relaxing our exclusionary criteria based on these variables and have not observed ill effects from doing so. Specific cutoff points for these variables, however, cannot be established without further study.

An important question yet to be answered is to what degree, if any, the declines in memory and frontal lobe functioning measured postoperatively affect real-world social skills and activities, as well as avocational and vocational endeavors. Patient complaints of a noticeable decline in cognitive abilities following pallidotomy are rare; and any decline, noted or not, probably does not substantially increase a patient's stress level or require any new adaptation beyond those needed preoperatively. The relation between significant statistical changes and the significance of these changes in terms of day-to-day adjustment are unknown. Delis and Massman (21) have questioned the meaningfulness of some statistically significant differences, noting that in within-subjects studies that use relatively large samples and reliable measures, "even small group differences will be statistically significant," but, they continue, "these effects might not be large enough to be of much importance." Their point is a valid one, and additional studies using patient and caregiver questionnaires and real-life observations are needed to address this question. At the present time, it appears that the risks associated with any cognitive changes are slight when compared with the consistent, substantial improvements in motor function and independence observed in patients with advanced and debilitating PD who undergo unilateral posteroventral pallidotomy.

Acknowledgments. The authors express their appreciation to Paul Swank, Ph.D., Professor of Research, Statistics, and Management, Department of Educational Psychology, University of Houston, for his assistance in analyzing the data; Paul J. Massman, Ph.D., Associate Professor of Psychology, University of Houston, for review of the neuropsychological measures and their presentation; and Harvey S. Levin, Ph.D., Professor, Department of Physical Medicine and Rehabilitation, Baylor College of Medicine, and Winifred J. Hamilton, Ph.D., Department of Neurosurgery, Baylor College of Medicine, for their review of the manuscript and helpful suggestions.

REFERENCES

1. Agid Y. Parkinson's disease: pathophysiology. *Lancet* 1991;337:1321–1324.
2. Albert ML. Subcortical dementia. In: Katzman R, Terry RD, Bick KL, eds. *Alzheimer's disease.* New York: Raven Press, 1994:173–196.
3. Albert ML, Feldman RG, Willis AL. The "subcortical dementia" of progressive supranuclear palsy. *J Neurol Neurosurg Psychiatry* 1974;37:121–130.
4. Alexander GE, DeLong MR, Strick PL. Parallel organization of functionally segregated circuits linking basal ganglia and cortex. *Annu Rev Neurosci* 1986;9: 357–381.
5. Baron MS, Vitek JL, Bakay RA, et al. Treatment of advanced Parkinson's disease by posterior GPi pallidotomy: 1-year results of a pilot study. *Ann Neurol* 1996;40:355–366.
6. Beck AT, Ward CH, Mendelson M, Mock J, Erbaugh J. An inventory for measuring depression. *Arch Gen Psychiatry* 1961;4:561–571.
7. Benton A, Hamsher K. *Multilingual aphasia examination,* 2nd ed. Iowa City: University of Iowa, 1989.
8. Boller F, Mizutani T, Roessmann U, Gambetti P. Parkinson's disease, dementia, and Alzheimer disease: clinicopathological correlations. *Ann Neurol* 1980;7: 329–335.
9. Bowers D, Crucian GP, Friedman WA, Triggs WJ, Behrman A, Greer M. Memory and neuropsychological status following computerized image guided stereotactic pallidotomy in Parkinson's disease. *Neurology* 1997;48:A233 (abst).
10. Brown RE, Marsden CD. "Subcortical dementia": the neuropsychological evidence. *Neuroscience* 1988;25: 363–387.
11. Brown RG, Marsden CD. Cognitive function in Parkinson's disease: from description to theory. *Trends Neurosci* 1990;13:21–29.
12. Cahn DA, Heit G, Sullivan EV, et al. Three-month followup of posterior ventral pallidotomy. *J Int Neuropsychol Soc* 1997;3:60 (abst).
13. Cronin-Golomb A. Abstract thought in aging and age-related neurological disease. In: Boller F, Grafman J, eds. *Handbook of neuropsychology,* vol 4. Amsterdam: Elsevier Science, 1990:279–309.
14. Cronin-Golomb A, Braun AE. Visuospatial dysfunction and problem solving in Parkinson's disease. *Neuropsychology* 1997;11:44–52.
15. Cullum CM, Lacritz LH, Frol AB, Brewer KK, Giller C, Dewey R. Effects of pallidotomy on cognitive function in Parkinson's disease. *J Int Neuropsychol Soc* 1997;3:61 (abst).
16. Cummings JL. Intellectual impairment in Parkinson's disease: clinical, pathological, and biochemical correlates. *J Geriatr Psychiatr Neurol* 1988;1:24–36.
17. Cummings JL, Benson DF. *Dementia: a clinical approach.* Boston: Butterworth, 1983.
18. Cummings JL, Benson DF. Subcortical dementia: review of an emerging concept. *Arch Neurol* 1984; 41:874–879.
19. Cummings JL, Benson FD. Subcortical mechanisms and human thought. In: Cummings JL, ed. *Subcortical dementia.* New York: Oxford University Press, 1990; 251–259.
20. Daum I, Schugens MM, Spieker S, Poser U, Schonle PW, Birbaumer N. Memory and skill acquisition in Parkinson's disease and frontal lobe dysfunction. *Cortex* 1995;31:413–432.
21. Delis DC, Massman PJ. The effects of dopamine fluctuation on cognition and affect. In: Huber SJ, Cummings JL, eds. *Parkinson's disease: neurobehavioral aspects.* New York: Oxford University Press, 1992;288–302.
22. Delis DC, Kramer JH, Kaplan E, Ober BA. *The California Verbal Learninq Test: Adult Version.* San Antonio, TX: The Psychological Corporation, 1987.
23. Dubois B, Pillon B. Cognitive deficits in Parkinson's disease. *J Neurol* 1997;244:2–8.
24. Dubois B, Boller F, Pillon B, Agid Y. Cognitive deficits in Parkinson's disease. In: Boller F, Grafman J, eds. *Handbook of neuropsychology,* vol 5. Amsterdam: Elsevier Science, 1991:195–240.
25. Dubois B, Pillon B, Sternic N, Lhermitte F, Agid Y. Age-induced cognitive disturbances in Parkinson's disease. *Neurology* 1990;40:38–41.
26. Folstein MF, Folstein SE, McHugh PR. Mini-Mental State: a practical guide for grading the mental state of patients for the clinician. *J Psychiatr Res* 1975;12: 189–198.
27. Freedman M, Oscar-Berman M. Selective delayed response deficits in Parkinson's and Alzheimer's disease. *Arch Neurol* 1986;43:886–890.
28. Freedman M, Oscar-Berman M. Spatial and visual learning deficits in Alzheimer's and Parkinson's disease. *Brain Cogn* 1989;11:114–126.
29. Gabrieli JDE, Singh J, Stebbins GT, Goetz CG. Reduced working memory span in Parkinson's disease: evidence for the role of a frontostriatal system in working and strategic memory. *Neuropsychology* 1996;10: 322–332.
30. Goldman-Rakic PS. Circuitry of the primate prefrontal cortex and regulation of behavior by representational knowledge. In: Plum F, Mountcastle V, eds. *Hiqher cortical function: handbook of physiology,* vol 5. Washington, DC: American Physiology Society, 1987; 373–417.
31. Gotham AM, Brown RG, Marsden CD. Depression in Parkinson's disease: a quantitative and qualitative analysis. *J Neurol Neurosurg Psychiatry* 1986; 49:381–389.
32. Heaton RK. *Wisconsin Card Sorting Test Manual (WCST).* Odessa, FL: Psychological Assessment Resources, 1981.
33. Hooper HE. *Hooper Visual Organization Test (VOT).* Los Angeles: Western Psychological Services, 1983.
34. Hornykiewicz O. Brain neurotransmitter changes in Parkinson's disease. In: Marsden CD, Fahn S, eds. *Movement disorders.* Boston: Butterworth, 1982:41–58.

35. Huber SJ, Freidenberg DL, Paulson GW, Stuttleworth EC, Christy JA. The pattern of depressive symptoms varies with progression of Parkinson's disease. *J Neurol Neurosurg Psychiatry* 1990;53:275–278.

36. Huber SJ, Freidenberg DL, Shuttleworth EC, Paulson GW, Christy JA. Neuropsychological impairments associated with severity of Parkinson's disease. *J Neuropsychiatry Clin Neurosci* 1989;1:154–158.

37. Jahanshani M, Brown RG, Limousin P, Rothwell JC, Quinn N. Posteroventral pallidotomy (PVP) in Parkinson's disease (PD). II. Effects on executive function and working memory. *Mov Disord* 1997;12[suppl 1]: 130 (abst).

38. Johnson TN, Rosvold HE, Mishkin M. Projections from behaviorally-defined sectors of the prefrontal cortex to the basal ganglia, septum, and diencephalon of the monkey. *Exp Neurol* 1968;21:20–34.

39. Kaplan E, Goodglass H, Weintraub S. *The Boston Naming Test,* 2nd ed. Philadelphia: Lea & Febiger, 1983.

40. Langston JW, Widner H, Goetz CG, et al. Core Assessment Program for Intracerebral Transplantations (CAPIT). *Mov Disord* 1992;7:2–13.

41. Levin BE, Llabre MM, Reisman S, Weiner WJ. Visuospatial impairment in Parkinson's disease. *Neurology* 1991;41:365–369.

42. Lund-Johansen M, Hugdahl K, Wester K. Cognitive function in patients with Parkinson's disease undergoing stereotaxic thalamotomy. *J Neurol Neurosurg Psychiatry* 1996;60:564–571.

43. Manning CA, Bennett JP, Wilkniss SM, Jones MG, Laws ER. Comprehensive neuropsychological assessment of cognitive functioning pre- and post-unilateral posteroventrolateral pallidotomy. *Neurology* 1997;48: A252 (abst).

44. Marsden CD. Parkinson's disease. *Lancet* 1990;335: 948–952.

45. Masterman DL, Bronstein J, DeSalles AF, Foti DF, Cummings JL. Cognitive and behavioral performance following unilateral ventroposterior pallidotomy. *Neurology* 1997;48:A252–A253 (abst).

46. Mayberg HS, Solomon DH. Depression in Parkinson's disease: a biochemical and organic viewpoint. *Adv Neurol* 1995;65:49–60.

47. Mayeux R, Stern Y. Intellectual dysfunction and dementia in Parkinson's disease. *Adv Neurol* 1983;38: 211–227.

48. Mayeux R, Stern Y, Rosen J, Benson FD. Is "subcortical dementia" a recognizable clinical entity? *Ann Neurol* 1983;14:278–283.

49. Milner B, Petrides M. Behavioral effects of frontal lobe lesions in man. *Trends Neurosci* 1984;7:403–407.

50. Morris RG, Downes JJ, Shakian BJ, Evenden JL, Heald A, Robbins TW. Planning and spatial working memory in Parkinson's disease. *J Neurol Neurosurg Psychiatry* 1988;51:757–766.

51. Mortimer AJ, Pirozzolo FJ, Hansch EC, Webster DD. Relationship of motor symptoms to intellectual deficits in Parkinson's disease. *Neurology* 1982;32:133–137.

52. Owens AM, James M, Leigh PN, et al. Fronto-striatal cognitive deficits at different stages of Parkinson's disease. *Brain* 1992;115:1727–1751.

53. Partiot A, Verin M, Pillon B, Teixeira-Ferreira C, Agid Y, Dubois B. Delayed response tasks in basal ganglia lesions in man: Further evidence for a striato-frontal cooperation in behavioural adaptation. *Neuropsychologia* 1996;34:709–721.

54. Pillon B, Ertle S, Deweer B, Bonnet AM, Vidailhet M, Dubois B. Memory for spatial location in "de novo" parkinsonian patients. *Neuropsychologia* 1997;35: 221–228.

55. Reid WG, Broe GA, Hely MA, et al. The neuropsychology of de novo patients with idiopathic Parkinson's disease: the effects of age of onset. *Int J Neurosci* 1989;48: 205–217.

56. Reitan RM. Validity of the Trail Making Test as an indication of organic brain damage. *Percept Mot Skills* 1958;8:271–276.

57. Riordan HJ, Flashman L, Carroll K, Roberts D. Neuropsychological functioning before and after stereotactic ventroposterolateral pallidotomy in Parkinson's patients: preliminary findings. *J Int Neuropsychol Soc* 1997; 3:60–61 (abst).

58. Riordan HJ, Flashman LA, Roberts DW. Neurocognitive and psychosocial correlates of ventroposteriorlateral pallidotomy surgery in Parkinson's disease. *Neurosurg Focus* 1997;2 (electronic publication). http://server400.aans.org/journals/online_j/mar497/402-403-407.htm.

59. Saint-Cyr JA, Taylor AE, Nicholson K. Behavior and the basal ganglia. *Adv Neurol* 1995;65:1–128.

60. Smith A. *Symbol Digit Modalities Test (SDMT) manual (revised).* Los Angeles: Western Psychological Services, 1982.

61. Soukup VM, Ingram F, Schiess MC, Bonnen JG, Nauta HJW, Calverley JR. Cognitive sequelae of unilateral posteroventral pallidotomy. *Arch Neurol* 1997;54: 947–950.

62. Starkstein SE. Cognition and hemiparkinsonism. In: Huber SJ, Cummings JL, eds. *Parkinson's disease: neurobehavioral aspects.* New York: Oxford University Press, 1992:107–116.

63. Starkstein SE, Perziosi TJ, Bolduc PL, Robinson RG. Depression in Parkinson's disease. *J Nerv Ment Dis* 1990;178:27–31.

64. Stebbins GT, Gabrieli JDE, Goetz CG, Shannon KM, Penn RD, Masciari F. Impaired fronto-striatal memory functioning following pallidotomy in advanced Parkinson's disease. *Neurology* 1997;48:A252 (abst).

65. Stern Y, Groves M, Sano M, Hoover K, Mayeux R. Decreased consistency of recall for verbal lists in Parkinson's disease. *J Clin Exp Neuropsychol* 1992;14:81 (abst).

66. Stroop M. Studies of interference in serial verbal reactions. *J Exp Psychol* 1935;18:643–662.

67. Stuss DT, Benson DF. *The frontal lobes.* New York: Raven Press, 1986.

68. Taylor AE, Saint-Cyr JA. The neuropsychology of Parkinson's disease. *Brain Cogn* 1995;28:281–296.

69. Taylor AE, Saint-Cyr JA, Lang AE. Frontal lobe dysfunction in Parkinson's disease. *Brain* 1986;109: 845–883.

70. Taylor AE, Saint-Cyr JA, Lang AE. Memory and learning in early Parkinson's disease: evidence for a "frontal lobe syndrome." *Brain Cogn* 1990;13:211–232.

71. Uitti RJ, Wharen RE Jr, Turk MK, et al. Neuropsychological and motor function outcome following medial pallidotomy for elderly Parkinson's disease patients. *Neurology* 1997;48:A358 (abst).

72. Wechsler D. *Wechsler memory scale: revised manual.* San Antonio, TX: The Psychological Corporation, 1987.

73. Whitehouse PJ. The concept of subcortical and cortical dementia: another look. *Ann Neurol* 1986;19:1–6.

APPENDIX: NEUROPSYCHOLOGICAL TEST BATTERY

Verbal Learning and Memory

California Verbal Learning Test

Two forms of the California Verbal Learning Test (CVLT) are used to avoid practice effects during subsequent retesting. The test is organized around a 16-word "shopping list" (List A). Different recall strategies and types of memory are measured using various indices.

The Total List A subtest consists of presenting List A orally to the patient for a total of five trials. After each presentation the patient is to recall as many of the items as he or she can in any order desired. The total number of words recalled during these five trials is referred to as Total List A. The list consists of four categories of items (clothing, tools, fruits, and spices) with four items in each category, but the patient is not given this clue.

Following the Total List A subtest, the patient is presented with an "interference list" (List B) one time. This list also consists of four categories of shopping items, two of which are the same as List A (fruits and spices) and two of which are new (fish and utensils).

Following the free recall trial of List B, there is another Short Delay Free Recall trial of List A, followed by a category-cued recall of List A. After a 20-minute delay, there is a Long Delay Free Recall trial of List A and another category-cued recall trial. Last is the Discrimination Memory subtest of List A using a yes/no paradigm, with List A words mixed with 28 distracter words, some of which are from List B and some of which are exemplar items from the same categories as used in List A.

Although computerized scoring of the CVLT results in standard scores for 25 variables, we chose only six subtests for analysis. They are (a) Total List A (the sum of words recalled for the five trials of List A); (b) Short Delay Free Recall of List A, following the presentation of List B; (c) Long Delay Free Recall of List A, which follows a 20-minute delay; (d) Semantic Cluster Score (the measure of the degree to which the patient reorganizes List A into the appropriate cat-egories, which is the most effective recall strat-egy; and (e) Serial Cluster Score (the measure of the degree to which the patient recalls List A in the same order as presented, which is a poor recall strategy and indicates a concrete conceptual style). Higher scores represent better perfor-mance on all CVLT subtests except the Serial Cluster Score, for which higher scores represent poorer performance.

Wechsler Logical Memory I and II:

For the Wechsler Logical Memory I and II tests the patient is told that he or she will be read a paragraph of a few lines. The patient is to re-member and repeat the paragraph using as many of the same words as possible. The paragraph contains so much detailed information that it exceeds the storage capacity of most people, so it is necessary for patients to be somewhat selective about what they choose to retain to convey the essential features of the paragraph. The immediate recall trial represents Scale I, and the 20-minute (warned) delay trial repre-sents Scale II. Each trial is analyzed and scored separately.

Verbal Expression

Boston Naming Test

The Boston Naming Test consists of 60 line drawings of objects, ranging in familiarity from common (e.g., bed and house) at the beginning of the test to rarely encountered words (e.g., protractor, trellis, and abacus) near the end. The test measures semantic retrieval (nominal abilities) and was retained in the battery to help identify patients undergoing a dementing process.

Multilingual Aphasia Examination— Controlled Oral Word Association

The Multilingual Aphasia Examination—Con-trolled Oral Word Association test (MAE-COWA) is a measure of verbal fluency that is sensitive to functional or structural changes in the language dominant frontal lobe.

Executive Abilities

Wisconsin Card Sorting Test

The Wisconsin Card Sorting Test (WCST) provides a way to evaluate "abstract behavior" and the "ability to shift sets." The computer version was used to administer and score this test.

There are four stimulus cards (key cards) at the top of the screen, which contain one of four symbols (triangle, star, cross, circle) each of which is red, green, yellow, or blue. The patient is shown how to choose any one of these key cards by placing an indicator arrow under it. Next the patient is instructed to select the key card at the top of the screen that he or she thinks matches a card at the bottom of the screen. The patient is never told how to match the cards—based on the principles of color, shape, or number—but the computer flashes "right" or "wrong" following each choice, and a new card appears in its place for a total of 128 trials. The principle changes without warning after ten successive correct choices.

Making this shift to a new principle is particularly difficult for PD patients, and they tend to perseverate by using the principle that was previously correct. For our study the test was scored on the basis of the number of categories achieved with a maximum score of 6 (the same three principles are used twice) and the number of perseverative errors incurred.

Trail Making B

The Trail Making B test is always administered following Trail Making A (see below). The patient is told that this test is more difficult than Trail Making A, because it is necessary to alternate connecting circles that contain a number and circles that contain a letter, all of which are arranged in a pseudorandom fashion. The score is the time (in seconds) required to complete the test in the correct order. If a mistake is made, the patient is immediately told to correct it, with the time running. Shifting between the two conceptual sets of numbers and letters is difficult for advanced PD patients, and they may take three to five times longer to complete the test than their age-matched controls.

Semantic Versus Serial Cluster Scales:

The Semantic and Serial Cluster CVLT Scales were used as an index of executive functioning because they involve "strategic memory," which is often impaired in patients with frontal lobe damage. The Semantic Cluster Scale measures a patient's ability to organize conceptually the CVLT's 16-item shopping list (List A) in terms of its four categories (clothing, tools, fruits, spices), which is an effective strategy for recalling the words. The Serial Cluster Scale measures the degree to which the word list is repeated in the same order in which it was presented.

Stroop Color/Word Test—Interference

The Stroop Color/Word Test—Interference is a subtest administered to determine information-processing speed and executive functioning. The patient is instructed to say the color of the ink in which the words "red," "green," and "blue" are printed. The color of the ink never matches the name of the color as printed. The score is based on the number of correct responses given during a 45-second interval and is used to measure mental control and the patient's ability to suppress the automatic reading response in favor of the color-naming response.

Visuospatial Abilities

Hooper Visual Organization Test

The Hooper Visual Organization Test (HVOT) measures the ability to identify verbally simple objects that have been cut up and rearranged in a jigsaw puzzle-like fashion. Correct identification requires visuospatial analysis and synthesis as well as acquired nominal abilities. This test has been shown to be sensitive to disease duration in PD patients.

Information-Processing Speed

Symbol Digit Modalities Test— Verbal Response

The Symbol Digit Modalities Test—Verbal Response was used primarily to examine the patient's speed of complex scanning and visual tracking. For this reason a verbal response mode was used to avoid contamination with manual speed and agility, which is required for the written mode of the test. Patients with visuospatial problems have great difficulty shifting visual fixation between the key located at the top of the page and the correct location in the work space below. The key gives the number that goes in the space below each symbol at the bottom of the page. The score is the number of symbols for which the patient provided the correct number during a 90-second interval.

Trail Making A

The Trail Making A test was used as a simple measure of speed and accuracy of visuomotor tracing, with sustained attention also playing an important part. The test consists of connecting circles numbered from 1 to 25. The circled numbers are arranged in a pseudorandom order on the page, and the patient simply draws a line to connect the circles in order of ascending numbers. The score is the number of seconds needed to connect all of the circles in the correct order.

Stroop Word and Color Test

The Stroop Word and Color Test measures the speed of reading the words "red," "green," and "blue" ordered randomly in vertical columns on a page during a 45-second period and the speed of saying the name of the color of XXXs printed in red, green, or blue ink.

Pallidal Surgery for the Treatment of Parkinson's Disease and Movement Disorders, edited by J. K. Krauss, R. G. Grossman, and J. Jankovic. Lippincott-Raven Publishers, Philadelphia © 1998.

15

Deep Brain Stimulation of the Pallidum

Steven B. Wilkinson and *William Koller

*Department of Surgery, Division of Neurosurgery, and *Department of Neurology Kansas University Medical Center, Kansas City, Kansas 66160-7383, USA*

Pallidotomy provides substantial benefit to motor function in severely affected Parkinson's disease (PD) patients (1,6,7,14). Because a lesion of the brain is created with pallidotomy, nuclear groups and white matter tracts in relation to the pallidum are at risk of being included in the lesion and causing subsequent complications. Possible complications include not only motor and visual deficits but there is a risk of cognitive dysfunction (12). These problems are often permanent when they do occur, adding extra disability to an already impaired patient. In addition to these risks there is some reluctance on the part of both patients and physicians to embrace the finality of a lesioning procedure.

Deep brain stimulation (DBS) may offer an alternative to destructive procedures. Because no brain tissue is destroyed, the risks of permanent side effects should therefore be lessened and the treatment reversible. Experience with DBS in the thalamus for the treatment of tremor has been generally safe and effective (4,5). There is good evidence that thalamic DBS offers the same benefits as thalamotomy (4,5). If this is the case, it seems that DBS could replicate the outcome seen with other destructive procedures. Pallidal stimulation (PS) may offer an alternative to pallidotomy analogous to that which thalamic stimulation offers for thalamotomy.

There are definite down sides to this technology. The stimulation hardware, like any implanted mechanical device, is subject to malfunction and infection (Fig. 15-1). At present there is a finite life of the battery in the stimulator, necessitating

another procedure to replace the generator. Also after implantation the device must be programmed to deliver the optimal stimulation parameters to that individual. This task is much more complex than when applying DBS for tremor in that in PS benefit must be optimized for both the "on" and "off" states associated with levodopa therapy. Given the theoretical and real risks associated with PS, the benefit ultimately comes down to the ability to provide the same results as pallidotomy without destroying a portion of the brain. This chapter discusses a pilot study of PS for PD that was performed at the University of Kansas Medical Center.

SELECTION OF PATIENTS

Criteria for patient selection are similar to those for pallidotomy. Selection is limited to patients with levodopa-responsive PD. Our selection was based primarily on patients with disabling levodopa-induced dyskinesias. Dyskinesias were present during most of their "on" time. As with pallidotomy, other aspects of PD (e.g., tremor, gait dysfunction, rigidity, and bradykinesia) could be alleviated. Dementia excluded a patient from the study, and for our purposes it was defined as a Mattis Dementia Rating Scale score of less than 124. Although we excluded these patients, PS may prove to be a better alternative to pallidotomy for them in terms of risks about cognitive function. Autonomic dysfunction, swallowing dysfunction, and disabling freezing would not be expected to respond to PS and

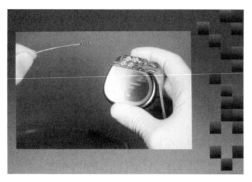

FIG. 15-1. Pallidal stimulation system: deep brain stimulation (DBS) electrode (left) and the stimulating generator. (Provided by Medtronics, Minneapolis, MN.)

should be considered at least relative contraindications.

Obviously, the patient must be fit enough to withstand the operation and to be able to cooperate during the procedure. Coagulopathy or other bleeding disorders must be identified and corrected prior to surgery. Previous contralateral pallidotomy may be another indication for PS, which would alleviate, at least theoretically, the risks of bilateral lesions.

The best candidate for this surgery (or any surgery) is a patient who understands the objective of the operation and all of the risks and complications involved. This point is especially important for PS, as the outcome may be related to the ability to control certain symptoms with the stimulation but not alleviate others. Also, the responses may change with the on–off status of the patient. The patient must understand that programming the device after surgery may be time-consuming and tedious.

SURGICAL PROCEDURE

All of our operations were unilateral implantations, with the second side implanted usually at least 3 months after the first. We perform most of the procedure under local anesthesia with sedation used during the incision, burr hole, and microelectrode recording. Midazolam was used for sedation because of its short half-life. All of the patients were given antibiotics prior to skin incision that provided *Staphylococcus aureus* coverage. On the day of the surgery the patient withheld any antiparkinsonian medications. The stereotactic head frame was positioned under local anesthesia, trying to angle the frame to approximate the angle of the anterior commissure–posterior commissure (AC-PC) plane in the sagittal plane and to avoid any pitch of the frame in the coronal plane. These precautions were used to avoid errors induced by angulation during the initial target calculations.

Computed tomography (CT) was used for the initial targeting in all of our patients. Initial scans are made with the gantry angled to approximate the AC-PC plane, and a thickness of 10 mm to localize the region of the AC-PC line. Then thin slices (1.0–1.5 mm in thickness) were made through the region of interest, and the slice that best depicted the AC-PC line was chosen. The target derived from the CT scan was 3 mm anterior to the AC-PC midline and 20 mm lateral to the midline. The vertical coordinate was usually 3 to 7 mm below the AC-PC line. It was determined by viewing the individual slices; the first slice below the AC-PC line in which the optic tract was clearly visible was chosen. Certainly magnetic resonance imaging (MRI) or ventriculography could also be used for targeting. We selected CT because of the speed of scanning, patient comfort, and noninvasiveness; and it is not susceptible to the field distortions as is MRI.

The patient was placed in a comfortable, semisitting position in the operating room (Fig. 15-2). Care was taken to ensure that there was no tension on the neck, which was accomplished by placing supportive padding behind the neck. This small point obviated many headaches later in the case: Invariably, unless these measures are taken the patient complains of severe neck pain usually near the end of the procedure. The burr hole is placed about 2.5 cm from the midline anterior to the coronal suture. A 14-mm perforator is needed to place the burr hole ring (Medtronics, Minneapolis, MN), which eventually holds the electrode. Alternatively, either a twist drill or larger opening may be made if methylmethacrylate is used to secure the electrode. The advantage of the burr hole ring and securing cap is that if the

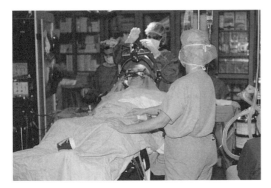

FIG. 15-2. Patient positioning and setup of the operating room. Note that space is provided for examination of the target extremities.

electrode needs to be revised later it is easy to remove and replace through the same opening. Working through a burr hole may be somewhat safer, as most intracranial hemorrhages from stereotactic procedures are due to cortical bleeding usually from a vessel in a sulcus. With a burr hole the cortical surface can be inspected and any bleeding controlled. The down side to this is cerebrospinal fluid (CSF) loss, which may lead to shifting of the brain and distortion of the target. We usually make a fairly small hole in the dura (2–3 mm) to minimize CSF loss and enlarge the opening if there is any evidence of bleeding.

Our approach has been to confirm the target using microelectrode recording to map the globus pallidus internus (GPi) and its boundaries. We used an electrode that is a platinum-iridium wire with a glass tip. The shaft diameter is 0.66 mm, and the recording tip is 10 to 15 µm. The electrode is electrically conditioned, once below the cortex, to an impedance between 0.3 and 1.0 MΩ. The angle of approach is dependent mostly on the angle of the placement of the frame; in our cases it varied usually between 40 and 75 degrees. Recordings began 15 to 20 mm above the target. The aim of the recordings was to: (a) define the nature of the individual recorded neuronal firings [i.e., differentiate the putamen, globus pallidus externus (GPe), and GPi]; (b) locate the posterior and inferior margins of the GPi; and (c) define GPi cells that were responsive to passive joint move-

ment or fired in synchrony with the resting tremor. This method is used to define the optimal location for placing the electrode in the same way that the optimal site of pallidotomy is defined (1,7,8).

As the microelectrode is advanced through the brain, each persistent neuronal impulse is observed for frequency, amplitude, pattern of spikes, and responsiveness to passive joint movement. White matter tracts are identified as being "quiet" areas without neuronal signals. The optic tract or internal capsule is usually encountered at the posteroinferior border of the GPi. The optic tract location can be defined precisely by producing phosphenes via microstimulation or observing an evoked response of light flash to the patient's appropriate visual field (6). Microstimulation of the capsule produces contraction of the face or extremity.

Parameters that we use for microstimulation are 330 Hz, 300 µs pulse width, and an amplitude that varies from 0 to 50 µA. All of this information was recorded on an acetate sheet that denoted the vertical position of each response and the areas of white matter. The acetate sheets were then compared to the Schatalbrand and Bailey atlas for the "best fit" location of the tract. Depending on the recorded information, the location of a parallel tract was chosen to define the most posterior extent of the GPi. Tracts were usually separated by 3 mm. Three to six tracts were usually made to complete the mapping process.

The final position was usually the most posterior tract with cells that responded to movement and in which an optic tract response was also recorded. A macroelectrode was then used for macrostimulation. We did not usually find any dramatic benefit from the macrostimulation but used it to ensure that there was no significant spread to the internal capsule or the optic tract with the usual range of stimulation. The macroelectrode (Radionics, Burlington, MA) has a diameter of 1.1 mm and an exposed tip of 3 mm. Stimulation parameters were 116 Hz, 120 µs pulse width, and voltage of 0 to 5 V. If this voltage range did not produce muscle contraction or persistent visual defects, the location was judged suitable for implantation. For patients who demonstrated these side effects, the electrode position was adjusted superiorly or another tract was selected.

The macroelectrode makes a tract through the brain that aids in accurate placement of the DBS electrode, which was placed next. This electrode has four individual contacts (model 3382 electrode, Medtronics) each separated over a distance of 10 mm. This electrode was tested with the same stimulation parameters. The stylet was removed and the electrode secured in the burr hole (Fig. 15-3). Stimulation was performed a final time. In most cases we then implanted the rest of the stimulating system, but on occasion (if there was any doubt about the usefulness of the stimulation or of side effects) the lead was externalized for a period of trial external stimulation (Fig. 15-4). Prior to leaving the operating room, stereotactic skull radiographs were obtained to confirm the X, Y, and Z coordinates of the lead tip.

Implantation of the pulse generator and its connection to the DBS lead is similar to that for dorsal column stimulation. We have used general anesthesia for this portion, though local anesthesia and sedation (particularly heavy sedation for the tunneling portion) is equally effective. A pocket was made subcutaneously in the infraclavicular area. One or two relaxing incisions between this and the cranial incision aid in passing the connecting extension, which is secured to the DBS electrode proximally and the pulse generator distally. The skin over the connector may erode from traction if the connector is placed over the superior temporal line. Ideally, the connector is placed

behind the ear or below, in the neck, to avoid this problem. The pulse generator should be secured to the pectoralis fascia to keep it from "flipping" over in the pocket. If flipping occurs, it may be impossible to turn the device on or off or to program it.

After the procedure, a CT scan was obtained to ensure placement of the electrode and to rule out intracranial hemorrhage. The patient was hospitalized overnight for observation. The next day the initial attempt at programming the device was made prior to the patient receiving antiparkinsonian medications. The pulse generator was programmed with a telemetric device held over the generator. Selecting the individual electrodes for cathode and anode, frequency, pulse width, and amplitude can be done with the programmer. Also, the device can be queried to determine the battery function and impedance of the system. After the device was programmed to obtain the most benefit in terms of rigidity and bradykinesia, the patient was medicated. With the patient in an "on" state, the programming was adjusted, if needed, to help control the dyskinesias. The device could be turned on or off with a magnet. The patient may turn the device off at night to conserve the battery life of the pulse generator (usually a 3- to 5-year life-span). Once the patient was stable, he or she was discharged from the hospital. During the first month after implantation, the effects of the stimulation vary from changes most likely related to edema or hemorrhage at the elec-

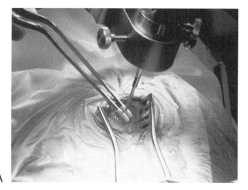
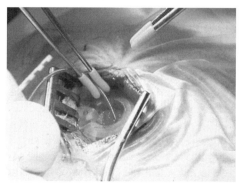

A   B

FIG. 15-3. Securing the DBS electrode. **A.** The electrode is grasped with protected forceps by an assistant as the introducing assembly and stylet are removed. **B.** After the stylet is removed, the electrode may be placed in one of the grooves of the burr hole ring and then secured with the burr hole cap (Medtronics) (not pictured).

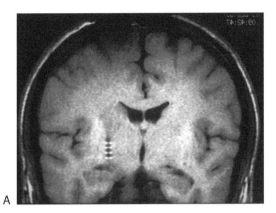
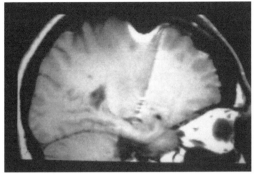

Fig. 15-4. A. Coronal T1-weighted MR scan after unilateral pallidal DBS electrode placement.
B. Sagittal T1-weighted MR scan after unilateral pallidal DBS electrode placement.

trode tip. Usually the parameters have stabilized after this time.

The procedure for the contralateral implant was done usually 3 months or so after the first implant. The second procedure was similar to that used for the initial implant.

RESULTS

Nine patients have undergone PS at the University of Kansas Medical Center. Six of them have had bilateral implants (in staged procedures). The average age was 44.6 years (32–71 years). PD had been present in these patients for an average of 10.8 years. Follow-up has ranged from 6 to 18 months (average 12.6 months). Six patients are men.

Overall the patients did well. Most of the benefit from the stimulation was seen in the contralateral extremities. A 5-point disability rating scale (0 = no disability to 4 = severe disability) was done at baseline and follow-up by both the examiner (a neurologist specializing in movement disorders) and the patient. The examiner's disability scores averaged 3 at baseline and at last follow-up averaged 1. The patients rating averaged 3.1 at baseline and 1.3 at last follow-up. No patient was worse at follow-up. The most significant change was in the dyskinesia, which was reported on an 11-point scale (0 = absent to 10 = severe disabling), measured with the patient "on."

Patients averaged 7.2 at baseline and at last follow-up 2.25. This score improved in all patients.

Patients recorded "on" and "off" time in diaries. The results at last follow-up are consistent with the findings from our previous study, which looked at the initial 3 months of follow-up (9). There were significant increases in "on" time and decreases in "off" time and "on" time with dyskinesias. "On" time increased 40% on average, and the "on" time with dyskinesias has decreased an average of 30%. The decrease in "off" time has averaged 15%.

There were a significant number of complications with this group, likely representing the novelty of the procedure. The most serious complication involved a hemorrhage that occurred during physiological mapping of the pallidum on the second side. This patient had a prominent hemiparesis and general decrease in level of functioning but has made a good recovery over a 6- to 8-month period. This patient was the oldest one in the series. Three patients required lead revisions because of internal capsular involvement from the stimulation (contralateral muscle contraction), and two are now doing well. The third patient is improved, but currently the stimulator has been turned off because the effect on her dyskinesias has been inconsistent. One other patient had the lead replaced because the lead fractured near the connector approximately 6 months after implantation. This patient developed an infection of the pulse generator pocket 1 month after the revision that was treated by explanting the generator and connecting extension and giving intravenous antibiotics.

One patient had an asymptomatic intraventricular hemorrhage that was discovered on the postoperative CT scan. One patient experienced seizures after implantation that were successfully treated with anticonvulsants. The pulse generator of two of the patients (both women) rotated in the pocket, and on revision the sutures tacking down the device had pulled through the fascia.

The most interesting complication has been mania associated with bilateral stimulation in one of our patients. This individual had an excellent motor response to the stimulation, but with both of the devices activated he developed a true mania with a marked increase in his energy level and a decrease in his sleep patterns. With additional medication and adjustments to the stimulation parameters his situation has improved. This effect raises some interesting questions about the frontostriatal connections and their role in affective disorders. This patient has been studied with H_2O^{15} position emission tomography (PET) scans. Without stimulation there is a decrement in the left parahippocampus and hippocampus and the right midcingulate gyrus. With bilateral stimulation there is increased activity in both insular regions, the precuneus, the left inferior frontal cortex, and the right dorsolateral prefrontal cortex (Miyawaki, personal communication). The significance of this finding and the relevance to other patients undergoing this procedure is not yet clear.

DISCUSSION

From our preliminary study PS seems to offer at least the same degree of improvement as pallidotomy (1,6–8,12,13,14). There were a large number of complications in our series, likely representative of the learning curve associated with any new procedure. As more of these procedures are done, the number of complications should decrease. There have been few reports outlining the specific complications associated with pallidotomy, so it is difficult to compare these two operations. Even in our own series of patients we cannot directly compare PS with pallidotomy, as the

selection criteria for these two groups are not the same and the patients were not randomly assigned to a specific procedure.

The programming of the device was initiated during the "off" state to minimize brakykinesia and rigidity. On the initial programming, one strategy was to make the pulse generator positive and then use unipolar stimulation of each of the four contacts to determine the effect of that one contact. Once this was known, a bipolar combination was tried, using the best contacts from unipolar stimulation. After these settings were accomplished, the patient was given his usual dose of medication. When the patient was "on," the device was adjusted to control dyskinesias, if present. Most of the time the optimal settings for each of the states were different, so a compromise between the two was selected. Our patients were selected primarily for severe dyskinesias, so the programming was geared toward the control of the dyskinesias. Most of the patients averaged 3 to 4.5 volts amplitude with a rate of 130 to 185. The pulse width was quite variable, ranging from 90 to 210 microseconds. The time and effort put into the programming of the device, as one would imagine, is enormous. Programming time varies between several hours to essentially the whole day. Certainly most of the time is spent letting the patient see if there are any side effects or changes in the effect over time (and with changes in the medication levels). This demands a great deal of patience on the part of the programmer. As time has gone on, the time taken to program has decreased, but it still exceeds that of the programming of the thalamic stimulator.

Currently there is little published on the use of PS. Siegfried and Lippitz reported on three patients treated with PS, all of whom had excellent results (11). In a larger series the outcome has continued to be excellent with no significant complications (Siegfried, personal communication).

In another report, seven patients implanted unilaterally all had significant and (for the most part) sustained improvement in the UPDRS motor scores and decrease in dyskinesias (3). Overall, the outcome was more pronounced in the upper extremity than in the lower extremity, and this was attributed to the position of the electrode tip in the region of the pallidum that somatotopically represents the arm (3). Tronnier reported on a series of six patients with bilateral PS (15). Though the patients benefited in respect to improvement in dyskinesias, this was offset by worsening in the "off" period from freezing (15). This, along with what was felt to be generally less benefit than was typically seen in that center with pallidotomy, led the authors to not recommend PS (15). In other trials, this decrement in "off" period function has not been seen. Also it should be pointed out that the benefit from pallidotomy was greater than what has been predominately published (1,8,13).

The mechanism of action of pallidal stimulation is currently unknown. Electrical stimulation in nuclear regions of the brain is felt to produce a depolarization block that inhibits firing of that nucleus. Conversely, stimulation in white matter tracts may propagate conduction and produce "positive" phenomena (i.e., motor movements from internal capsule stimulation). Because the benefits of stimulation occur when the stimulation is started and stop when it ceases, this suggests that this is not an effect of neurotransmitter release (3).

The most appealing aspect of PS is that it is not a destructive procedure and may not limit the patient's candidacy for other future therapies as they arise. There has been some question of the cognitive effects of pallidotomy (12). The damage caused by a lesion in a brain with an ongoing degenerative disease may accelerate the problem of cognitive dysfunction. We have looked at neuropsychological testing in the short term in our patients with unilateral stimulation (16). There were few if any significant changes in either cognition or memory in patients with unilateral PS (16), similar to our findings with thalamic stimulation (16). If after bilateral stimulation the results are similar, a strong argument can be made for the use of PS. Certainly this study is small and may not be large enough to detect some cognitive changes. Moreover, patients with dementia were specifically excluded, and the average age of the patients was rather young, which would also decrease the incidence of cognitive dysfunction. Lang and Lozano have used PS contralateral to an existing pallidotomy as an alternative to bilateral pallidotomy, and they have not found it to be associated with any significant cognitive dysfunction (Lozano, per-

sonal communication). This indication may be the most justifiable use of PS. It would decrease the expense of the hardware for both sides and decrease the risk of cognitive problems associated with bilateral lesions.

Deep brain stimulation has now been used in the subthalamic nucleus (STN) for akineto-rigid forms of PD with encouraging results (2,10). The advantage of STN stimulation is that the STN outflow is mostly glutaminergic. By decreasing the release of glutamate and therefore stimulation of *N*-methyl-D-aspartate receptors, STN stimulation may be a protective therapy. Moreover, these patients have been able to have their levodopa doses decreased over time. All of these factors point to the STN as an alternative target for PD. So far, comparative studies of the benefits of pallidotomy, pallidol stimulation, and STN stimulation are not available.

Currently, the cost of the hardware for one side is about ten thousand dollars (U.S.). Currently in the U.S., the device is FDA approved for unilateral use in the thalamus for tremor. Some insurance carriers and Medicare may cover its use in the pallidum, especially for stimulation contralateral to a pallidotomy. Overall, though, it is extremely difficult to get insurance coverage for this procedure. Hopefully, as more is published and long term outcome studies are also positive, this should not be as much of an obstacle.

Overall, PS is a viable alternative to pallidotomy as either the primary therapy or an alternative to bilateral pallidotomy. More study is needed to define the best electrode placement (as for lesion location with pallidotomy), the true rate of complications, and the long-term outcome. If STN stimulation continues to be as promising, there may be some instances where STN stimulation is superior. At least for patients who have undergone unilateral pallidotomy, PS would then be a reasonable choice.

Acknowledgments. Funding for the reported study was provided by Medtronics, Inc.

REFERENCES

1. Baron MS, Vitek JL, Bakay RAE, et al. Treatment of advanced Parkinson's disease by posterior GPi pallidotomy. *Ann Neurol* 1996;40:355–366.
2. Benabid AL, Pollack P, Gross C, et al. Acute and long-term effects of subthalamic nucleus stimulation in

Parkinson's disease. *Stereotact Funct Neurosurg* 1994; 62:76–84.

3. Gross C, Rougier A, Guehl D, Boraud T, Julien J, Bioulac B. High-frequency stimulation of the globus pallidus internalis in Parkinson's disease: a study of seven cases. *J Neurosurg* 1997;87:491–498.

4. Hubble JP, Busenbark KL, Wilkinson S, Penn RD, Lyons KE, Koller WC. Deep brain stimulation for essential tremor. *Neurology* 1996;46:1150–1153.

5. Hubble JP, Busenbark KL, Wilkinson S, et al. Effects of thalamic deep brain stimulation based on tremor type and diagnosis. *Mov Disord* 1997;12:337–341.

6. Iacono RP, Shima F, Lonser FF, Kuniyoshi S, Maeda G, Yamada S. The results, indications, and physiology of posteroventral pallidotomy for patients with Parkinson's disease. *Neurosurgery* 1995;36:1118–1127.

7. Laitinen LV, Hariz MI, Bergenheim AT. Ventroposterolateral pallidotomy in the treatment of Parkinson's disease. *J Neurosurg* 1992;76:53–61.

8. Lozano A, Hutchison W, Kiss Z, Tasker R, Davis K, Dostrovsky J. Methods for microelectrode-guided posteroventral pallidotomy. *J Neurosurg* 1996;84:194–202.

9. Pahwa R, Wilkinson S, Smith D, Lyons K, Miyawaki E, Koller WC. High frequency stimulation of the globus pallidus for the treatment of Parkinson's disease. *Ann Neurol* 1996;40:533.

10. Pollak P, Benabid AL, Limousin P, et al. Subthalamic nucleus stimulation alleviates akinesia and rigidity in parkinsonian patients. *Adv Neurol* 1996;69:591–594.

11. Siegfried J, Lippitz B. Chronic electrical stimulation of the VL-VPL complex and of the pallidum in the treatment of movement disorders: personal experience since 1982. *Stereotact Funct Neurosurg* 1994;62:71–75.

12. Stebbins GT, Gabrieli JDE, Goetz CG, Shannon KM, Penn RD, Masciari F. Impaired fronto-striatal memory functioning following pallidotomy in advanced Parkinson's disease. *Neurology* 1997;48:A252 (abst).

13. Sterio D, Beric A, Dogali M, Fazzini E, Alfaro G, Devinsky O. Neurophysiological properties of pallidal neurons in Parkinson's disease. *Ann Neurol* 1994;35: 586–591.

14. Sutton JP, Couldwell W, Lew MF, et al. Ventroposterior medial pallidotomy in patients with advanced Parkinson's disease. *Neurosurgery* 1995;36:1112–1117.

15. Tronnier VM, Fogel W, Kronenbuerger W, Steinvorth S. Pallidal stimulation: an alternative to pallidotomy? *J Neurosurg* 1997;87:700–705.

16. Troster AI, Fields JA, Wilkinson SB, et al. Unilateral pallidal stimulation for Parkinson's disease: neurobehavioral functioning before and three months after electrode implantation. *Neurology* 1997;49:1078–1083.

Pallidal Surgery for the Treatment of Parkinson's Disease and Movement Disorders, edited by
J. K. Krauss, R. G. Grossman, and J. Jankovic.
Lippincott-Raven Publishers, Philadelphia © 1998.

16

Gamma Knife Pallidotomy for Parkinson's Disease

Gerhard M. Friehs, Joseph H. Friedman, Mel H. Epstein,
and Georg Norén

*Department of Clinical Neurosciences, Brown University School of Medicine,
Providence, Rhode Island 02905, USA*

When Lars Leksell began developing the gamma knife during the early 1950s it was his desire to use this radiosurgical tool for the treatment of functional disorders (9,10). The first functional radiosurgical procedure was undertaken in 1955 by the "father" of radiosurgery himself with a 200-kV x-ray source prototype version of a radiosurgical apparatus (8). Since 1967 the gamma knife has existed more or less as we know it today.

When it became evident how appealing this new technique was for treating other disorders of the brain, the use of the gamma knife for functional radiosurgery was overshadowed by its use for brain tumors and arteriovenous malformations. Only since the late 1980s has interest reemerged in taking advantage of the high precision and non-invasiveness of the gamma knife for the treatment of parkinsonism (3,4,11–15,17–19), psychiatric disorders (5), tic doloreux (6), and other forms of intractable pain (16,17) in accordance with Leksell's original vision. Several gamma knife thalamotomies and anterior capsulotomies were performed during the early years of the gamma knife (9, 10), but the first radiosurgical pallidotomy was not done until about 1991 (15). Leksell never used the *StrÁhlknifen* to target the pallidum internum, although the coordinates employed even today to perform posteroventral pallidotomy also carry his name (7).

GAMMA KNIFE

The gamma knife is a radiosurgical instrument that uses 201 cobalt-60 gamma ray emitters aligned in a hemispherical array. The emitted radiation sources intersect at a fixed focus. To reach any given point within the coordinate system the stereotactic frame must be adjusted with respect to the focus. The geometrical accuracy of the gamma knife is in the submillimeter range, and several studies have confirmed that the gamma knife provides millimeter accuracy in biological systems. The radiation can be modified in several ways. Four collimator sizes are available (18, 14, 8 and 4mm), although only the 4-mm collimator is currently used for functional radiosurgery. Each of the 201 sources can be blocked with a plug, which allows adaptation of the isodose distribution to specific needs. Furthermore, when combining isocenters to form a radiation field, the relative weight ratio between these "shots" can be altered, which in turn makes possible changes in the shape and configuration of isodose distribution. A gamma knife with new cobalt-60 sources has an output of approximately 3 Gy per minute. Based on animal experiments and experience in humans it is known that radiation of less than 90 to 100 Gy does not produce necrosis in white or gray matter and therefore does not result in a visible lesion. From the time of exposure in the gamma knife it takes a minimum of 4 weeks for a necrotic lesion to form. The size of the lesion created can be estimated based on the isodose distribution (Fig. 16-1). If, for example, the 50% isodose line receives a necrotizing dose, the expected lesion size is approximately 5 mm in diameter, which translates into a lesion volume of approximately 65 mm^3.

PROCEDURE

Step 1: Application of the Stereotactic Frame

The Leksell stereotactic frame is applied under local anesthesia. Because the stereotactic frame is typically placed in the anatomical midline, many neurosurgeons prefer to use earpins for symmetrical positioning. It is desirable to approximate the frame angle to the plane of the anterior commissure and posterior commissure (AC-PC). For that purpose the anterior margin of the frame is angled superiorly with respect to the posterior frame margin. The imaginary line between the lateral canthus and external auditory canal is a good external landmark for this angulation. Thus, the imaging studies performed are aligned parallel to the AC-PC plane without having to change the gantry angle.

Step 2: Imaging Studies

For radiosurgical pallidotomy it is advisable to use magnetic resonance imaging (MRI) for target localization, as the target can be visualized directly. It is of utmost importance to ensure that the distortion generated by any given MRI machine in combination with a stereotactic frame is within acceptable limits. As in most gamma knife centers we perform this quality assurance process on a daily basis. It involves obtaining MRI images of a phantom in at least two planes and shimming of the MRI magnet if the inaccuracy is found to be out of limits. Typically, the highest geometrical accuracy is found on axial images where the distortion is in the 1-mm range. Coronal images have a slightly higher tendency for distortion especially in the X-Z direction. At our gamma knife center the typical geometrical error is 1 mm. Sagittal images are not recommended as a basis for treatment planning. Although various MRI sequences can be helpful, we found that inversion recovery sequences in the axial and coronal plane with a slice thickness of 2 mm or less without interslice gap are most useful for delineating the globus pallidum internum (GPi) target area with its surrounding structures (Fig. 16-2).

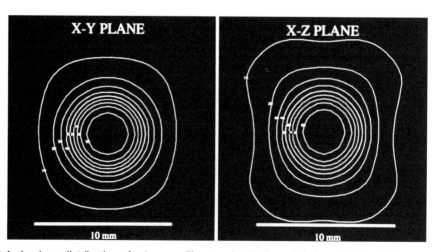

FIG. 16-1. Isodose distribution of a 4-mm collimator shot in the axial plane (*left*) and the coronal plane (*right*). The 10%, 20%, 30%, 40%, 50%, 60%, 70%, 80%, and 90% isodose lines are shown with a reference bar below.

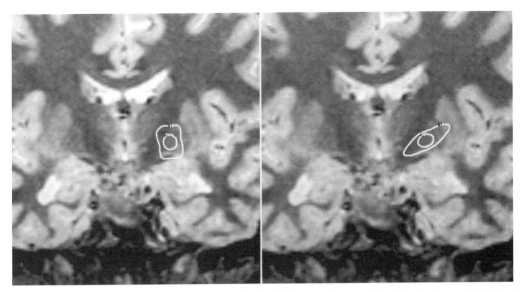

FIG. 16-2. Sample dose planning for radiosurgical pallidotomy. A coronal section is shown at the level of the posteroventral pallidum internum. The left image depicts a single 4-mm collimator shot without plugging; on the right side the same 4-mm shot is shown with heavy plugging. The 10% and 50% isodose lines are depicted. Note the shift of the 10% isodose line away from the optic tract after a collimator plugging patter was used (*right*). If a dose of 140 Gy were to be delivered, the optic tract would be outside the 14-Gy isodose (= 10% isodose line).

Step 3: Treatment Planning

The GPi is located in a triangle described by the internal capsule medially, the optic tract inferiorly, and the globus pallidum externum (GPe) laterally. These structures are all visualized on coronal images. Another method of finding the target area is to follow the guidelines given for open stereotactic pallidotomy, described in detail elsewhere (7). Briefly, the approximate coordinates are 3 mm anterior to the mid-AC-PC planes 18 to 21 mm lateral of midline, and 3 to 6 mm inferior to the AC-PC plane. Today, only single 4-mm collimator shots are used for radiosurgical pallidotomy. A maximum dose of 140 to 160 Gy is prescribed, and care is taken that the optic tract is not exposed to more than 8 to 12 Gy. If necessary, the isodose configuration can be changed by introducing certain plugging patterns in an attempt to drive the isodose lines away from the optic tract, which is the most radiosensitive structure adjacent to the GPi (Fig. 16-2).

Step 4: Treatment

Using a gamma knife with new cobalt-60 sources, treatment time for a typical pallidotomy is around 60 minutes. Aging of the cobalt sources naturally increases the treatment time; it is doubled after 5 years of operation, which is the approximate half-life of cobalt-60. Treatment itself is pain-free. There are no immediate side effects, and there is also no immediate primary effect, as the development of a radionecrotic lesion requires several weeks. After treatment and removal of the stereotactic frame, patients are typically kept in the hospital overnight. There is no evidence that any medication (e.g., dexamethasone) is necessary or helpful during the immediate perioperative period.

Step 5: Postoperative Follow-Up

The gamma knife pallidotomy procedure is typically performed on an inpatient, same-day admittance basis with 1 night of hospitalization. Patients are seen for follow-up several weeks after gamma knife treatment. It is during this period that patients may experience the onset of relief from symptoms of parkinsonism. A follow-up MRI scan with contrast enhancement most likely reveals a ring-enhancing lesion in the target area that is larger than the expected lesion volume. It is important to distinguish between the enhancement (i.e., disrupted blood–brain barrier) and the true zone of necrosis, which is much smaller than the enhancing area. If a T2-weighted MRI scan is obtained, dramatic signal changes may be found that extend into the internal capsule, thalamus, or even putamen, which surprisingly does not result in neurological deficits. Whether this abnormal signal represents radiogenic edema or reactive gliosis remains to be determined. Both the T1-weighted contrast enhancement and T2-weighted signal changes reach a maximum around 6 months after treatment and slowly disappear 1 to 2 years after radiosurgery (Fig. 16-3).

Gamma knife pallidotomy is a noninvasive procedure, so there is no risk of associated infection or hemorrhage. Possible treatment complications include damage to the optic tract, resulting in visual field cuts, or damage to the internal capsule with consequent hemiparesis or dysarthria.

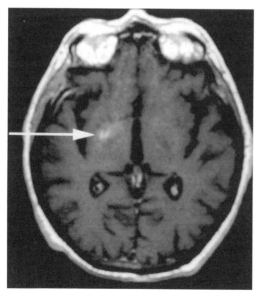

FIG. 16-3. T1-weighted MRI image with gadolinium enhancement, axial plane 1 year after gamma knife pallidotomy on the right side (*white arrow*).

CLINICAL EXPERIENCE

Several concerns have been raised when it comes to performing functional procedures with noninvasive means. For one, radiosurgical destruction of the target relies purely on anatomical localization. By definition, electrophysiological confirmation of the target is not possible. One publication has specifically addressed the question of whether electrophysiological target identification is necessary (19). To date no study has proven the need for invasive target confirmation, and the increasing experience with functional radiosurgery argues against it. The limiting factor for functional radiosurgery is the quality of the stereotactic MRI and not the accuracy of the gamma knife, which is, without doubt, an instrument of superb precision. A second question of possible concern is related to the fact that radiosurgical lesion sizes have been thought to be somewhat variable and unpredictable. This issue was addressed in a multicenter retrospective analysis of lesion sizes after functional radiosurgical procedures (2). Briefly, the study showed that the unpredictability of lesions increases dramatically if more than one isocenter is used to create the lesion. Furthermore, unexpectedly large lesion volumes were found when doses of 160 Gy or more were used. With single isocenter 4-mm collimator exposures of less than 160 Gy, without exception the lesion volumes were predictable.

As of February 1998 a total of 29 centers worldwide have reported using the gamma knife to treat Parkinson's disease, at least three of which have performed gamma knife pallidotomy for Parkinson's disease (Table 16-1). A MEDLINE literature search for the years 1993 to the present conducted on the key words "gamma knife or radiosurgery" and "pallidotomy" revealed six hits, three of which are valid. The first study (15) reported the authors' experience with gamma knife pallidotomy starting in 1991. Eight patients were treated with unilateral pallidotomy using a single 4-mm collimator shot with maximum doses ranging from 140 to 165 Gy. The follow-up intervals are not reported. Fifty percent (four of eight patients) showed definite alleviation of bradykinesia, rigidity, or tremor. The authors did not report any complications associated with the treatment.

TABLE 16-1. *Centers that have performed gamma knife treatment for Parkinson's disease*

2nd Affiliated Hospital of China Medical University, Shenyang City, Liaoning, China
2nd Affiliated Hospital of Tianjin Medial University, Tianjin, China
150th P.L.A. Central Hospital, Luo Yang, Henan Province, China
Beijing Neurosurgical Institute, Beijing, China
Canossa Hospital Gamma Unit Center, Hong Kong, China

Guangzhou Gamma Knife Center, Guangzhou, China
Liu Hua Qiao Hospital, Guangzhou, China
Shanghai Gamma Knife Hospital, Shanghai, China
Union Hospital of Tonji Medical University, Wuhan, China

Zibo Wan Dresher Hospital, Zibo, Shandong Province, China
Asian Medical Center, Seoul, Korea
Singapore Gamma Knife Center, Singapore
Furukawa Seiryo Hospital, Furukawa, Japan
Hidaka Hospital Gunma University, Takasaki City, Japan
Hisei Memorial Hospital, Fujieda, Japan
AKH Wien, Vienna, Austria
Karolinska Sjukhuset, Stockholm, Sweden
Na Homolce Hospital, Prague, Czech Republic
Ruber Hospital Internacional, Madrid, Spain
Universitätskliniken Graz, Graz, Austria
Piedmont Hospital, Atlanta, GA, USA
Miami Neuroscience Center, Coral Gables, FL, USA
Cleveland Clinic Health System, Cleveland, OH, USA

Good Samaritan Hospital, Los Angeles, CA, USA
The Neurosensory Institute, Wills Eye Hospital, Philadelphia, PA, USA
Presbyterian University Hospital, Pittsburgh, PA, USA
New England Gamma Knife Center, Rhode Island Hospital, Providence, RI, USA

Northwest Gamma Knife Center, Northwest Hospital, Seattle, WA, USA
San Diego Gamma Knife Center, Scripps Hospital, San Diego, CA, USA

Centers in bold typeface have performed more than 50 procedures.

The second report (1) summarized our own experience and is comprised of four patients with severe parkinsonism. All patients had failed multiple trials of antiparkinsonian medication after having a good response to L-dopa during the early stages of their disease. Two patients had severe fluctuations in response to medications (Hoehn and Yahr stages 3.0–5.0). The other two patients were dependent on assistance (stage 4) and were wheelchair-bound (stage 5); they had basically lost their responsiveness to L-dopa

therapy. The four patients were treated with a single 4-mm collimator shot with heavy plugging. In all cases a maximum dose of 180 Gy was used. One patient (25%) showed alleviation of dyskinesias starting 3 months after treatment. He developed dementia and psychosis 7 months after treatment. Serial MRI images obtained during that time did not show any correlation between the T2-weighted signal changes and the onset or severity of his psychosis. He fully recovered from his symptoms 6 months later and continued to improve from his parkinsonism with early relief of bradykinesia. He died suddenly of an unknown cause at a time of maximum improvement 31 months after gamma knife treatment. The brain-only autopsy specimen, shown in Fig. 16-4, depicts a radiosurgical lesion in the GPi. In addition, a lacunar infarct was found in the putamen, which was believed to be related to radiosurgery-induced occlusion of a small perforating arteriole. The other three

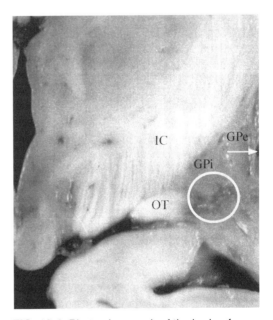

FIG. 16-4. Photomicrograph of the brain of a patient 31 months after gamma knife pallidotomy (see text). A coronal section through the target area is shown. The gamma knife lesion is seen in the globus pallidus internus (*white circle*) without affecting the optic tract (*OT*). Note also the lacunar infarct in the globus pallidus externus (*white arrow*). *IC*, internal capsule.

patients had not experienced any benefit or side effects 1 year after treatment. In retrospect, patient selection was thought to be suboptimal, which is likely responsible for the low response rate. Also, our treatment doses of 180 Gy are too high and may be the cause of the occluded artery. These findings further underline the fact that patients with severe parkinsonism and lack of L-dopa response generally are not the best candidates for pallidotomy.

The largest experience with functional radiosurgery was summarized by Young and co-authors in three publications (17–19), the most recent of which reported on 124 functional stereotactic procedures with the Leksell gamma knife on 117 patients (18). This series also included 11 patients with unilateral radiosurgical pallidotomy and 4 with bilateral gamma knife pallidotomy. A single isocenter exposure with the 4-mm collimator was used, a maximum dose of 140 to 160 Gy was given. On follow-up 77% of patients were found to have relief of their bradykinesia or rigidity. Radiosurgical pallidotomy relieved symptoms in all patients who exhibited dyskinesia. There were no complications reported in this publication, but a follow-up report indicates the occurrence of visual field cuts in one patient (17).

CONCLUSIONS

Radiosurgical pallidotomy has been performed in small numbers unilaterally and bilaterally. The success rate after radiosurgical pallidotomy can be as high as 77% and therefore is similar to the likelihood of improvement after conventional stereotactic pallidotomy. Treatment-related complications are rare, typically involve visual field defects, and have been reported in the literature (17) and by personal communication. It is recommended that a single 4-mm collimator shot be used with a maximum dose of less than 160 Gy. In 1998 at least three methods are acceptable for treating patients with parkinsonism by interfering with hyperactivity in the GPi: conventional stereotactic pallidotomy with thermal (radiofrequency) lesioning, pallidal deep brain stimulation, and radiosurgical pallidotomy. The obvious attractiveness of chronic stimulation is its

TABLE 16-2. *Advantages and disadvantages of gamma knife pallidotomy*

Advantages
  Noninvasive treatment
  No risk of infection, hemorrhage
  Lesioning effect still visible after months (? years)
  Relatively short procedure
Disadvantages
  Ablative procedure
  Electrophysiological target confirmation not
    possible
  Delayed onset of effect
  Limited experience worldwide

nondestructive, neuroaugmentative nature, but enormous experience speaks in favor of conventional pallidotomy. The gamma knife pallidotomy is the only noninvasive method, although it is an ablative procedure (Table 16-2). In the authors' opinion, there are at least two absolute indications for choosing the gamma knife over the other methods: (a) contraindications to invasive surgery and (b) unwillingness of the patient to undergo invasive surgery. It allows us to treat patients who would otherwise be excluded from the benefits of modern functional neurosurgery.

REFERENCES

1. Friedman JH, Epstein M, Sanes JN, et al. Gamma knife pallidotomy in advanced Parkinson's disease. *Ann Neurol* 1996;39:535–538.
2. Friehs GM, Norén G, Ohye C, et al. Lesion sizes following gamma knife treatment for functional disorders. *Stereotact Funct Neurosurg* 1996;66[suppl 1]:320–328.
3. Friehs GM, Ojakangas CL, Pachatz P, Schröttner O, Ott E, Pendl G. Thalamotomy and caudatotomy with the gamma knife as a treatment for parkinsonism with a comment on lesion sizes. *Stereotact Funct Neurosurg* 1995;64[suppl 1]:209–221.
4. Hirato M, Ohye C, Shibasaki T, Nakamura M, Inoue HK, Andou Y. Gamma knife thalamotomy for the treatment of functional disorders. *Stereotact Funct Neurosurg* 1995;54[suppl 1]:164–171.
5. Kihlström L, Guo WY, Lindquist C, Mindus P. Radiobiology of radiosurgery for refractory anxiety disorders. *Neurosurgery* 1995;36:294–302.
6. Kondziolka D, Lundsford LD, Flickinger JC, et al. Stereotactic radiosurgery for trigeminal neuralgia: a multi-institutional study using the gamma unit. *J Neurosurg* 1996;84:940–945.
7. Laitinen LV, Bergheim R, Hariz MI. Leksell's posteroventral pallidotomy in the treatment of Parkinson's disease. *J Neurosurg* 1992;76:53–61.
8. Larsson B. The history of radiosurgery: the early years (1950–1970). In: Kondziolka D, ed. *Radiosurgery.* Basel: Karger, 1996:1–10.

9. Leksell L. Cerebral radiosurgery. I. Gamma thalamotomy in two cases of intractable pain. *Acta Chir Scand* 1968;134:585–595.

10. Leksell L. The stereotactic method and radiosurgery of the brain. *Acta Chir Scand* 1951;102:316–319.

11. Lindquist C, Steiner, L, Hindmarsh, T. Gamma knife thalamotomy for tremor: report of two cases. In: Steiner L, ed. *Radiosurgery: baseline and trends.* New York: Raven Press, 1992:237–243.

12. Ohye C, Shibazaki T, Hirato M, Inoue H, Andou Y. Gamma thalamotomy for parkinsonian and other kinds of tremor. *Stereotact Funct Neurosurg* 1996;66[suppl 1]:333–342.

13. Otsuki T, Jokura H, Takahashi K, et al. Stereotactic gammathalamotomy with a computerized brain atlas: technical case report. *Neurosurgery* 1994;35:764-767; discussion 767–768.

14. Pan Li, Jia-Zhong Dai, Bin-Jiang Wang, Wei-min Xu, Liang-fu Zhou, Xing-Rong Chen. Stereotactic gamma thalamotomy for the treatment of parkinsonism. *Stereotact Funct Neurosurg* 1996;66[suppl 1]:329–332.

15. Rand RW, Jacques DB, Melbye RW, Copcutt BG, Fisher MR, Levenick MN. Gamma knife thalamotomy and pallidotomy in patients with movement disorders: preliminary results. *Stereotact Funct Neurosurg* 1993;61[suppl 1]:65–92.

16. Steiner L, Forster D, Leksell L, Meyerson BA, Boethius J. Gamma thalamotomy in intractable pain. *Acta Neurochir (Wien)* 1980;52:173–184.

17. Young RF. Functional disease of the brain: treatment by gamma knife radiosurgery. In: De Salles AAF, Lufkin RB, eds. *Minimally invasive therapy of the brain.* Stuttgart: Thieme Medical Publishers, 1997: 225–234.

18. Young RF. Functional neurosurgery with the Leksell gamma knife. *Stereotact Funct Neurosurg* 1996;66: 19–23.

19. Young RF, Vermeulen SS, Grimm P, Posewitz A. Electrophysiological target localization is not required for the treatment of functional disorders. *Stereotact Funct Neurosurg* 1996;66[suppl 1]:309–319.

Pallidal Surgery for the Treatment of Parkinson's Disease and Movement Disorders, edited by J. K. Krauss, R. G. Grossman, and J. Jankovic. Lippincott-Raven Publishers, Philadelphia © 1998.

17

Parkinson's Disease and Stereotactic Pallidal Surgery: Studies with Positron Emission Tomography

Angelo Antonini and David Eidelberg

Movement Disorders Center, North Shore University Hospital, Manhasset, New York 11030, USA

Positron emission tomography (PET) is an imaging technique that employs small amounts of positron-emitting radioligands to measure physiological and biochemical processes in the brain and other organs. In a PET experiment, a subject is given trace quantities of a compound of biological interest. The spatial and temporal distribution of the radiotracer is measured quantitatively during the course of the PET study, providing a tomographical representation of regional radioactivity concentration (Table 17-1).

In patients with Parkinson's disease (PD) PET has been applied to the investigation of striatal dopaminergic nerve terminals using [^{18}F]fluorodopa (7,14,20,37) and dopamine transporter ligands (8,16,31,40,51) as well as the postsynaptic dopamine D2 receptor system using [^{11}C]raclopride (5,7,13) and [^{18}F]spiperone (66). PET has also been used to study regional cerebral blood flow with [^{15}O]H$_2$O (15,32,33) and glucose metabolism with [^{18}F]fluorodeoxyglucose (7,20, 21,23,25). Particularly, studies of brain metabolism and blood flow have contributed considerably to our understanding of the pathophysiology of PD and other movement disorders.

In this review, we summarize recent PET studies in patients with PD. We additionally focus on the application of PET to the selection of suitable candidates for stereotactic surgical interventions, such as pallidotomy, and for the assessment of their outcome after surgery.

POSITRON EMISSION TOMOGRAPHY STUDIES OF THE STRIATAL DOPAMINERGIC SYSTEM

Presynaptic Dopaminergic Function

[^{18}F]fluorodopa FDOPA is probably the most commonly applied radiotracer for studying striatal dopaminergic nerve terminals in PD. PET studies with this tracer measure the rate of decarboxylation of FDOPA to [^{18}F]fluorodopamine by the enzyme dopa decarboxylase (DDC) and its subsequent storage in the striatal dopaminergic nerve terminals. In the plasma, FDOPA is metabolized by catechol-*O*-methyltransferase to 3-*O*-methylfluorodopa and by DDC (18,37,39). In the PET experiments, peripheral DDC can be blocked by the administration of the DDC inhibitor carbidopa before tracer administration. FDOPA transport across the blood–brain barrier follows the same channel as large neutral amino acids (9).

The FDOPA/PET data can be analyzed using simple target-to-background ratios obtained by dividing striatal count rates by those in a neutral brain region such as the occipital cortex (20,38), or, alternatively, by multiple time graphical analysis (MTGA) (28,37,62). With MTGA the gradient of the linear regression of the data, described as the net influx constant (K$_i$), reflects the rate of FDOPA decarboxylation and storage (65). Compartmental models have also been developed to estimate the specific kinetic rate constant for striatal DDC activity (k$_3$) (18,34,37,43).

TABLE 17-1. *Most common PET tracers for assessing movement disorders*

Biological behavior	Tracer	Application
Regional synaptic activity		
Regional metabolic rate for glucose (rCMRGlc)	[^{18}F]FDG	Differential diagnosis (parkinsonism); selection of candidates for stereotactic surgery; research
Regional cerebral blood flow (rCBF)	[^{15}O]H$_2$O	Research
Markers of nigrostriatal dopaminergic nerve terminals		
Dopamine precursor	[^{18}F]FDOPA [^{18}F]tyrosine	Diagnosis of parkinsonism; assessment of severity, progression, and post-transplantation changes
Dopamine transporter (reuptake site)	[^{11}C]-, [^{18}F]-, or [^{123}I]*-labeled cocaine derivatives	
Markers of the striatal postsynaptic dopaminergic system		
D$_2$ receptor	[^{11}C]raclopride [^{11}C] or [^{18}F] spiperone derivatives	Research; Differential diagnosis of parkinsonism, other movement disorders

A number of studies have shown that the assessment of nigrostriatal dopaminergic function using FDOPA/PET yields quantitative parameters that correlate with independent disease severity measures (7,14,20,37,38) and can discriminate early-stage PD patients from normal control subjects (7,48,69). More importantly, it has been shown that in vivo striatal FDOPA measurements correlate with dopamine cell counts and levels measured postmortem (61,68).

The development of radiotracers binding to the striatal dopamine transporter has led to another means for directly imaging the nigrostriatal dopaminergic nerve terminals with PET, or single-photon emission computed tomography (SPECT) (16,49,66,71). The most extensively studied agents in this category are the cocaine analogues, such as 2β-carbomethyl-3β-(4-iodophenyl)tropane (βCIT) and its fluoroalkyl esters (16,57). Like FDOPA, βCIT and FP-βCIT are effective markers of nigrostriatal degeneration in parkinsonism (8,31,36,45, 51,66). In contrast to FDOPA/PET (28,36), FP-βCIT/SPECT studies have shown a decline of striatal dopaminergic nerve terminals with normal aging (38,70). Our laboratory has reported that PET imaging with [^{18}F]FP-βCIT can provide images with higher resolution and better quantification than SPECT images acquired with the radioiodinated version of the same ligand (16).

Postsynaptic Dopaminergic Function

Dopamine receptor-bearing neurons constitute approximately 80% of the neuronal population in the striatum (59,60). In the striatum, dopamine receptors are located mainly on γ-aminobutyric acid (GABA) ergic neurons projecting to the globus pallidus. In normal subjects [^{11}C]raclopride/PET studies have demonstrated a decrement of dopamine D$_2$ receptor binding of approximately 0.6% per year, suggesting that the striatal projection neurons may also progressively decline with normal aging (4). By contrast, in PD the postsynaptic response to nigrostriatal deafferentation is likely to differ from that of normal aging. It has been suggested that loss of dopaminergic nerve terminals in association with changes in dopamine D$_2$ receptors may underlie motor complications that occur during the course of treatment of PD (14). A relative increase of striatal dopamine D2 receptors binding has been reported in early untreated parkinsonian patients, particularly in the putamen contralateral to the more affected body side (5). Relative dopamine D2 receptor up-regulation has also been demonstrated in the striatum of subjects with *N*-methyl-4-phenyl-1,2,3,6-tetrahydropyridine (MPTP)-induced parkinsonism (63). However, the initial dopamine D2 receptor up-regulation in the putamen may reverse with increasing disease severity, and binding values are in the range of those in control subjects or lower than those in advanced PD patients (6,13). Because [^{11}C]raclopride and FDOPA changes are associated throughout the disease course, it is likely that dopamine D2 receptor changes result from the decline in presynaptic dopaminergic drive (7).

Studies of Brain Metabolism: Quantification of the Parkinsonian Network

Studies of presynaptic and postsynaptic striatal function may not fully describe the complexities of neural systems involved in a neurodegenerative process and their modulation with treatment. By contrast, measurements of regional rates of glucose utilization with [^{18}F]fluorodeoxyglucose (FDG) and PET in PD can be used to quantify the effect of nigrostriatal degeneration on brain regions functionally related to the dopaminergic system.

We have developed and applied a statistical model of regional metabolic covariation to identify abnormal brain topography in PD and related disorders (20,21,23,25,26). This algorithm, known as the Scaled Subprofile Model (SSM) (1,55,56) is a form of principal component analysis (PCA) and can be applied to identify patterns of regional covariation in brain metabolism data. Through modifications of the functional imaging data prior to performing the PCA, SSM analysis characterizes the regional covariance structure of subject groups and measures the expression of the obtained regional covariance patterns in individual subjects (subject scores). SSM provides a means of comparing the expression of these patterns in different populations and of examining their relation with independent clinical descriptors such as disease severity or subject age.

In PD patients SSM analysis revealed a reproducible pattern of regional metabolism characterized by increased lentiform and thalamic metabolism associated with reduced metabolism in the lateral frontal, paracentral, and parieto-occipital areas (20,21,23–27). In addition, the degree of individual expression of this covariance pattern correlates with disease severity ratings (Fig. 17-1) and independent PET measurements of striatal FDOPA uptake in PD patients (20,21,23,25). These results agree with those from experimental animal models, in which parkinsonian signs are associated with excessive pallidofugal inhibitory outflow with concomitant suppression of brain function in primary and association motor cortical regions (2). A reduction of nigrostriatal dopaminergic activity leads to increased functional activity in the putamen and the subthalamic nucleus (STN) (72). Increased activity in the STN results in overactivity of the pallidothalamic pathway with concomitant suppression of thalamocortical excitatory inputs.

FDG/PET is also a powerful tool in the differential diagnosis of parkinsonism (3,21,23, 25, 29,64). Atypical parkinsonian syndromes (APDs) can account for up to 10% of patients with parkinsonism and are characterized clinically by progressive rigidity and minimal or absent response to dopaminergic therapy (65). A reliable clinical diagnosis of APD can be made only when patients present with a combination of parkinsonism, autonomic dysfunction, and cerebellar and pyramidal signs (65). The recognition of patients with possible APD manifesting with predominant parkinsonism and only marginal atypical signs is a more challenging task. Although the presence of resting tremor or levodopa responsiveness is commonly considered to be diagnostic of classic PD, these signs have been recognized in parkinsonian patients ultimately found to have APD at neuropathological examination. Therefore an adjunctive diagnostic test, such as FDG/PET, may be helpful for supporting the clinical suspicion of APD even in the presence of minimal atypical features.

We have reported FDG/PET data from a cohort of 43 patients suspected to have possible APD based on the development of diminished levodopa responsiveness, orthostatic hypotension, or both (3). All patients had convincing levodopa responses without autonomic dysfunction or other atypical features at the time of the orig-

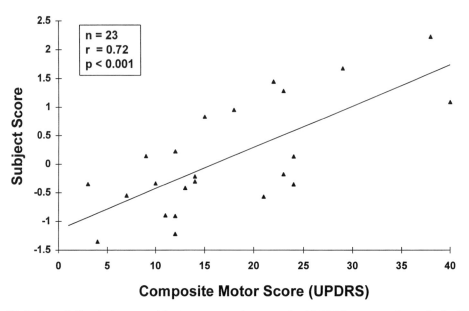

FIG. 17-1. Correlation between subject scores and composite UPDRS motor ratings. A significant positive correlation (*p* < 0.001) was found between these two variables (25).

inal clinical presentation. We used 56 other patients without atypical features as a reference population with likely idiopathic PD. We found significant reductions in the striatum and thalamus of the APD suspects relative to the group with likely PD. Indeed, a linear combination of caudate, lentiform, and thalamic metabolic values accurately discriminated typical and atypical patients. This finding was reproduced in two independent APD and PD populations scanned on different PET cameras (3). These results indicate that FDG/PET can be a helpful adjunct to the clinical examination for the differential diagnosis of parkinsonism. Indeed, this discrimination may be critical to the assessment of patients for possible surgical intervention.

SURGICAL TREATMENT OF PARKINSONIAN SYMPTOMS

Stereotactic Pallidotomy: Operative Changes in Network Modulation

Leksell's posteroventral pallidotomy has been shown to alleviate significantly the akinetic symptoms of Parkinson's disease and the dyskinesia associated with levodopa administration (10,19,35,

44,46,50,58). The pathophysiology of pallidal ablation for the relief of parkinsonism is not completely understood. The ameliorative effects of pallidotomy have been attributed to the reduction of excessive inhibitory outflow from the internal segment of the globus pallidus (GPi) (52).

We originally reported eight PD patients undergoing pallidotomy who were scanned with FDG/PET preoperatively and 6 months postoperatively (29). We found that pallidotomy resulted in a metabolic decline in the thalamus that occurred in conjunction with a metabolic increase in primary and associative motor cortical regions. Indeed, the improvement in limb performance (CAPIT: Core Assessment Protocol for Intracerebral Transplantation) (47) at 6 months after surgery was significantly correlated with the operative metabolic declines in the thalamus and the accompanying increases in lateral premotor cortex. To quantify potential modulations in the expression of motor networks by pallidotomy, we applied SSM analysis to operative differences in regional glucose metabolism. We found that the topography identified in this analysis closely resembled the PD-related profile identified previously (20,23) and was characterized by postoperative *declines* in the lentiform and thalamic metabolism ipsilateral to the surgical side associated with bilateral *increases* in SMA metabolism. Subject scores for this pattern of metabolic operative change correlated significantly with improvements in both contralateral and ipsilateral limb CAPIT scores (Fig. 17-2). These findings indicate that metabolic brain networks comprising functionally and anatomically interconnected brain regions remote from the lesion site may be modulated by pallidotomy, including motor cortical regions of the hemisphere contralateral to the surgery.

A variety of experimental data have indicated that the rate of glucose consumption in a region is determined by the activity of its afferent projections, rather than local cell body activity (40,42,53). In accord with these observations, we found that in PD glucose utilization in the ventral thalamus was reproducibly correlated with recorded spontaneous neuronal activity in the GPi (27). In this vein it was expected that internal pallidal ablation would give rise to postoperative reduction in thalamic metabolism noted in

our PET study of pallidotomy (24). Moreover, we found that GPi firing rates were also significantly correlated with the expression of an SSM network related to the pallidum and its major efferent projections (Fig. 17-3). It is therefore likely that pallidal ablation exerts its primary metabolic effect in spatially distributed projection fields lying in the ventral and intralaminar thalamus as well as the brainstem.

The PET activation studies using [¹⁵O]H_2O have also supported the notion of pallidotomy-induced modulation of the cortico-striato-pallido-thalamo-cortical (CSPTC) motor circuit. Subtraction of resting state from task-specific data allows isolation of changes in regional cerebral blood flow (rCBF) relating to various motor tasks (30). Grafton et al. reported postpallidotomy increases in rCBF in the ipsilateral premotor and supplementary motor areas with movement (33). In another study employing network analysis of motor system connectivity, Grafton and colleagues found significant postoperative reductions in the strength of interactions between the

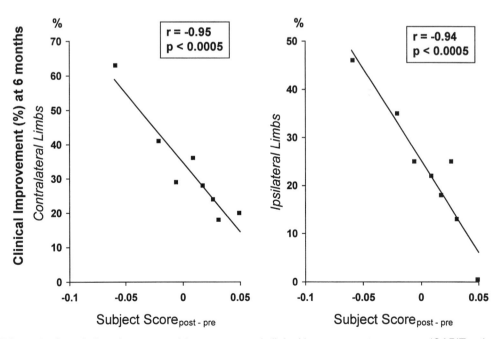

FIG. 17-2. Correlations between subject scores and clinical improvement measures (CAPIT ratings, see text) for limbs contralateral (*left*) and ipsilateral (*right*) to the lesion site. Highly significant ($p < 0.0005$) negative correlations were evident between pattern expression and clinical outcome (24).

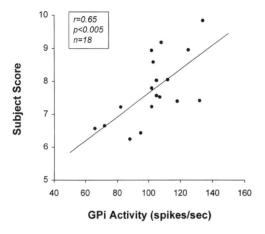

FIG. 17-3. Correlation between the subject scores and spontaneous internal pallidal (GPi) firing rates recorded intraoperatively in Parkinson's disease patients. A significant positive correlation ($r = 0.65$, $p < 0.005$) was found between these two variables (27).

globus pallidus and thalamus and the thalamus and mesial frontal motor area (32). These findings are consistent with the notion that pallidal ablation induces alterations in the normal functioning of CSPTC motor networks (11,17,52).

Stereotactic Pallidotomy: Functional Predictors of Clinical Outcome

In addition to adding to our understanding of the network modulations occurring with pallidotomy, FDG/PET may be used to select optimal candidates for pallidotomy. In our original study of ten patients undergoing pallidotomy, we found that preoperative FDG/PET measurements of lentiform metabolism in the "off" state correlated with clinical outcome up to 6 months after surgery (Fig. 17-4A) (24). We subsequently studied an additional 22 PD patients to assess the effectiveness of preoperative FDG/PET, quantitative motor performance indices, and magnetic resonance imaging (MRI) measurements of lesion size and location as potential predictors of surgical outcome (41). We found that the pallidotomy lesions were comparable in location and size in all patients and therefore did not uncorrelate with individual differences in surgical outcome. Nonetheless, in this series we

confirmed that preoperative measures of lentiform glucose metabolism offered an accurate prediction of ultimate surgical improvement ($R^2 \approx 50\%$) (Fig. 17-4B).

The finding of a significant correlation between levodopa response and clinical outcome following surgery suggests that the dynamic range of the CSPTC motor loop with pallidal suppression may be clinically estimated using a levodopa challenge. These findings have been supported by FDG/PET experiments in PD patients showing reduction of pallidal hypermetabolism during levodopa infusion (12). To the extent that the severity of clinical manifestations is correlated with the expression of abnormal CSPTC metabolic networks, the measured clinical benefit with levodopa administration may provide a simple indicator of the dynamic range of network modulation that can occur with either pharmacological or surgical pallidal suppression. In this vein we found that preoperative measurements of lentiform metabolism with FDG/PET reproducibly predict 50% of operative improvement in "off-"state CAPIT scores. The preoperative levodopa responsiveness index, though simpler to measure, predicted approximately 36% of individual differences in outcome. Together, however, both preoperative measures predicted approximately 70% of the pallidotomy response. Thus, preoperative FDG/PET measurements of the functional set-point of the CSPTC network combined with an independent clinicopharmacological estimate of the patient's individual capacity for network modulation can provide useful and complementary criteria for patient selection.

In summary, we propose that the following criteria may determine the clinical outcome of pallidotomy for PD.

1. The pallidum should be anatomically intact. Parkinsonian patients who present with coexisting vascular lesions of the basal ganglia may not be ideal candidates for pallidotomy. Similarly, patients with parkinsonism secondary to other forms of pallidal pathology (i.e., manganese intoxication) may not benefit from this procedure.

2. The pallidum should be functionally overactive. Parkinsonian patients who present pre-

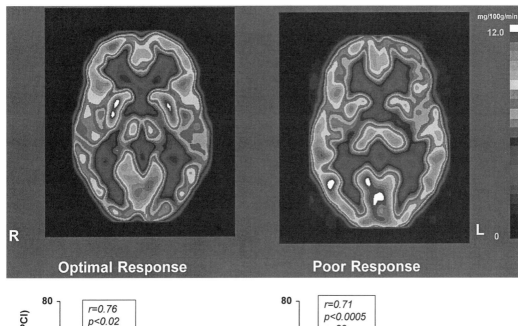

A

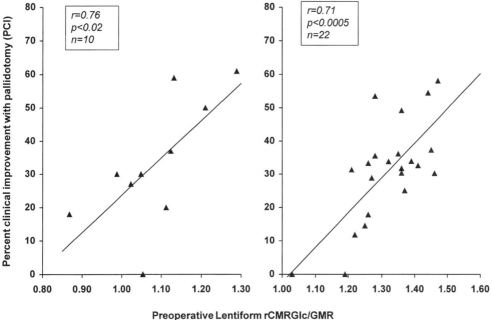

B   **Preoperative Lentiform rCMRGlc/GMR**

FIG. 17-4. A. Preoperative [¹⁸F]FDG/PET images from two patients with idiopathic Parkinson's disease who underwent right unilateral pallidotomy. *Left.* A patient with preoperative lentiform glucose hypermetabolism had an optimal surgical outcome. *Right.* A patient with a lower rate of metabolism in the lentiform nucleus had no therapeutic response to surgery. The two pallidotomy lesions were comparable in size and location. *Color stripe* represents regional rates of glucose metabolism, in milligrams per minute per 100 g. **B.** Correlation between preoperative lentiform glucose metabolism normalized by the global mean (*rCMRGlc/GMR*) and percent clinical improvement (*PCI*) in contralateral limb CAPIT scores measured 3 months after pallidotomy. Preoperative lentiform metabolism correlated significantly with PCI in two independent patient cohorts scanned on different tomographs [*left:* SuperPET 3000, full width at half-maximum (FWHM) = 7.5 mm; right: GE Advance, FWHM = 4.3 mm].

operatively with lentiform hypermetabolism are likely to be good candidates. Indeed patients with atypical parkinsonism presenting with lentiform hypometabolism are less likely to improve after pallidal ablation (3).

3. The pallidum should be functionally suppressible. Parkinsonian patients who present preoperatively with a good response to levodopa may be optimal candidates. We believe that the measurement of levodopa responsiveness provides an estimate of the individual's capacity to reduce baseline pallidal overactivity and to modulate the CSPTC motor circuit. Indeed, a prior PET study demonstrated reduction in pallidal hypermetabolism with levodopa infusion (12). As mentioned above, patients with blunted levodopa responses, as in atypical parkinsonism, are therefore unlikely to have a significant improvement from pallidotomy.

In conclusion, the combination of preoperative FDG/PET measurements of lentiform metabolism together with clinicopharmacological estimates of the patient's individual capacity for network modulation can provide useful and complementary criteria for patient selection for pallidotomy.

Deep Brain Stimulation of the Globus Pallidus

Deep brain high-frequency stimulation (DBS) has the advantage of avoiding permanent side effects due to the ablative lesion, thereby inducing the possibility of reversible amelioration of parkinsonian symptoms. In addition, this technique is adaptable, as the stimulation frequency can be increased or decreased. DBS of the ventral portion of the thalamus, usually the ventral intermedius nucleus (Vim), has been employed originally for the control of parkinsonian resting tremor. More recently DBS has been applied to the GPi to relieve the rigidity and bradykinesia of PD (67). We have investigated the effect of GPi stimulation on clinical scores and rCBF/PET in two parkinsonian patients. GPi stimulation resulted in an approximately 30% improvement in patient Unified Parkinson's Disease Rating Scale (UPDRS) scores, particu-

larly those for bradykinesia. Concurrently, GPi stimulation resulted in significant rCBF increases in the anterior cingulate area and in the right dorsolateral prefrontal cortex during movement execution (22). These findings are similar to those from our previous FDG/PET studies of pallidotomy and confirm that physiological suppression of GPi may result in improved motor planning as expressed by rCBF increases in auxiliary motor cortical areas.

CONCLUSIONS

Reliable in vivo markers of neuronal activity are needed to assess surgical outcome. Currently available clinical scales are relatively insensitive, are inherently variable, and may not accurately reflect the extent of neuropathological change. By contrast, quantitative functional brain imaging markers may be suitable as outcome measures for the surgical treatment of PD. Indeed, we have found that PET may be a useful tool for predicting optimal candidates for certain surgical interventions.

Considerable attention has been dedicated to the development of novel data analytical methods for the characterization and quantification of neural networks in functional brain imaging data. Moreover, new radiotracers have been developed to quantify neurochemical deficits associated with neurodegenerative processes. A major contribution of this research has been a combined approach utilizing both network analytical strategies and in vivo neurochemical measurements to investigate the relations between localized neuronal attrition and the expression of widely distributed functional brain networks. These complementary PET techniques may greatly advance our understanding of the pathophysiology of PD and the functional changes that occur with surgical treatment.

Acknowledgments. This work was supported by NIH NS RO1 32368 and 35069 and by the National Parkinson Foundation. Dr. Angelo Antonini is a faculty fellow of the Parkinson Disease Foundation and the United Parkinson Foundation. Dr. David Eidelberg is supported by the Cotzias Fellowship of the American Parkinson Disease Foundation.

REFERENCES

1. Alexander GE, Moeller JR. Application of the scaled subprofile model to functional imaging in neuropsychiatric disorders: a principal component approach to modeling brain function in disease. *Hum Brain Mapp* 1994;2:1–16.
2. Alexander GE, Crutcher MD, DeLong MR. Basal ganglia thalamo-cortical circuits; parallel substrates for motor, oculomotor, "prefrontal" and "limbic" functions. *Prog Brain Res* 1990;85:119–146.
3. Antonini A, Kazumata K, Feigin A, et al. Differential diagnosis of parkinsonism with [^{18}F]fluorodeoxyglucose and PET. *Mov Disord* 1998;13:268–274.
4. Antonini A, Leenders KL, Reist H, et al. Effect of age on D2 dopamine receptors in normal human brain measured by positron emission tomography and [^{11}C]raclopride. *Arch Neurol* 1993;50:474–480.
5. Antonini A, Schwarz J, Oertel WH, Beer HG, Madeja UD, Leenders KL. [^{11}C]Raclopride and positron emission tomography in previously untreated patients with Parkinson's disease: influence of L-dopa and lisuride therapy on striatal dopamine D2 receptors. *Neurology* 1994;44:1325–1329.
6. Antonini A, Schwarz J, Oertel WH, Pogarell O, Leenders KL. Long-term changes of striatal dopamine D2 receptors in patients with Parkinson's disease: a study with positron emission tomography and [^{11}C]raclopride. *Mov Disord* 1997; 12:33–38.
7. Antonini A, Vontobel P, Psylla M, et al. Complementary positron emission tomographic studies of the striatal dopaminergic system in Parkinson's disease. *Arch Neurol* 1995;52:1183–1190.
8. Assenbaum S, Brucke T, Pirker W, et al. Imaging of dopamine transporters with iodine-123-βCIT and SPECT in Parkinson's disease. *J Nucl Med* 1997;38:1–6.
9. Banos G, Daniel PM, Pratt OE. The effect of age upon the entry of some amino acids into the brain, and their incorporation into cerebral protein. *Dev Med Child Neurol* 1978;20:335–346.
10. Baron MS, Vitek JL, Bakey RAE, et al. Treatment of advanced Parkinson's disease by internal globus pallidotomy: 1-year results of a pilot study. *Ann Neurol* 1996;40:355–366.
11. Bathia KP, Marsden CD. The behavioral and motor consequences of focal lesions of the basal ganglia in man. *Brain* 1994;117:859–876.
12. Blesa R, Blin J, Miletich R, et al. Levodopa-reduced glucose metabolism in striatopallido-thalamocortical circuit in Parkinson's disease. *Neurology* 1991;41[suppl 1]:359.
13. Brooks DJ, Ibanez V, Sawle GV, et al. Striatal D2 receptor status in patients with Parkinson's disease, striatonigral degeneration, and progressive supranuclear palsy, measured with [^{11}C]raclopride and positron emission tomography. *Ann Neurol* 1992;31:184–192.
14. Brooks DJ, Salmon EP, Mathias CJ, et al. The relationship between locomotor disability, autonomic dysfunction, and the integrity of the striatal dopaminergic system in patients with multiple system atrophy, pure autonomic failure, and Parkinson's disease, studied with PET. *Brain* 1990;113:1539–1552.
15. Ceballos-Baumann AO, Obeso JA, Vitek JL, et al. Restoration of thalamocortical activity after posteroventral pallidotomy in Parkinson's disease. *Lancet* 1994; 344:814.
16. Chaly T, Dhawan V, Kazumata K, et al. Radiosynthesis of [^{18}F] *N*-3-fluoropropyl-2—β-carbomethoxy-3-β-(4-iodophenyl)nortropane and the first human study with positron emission tomography. *Nucl Med Biol* 1996; 23:999–1004.
17. DeLong M. Primate models of movement disorders of basal ganglia origin. *Trends Neurosci* 1990;13: 281.
18. Dhawan V, Ishikawa T, Patlak C, et al. Combined FDOPA and 3OMFD PET studies in Parkinson's disease. *J Nucl Med* 1996;37:209–216.
19. Dogali D, Fazzini E, Kolodny E, et al. Stereotactic ventral pallidotomy for Parkinson's disease. *Neurology* 1995;45:753–761.
20. Eidelberg D, Moeller JR, Dhawan V, et al. The metabolic anatomy of Parkinson's disease: complementary ^{18}F-fluorodeoxyglucose and ^{18}F-fluorodopa positron emission tomography studies. *Mov Disord* 1990;5: 203–213.
21. Eidelberg D, Moeller JR, Dhawan V, et al. The metabolic topography of parkinsonism. *J Cereb Blood Flow Metab* 1994;14:783–801.
22. Eidelberg D, Moeller JR, Dhawan V, et al. Patterns of brain activation in motor sequence learning: ^{15}O-H$_2$O/PET studies. *J Nucl Med* 1996;37:281P.
23. Eidelberg D, Moeller JR, Ishikawa T, et al. Early differential diagnosis of Parkinson's disease with ^{18}F-fluorodeoxyglucose and positron emission tomography. *Neurology* 1995;45:1995–2004.
24. Eidelberg D, Moeller JR, Ishikawa T, et al. Regional metabolic correlates of surgical outcome following unilateral pallidotomy for Parkinson's disease. *Ann Neurol* 1996;39:450–459.
25. Eidelberg D, Moeller JR, Ishikawa T, et al. The assessment of disease severity in parkinsonism with ^{18}F-fluorodeoxyglucose and positron emission tomography. *J Nucl Med* 1995;36:378–383.
26. Eidelberg D, Moeller JR, Ishikawa T, et al. The metabolic topography of idiopathic torsion dystonia. *Brain* 1995;118:1473–1484.
27. Eidelberg D, Moeller JR, Kazumata K, et al. Metabolic correlates of pallidal neuronal activity in Parkinson's Disease. *Brain* 1997;120:1315–1324.
28. Eidelberg D, Takikawa S, Dhawan V, et al. Striatal ^{18}F-dopa uptake: absence of an aging effect. *J Cereb Blood Flow Metab* 1993;13:881–888.
29. Eidelberg D, Takikawa S, Moeler J, et al. Striatal hypometabolism distinguishes striatonigral degeneration from Parkinson's disease. *Ann Neurol* 1993;33: 518–527.
30. Friston KJ, Holmes KJ, Worsely KJ. Statistical parametric maps in functional imaging: a general linear approach. *Hum Brain Mapp* 1995;2:189–210.
31. Frost JJ, Rosier AJ, Reich SG, et al. Positron emission tomographic imaging of the dopamine transporter with ^{11}C-WIN 35,428 reveals marked declines in mild Parkinson's disease. *Am J Neurol* 1993;34:423–431.
32. Grafton ST, Sutton J, Couldwell W, et al. Network analysis of motor system connectivity in Parkinson's disease: modulation of thalamocortical interactions after pallidotomy. *Hum Brain Mapp* 1994;2:45–55.
33. Grafton ST, Waters C, Sutton J. Pallidotomy increases activity of motor association cortex in Parkinson's disease: a positron emission tomographic study. *Ann Neurol* 1995;37:776–783.

34. Huang SC, Yu DC, Barrio JR, et al. Kinetics and modeling of L-6-[¹⁸F]fluoro-dopa in human positron emission tomographic study. *J Cereb Blood Flow Metab* 1991; 11:898–913.

35. Iacono RP, Shima F, Lonser RP, Kuniyoshi S, Maeda G, Yamada S. The results, indications, and physiology of posteroventral pallidotomy for patients with Parkinson's disease. *Neurosurgery* 1995;36:1118–1127.

36. Innis RB, Seibyl JP, Scanley BE, et al. Single-photon emission computed tomographic imaging demonstrates loss of striatal dopamine transporters in Parkinson's disease. *Proc Natl Acad Sci USA* 1993;90:11965–11969.

37. Ishikawa T, Dhawan V, Chaly T, et al. Clinical significance of striatal dopa decarboxylase activity in Parkinson's disease. *J Nucl Med* 1996;37:216–222.

38. Ishikawa T, Dhawan V, Kazumata K, et al. Comparative nigrostriatal dopaminergic imaging with iodine-123-βCIT-FP/SPECT and fluorine-18-Fdopa/PET. *J Nucl Med* 1996;37:1760–1765.

39. Ishikawa T, Dhawan V, Patlak C, et al. Fluorodopa positron emission tomography with an inhibitor of catechol-*O*-methyltransferase: effect of the plasma 3-*O*-methyldopa fraction on data analysis. *J Cereb Blood Flow Metab* 1996;5:854–863.

40. Kadekaro M, Crane AM, Sokoloff L. Differential effects of electrical stimulation of sciatic nerve on metabolic activity in spinal cord and dorsal root ganglion in the rat. *Proc Natl Acad Sci USA* 1985;82:6010–6013.

41. Kazumata K, Antonini A, Dhawan V, et al. Preoperative indicators of clinical outcome following stereotaxic pallidotomy. *Neurology* 1997;49:1083–1090.

42. Kozlowski M, Marshall JF. Plasticity of [¹⁴C]2-deoxy-D-glucose incorporation into neostriatum and related structures in response to dopamine neuron damage and apomorphine replacement *Brain Res* 1980;197:167–183.

43. Kuwabara H, Cumming P, Reith J, et al. Human striatal L-dopa decarboxylase activity estimated in vivo using 6-[¹⁸F]fluoro-dopa and positron emission tomography: error analysis and application to normal subjects. *J Cereb Blood Flow Metab* 1993;13:43–56.

44. Johansson F, Malm J, Nordh E, Hariz M. Usefulness of pallidotomy in advanced Parkinson's disease. *J Neurol Neurosurg Psychiatry* 1997;62:125–132.

45. Laihinen AO, Rinne JO, Nagren KA, et al. PET studies on brain monoamine transporters with carbon-11-βCIT in Parkinson's disease. *J Nucl Med* 1996;36:1263–1267.

46. Laitinen LV, Bergenheim AT, Hariz MI. Leksell's posterolateral ventral pallidotomy in the treatment of Parkinson's disease. *J Neurosurg* 1992;76:53.

47. Langston JW, Widner H, Goetz CG, et al. Core assessment program for intracerebral transplantations (CAPIT). *Mov Disord* 1992;7:2–13.

48. Leenders KL, Salmon EP, Tyrrell P, et al. The nigrostriatal dopaminergic system assessed in vivo by positron emission computed tomography in healthy volunteer subjects and patients with Parkinson's disease. *Arch Neurol* 1990;47:1290–1298.

49. Logan J, Fowler JS, Volkow ND, et al. Graphical analysis of reversible radioligand binding from time activity measurements applied to *N*-¹¹C-methyl-(–)cocaine PET studies in human subjects. *J Cereb Blood Flow Metab* 1989;10:740–747.

50. Lozano AM, Lang AE, Galvez-Jiminez N, et al. GPi pallidotomy improves motor function in patients with Parkinson's disease. *Lancet* 1995;346:1383–1386.

51. Marek KL, Seibyl JP, Zoghbi SS, et al. [¹²³I]β-CIT/SPECT imaging demonstrates bilateral loss of dopamine transporters in hemi-Parkinson's disease. *Neurology* 1996;46:231–237.

52. Marsden CD, Obeso JA. The functions of the basal ganglia and the paradox of stereotaxic surgery in Parkinson's disease. *Brain* 1994;117:877–897.

53. Mata M, Fink DJ, Gainer H. Activity-dependent energy metabolism in rat posterior pituitary primarily reflect sodium pump activity. *J Neurochem* 1980;34:213–215.

54. Mitchell IJ, Boyce S, Sambrook MA, et al. A 2-deoxyglucose study of the effects of dopamine agonists on the parkinsonian primate brain. *Brain* 1994;115:809–824.

55. Moeller JR, Strother SC. A regional covariance approach to the analysis of functional patterns in positron emission tomographic data. *J Cereb Blood Flow Metab* 1991;11:A121–135.

56. Moeller JR, Strother SC, Sidits JJ, Rottenberg DA. Scaled subprofile model: a statistical approach to the analysis of functional patterns in positron emission tomographic data. *J Cereb Blood Flow Metab* 1987;7:649–658.

57. Neumeyer JL, Wang S, Gao Y, et al. *N*-W-fluoroalkyl analogs of (1R)-2β-carbomethoxy-3β-(4-iodophenyl) tropane (βCIT) radiotracers for PET and SPECT imaging of dopamine transporters. *J Med Chem* 1994;37:1558–1561.

58. Olanow CW. GPi pallidotomy: have we made a dent in Parkinson's disease [Editorial]. *Ann Neurol,* 1996;40:341–343.

59. Parent A, Hazrati LN. Functional anatomy of the basal ganglia. I.The cortico-basal ganglia-thalamo-cortical loop. *Brain Res Brain Res Rev* 1995;20:91–127.

60. Parent A, Hazrati LN. Functional anatomy of the basal ganglia. II. The place of subthalamic nucleus and external pallidum in basal ganglia circuitry. *Brain Res Brain Res Rev* 1995;20:128–154.

61. Pate BD, Kawamata T, Yamada T, et al. Correlation of striatal fluorodopa uptake in the MPTP monkey with dopaminergic indices. *Ann Neurol* 1993;34:331–338.

62. Patlak CS, Blasberg RG. Graphical evaluation of blood-to-brain transfer constants from multiple-time uptake data: generalizations. *J Cereb Blood Flow Metab* 1985;5:584–590.

63. Perlmutter JS, Kilbourn MR, Raichle ME, Welch MJ. MPTP-induced up-regulation of in vivo dopaminergic radioligand-receptor binding in humans. *Neurology* 1987;37:1575–1579.

64. Przedborski S, Giladi N, Takikawa S, et al. The metabolic topography of the hemiparkinsonism-hemiatrophy syndrome. *Neurology* 1994;44:1622–1628.

65. Quinn N. Multiple system atrophy: the nature of the beast. *J Neurol Neurosurg Psychiatry* 1989;52:78–89.

66. Seibyl JP, Marek KL, Quilan D, et al. Decreased single-photon emission computed tomographic [¹²³I]β-CIT striatal uptake correlates with symptoms severity in Parkinson's disease. *Ann Neurol* 1995;38:589–598.

67. Siegfried J, Lippitz B. Bilateral chronic electrostimulation of ventroposterolateral pallidum: a new therapeutic approach for alleviating all parkinsonian symptoms. *Neurosurgery* 1994;35:1126–1130.

68. Snow BJ, Tooyama I, McGeer EG, et al. Human positron emission tomographic [¹⁸F]fluorodopa studies correlate with dopamine cell counts and levels. *Ann Neurol* 1993;34:324–330.

69. Takikawa S, Dhawan V, Chaly T, et al. Input functions for 6-[fluorine-18]fluorodopa quantitation in parkinsonism: comparative studies and clinical correlations. *J Nucl Med* 1994;35:955–963,

70. Van Dyck CH, Seibyl JP, Malison RT, et al. Age-related decline in striatal dopamine transporter binding with iodine-123-β-CIT SPECT. *J Nucl Med* 1995;36: 1175– 1181.

71. Volkow ND, Ding YS, Fowler JS, et al, [^{11}C]D-threo-methylphenidate: a new PET ligand for the dopamine transporter. II. Studies in the human brain. *J Nucl Med* 1995;36:2162–2168.

72. Wooten GF, Collins RC. Metabolic effects of unilateral lesions of the substantia nigra. *J Neurosci* 1981; 1:285–291.

Pallidal Surgery for the Treatment of Parkinson's Disease and Movement Disorders, edited by
J. K. Krauss, R. G. Grossman, and J. Jankovic.
Lippincott-Raven Publishers, Philadelphia © 1998.

18

Contemporary Pallidal Surgery for Treatment of Other Parkinsonian Syndromes

Ron L. Alterman and Patrick J. Kelly

*Department of Neurological Surgery, New York University Center for Movement Disorders,
New York, New York 10016, USA*

The population of parkinsonian patients who currently undergo posteroventral pallidotomy (PVP) are distinct from those operated during the pre-dopa era. In their classic 1967 monograph, Hoehn and Yahr (16) mentioned a small subset of patients with secondary parkinsonism, some of whom had evidence of "diffuse central nervous system degenerative disease." However, terms such as striatonigral degeneration, multiple system atrophy, progressive supranuclear palsy, and cortical basal ganglionic degeneration were yet to become engrained in the neurological lexicon.

To be sure, 30 years of clinical experience and careful pathological study have led to a purer definition of Parkinson's disease (PD) and the description of related syndromes of which parkinsonism is only a partial manifestation. Positron emission tomography (PET) has emerged as a buttress to the clinical examination, enhancing diagnostic accuracy in the living patient (1,3,7–10). Finally, the passage of time has all but eliminated postencephalitic parkinsonism as a clinical consideration. The contemporary pallidotomy population is more extensively evaluated and more likely to have true idiopathic PD than those operated a generation ago. This chapter considers the role of contemporary pallidotomy for treatment of the "Parkinson's plus" syndromes. As little has been published concerning this subject, the chapter is succinct but includes brief descriptions of each of these syndromes and important features that distinguish them from idiopathic PD.

PARKINSON PLUS SYNDROMES

Progressive Supranuclear Palsy

Described by Steele and colleagues in 1964 (30), progressive supranuclear palsy (PSP) is considered the second most common cause of parkinsonism and is frequently misdiagnosed as idiopathic PD, even by movement disorder specialists (17,24,26). Typical onset of the disease is after the age of 55; median survival is 6 to 7 years (24). Patients commonly suffer postural instability due to axial parkinsonism and multiple falls early in the course of their illness. Their parkinsonism is symmetrical, unlike idiopathic PD, which tends to be asymmetrical (4,24,32).

Supranuclear ophthalmoplegia, particularly paresis of vertical gaze, is the hallmark of the disease (22,32). The "dirty tie" sign derives from patients' inability to look down at their food while eating and incoordination of chewing, both of which result in food spillage (24). Corticobulbar and corticospinal dysfunction are common, resulting in dysarthria, dysphagia, hyperreflexia, and spastic gait. Tremor occurs in just 12% to 16% (4). Frontal lobe deficits are common, but the severity of dementia is variable.

The PET studies reveal reduced ^{18}F-fluorodopa binding in the caudate and putamen, distinguishing PSP from PD, in which fluorodopa binding in the caudate is preserved (3,4). ^{18}F-Fluorodeoxyglucose utilization PET (FDG/PET) demonstrates striatal hypometabolism, again distinguishing PSP from PD, where striatal metabolism is preserved or hyperactive (3). Frontal hypometabolism in PSP is postulated to arise from the loss of pallidal neurons, which project to the frontal lobes, and may account for the cognitive deficits associated with this syndrome. These functional imaging features permit PSP to be distinguished from PD in 90% of cases (3).

Pathological examination reveals atrophy of the midbrain and pontine tegmentum (4,30). The cerebral cortex is preserved. Histopathological examination reveals neurofibrillary tangles, granulovacuolar degeneration, neuronal loss, and gliosis most notably in the globus pallidus, subthalamic nucleus, substantia nigra pars compacta, periaqueductal gray matter, superior colliculi, and pretectal areas. Other brainstem nuclei may be involved as well.

On the whole, medical therapy for PSP is disappointing. Response to levodopa is seen in just 25% to 50% of PSP patients (24), and the duration is short-lived. As evidenced by the short median survival, disease progression is rapid. Pseudobulbar symptomatology typically leads to recurrent aspiration, pneumonia, and death. For more extensive reviews of this syndrome, the reader is directed to the reference list (4,13,17,20).

Multiple System Atrophy

Multiple system atrophy (MSA) is a term introduced by Graham and Oppenheimer in 1969 (15) to describe a "collection of overlapping, progressive, presenile multisystem degenerations." All forms of MSA are characterized by cell loss and gliosis, without Lewy bodies, in the substantia nigra and a variety of other structures, which may include the striatum, olives, pons, cerebellum, and Onuf's nucleus of the spinal cord (23–25,29,33,34).

Terminological discrepancies are still noted when reading this literature. According to Quinn (24), MSA is a general term that is subgrouped into striatonigral degeneration (SND) when extrapyramidal signs predominate, Shy-Drager syndrome (SDS) when autonomic failure is prevalent, and olivopontocerebellar atrophy (OPCA) when cerebellar signs are paramount. In contrast, Mathias and Williams (21) noted that Shy-Drager syndrome is the general term describing a group

of diseases marked by autonomic dysfunction. Shy-Drager syndrome can then be subgrouped into SND when extrapyramidal signs are primary, OPCA when cerebellar/pyramidal findings are prevalent, and MSA when all three are present.

In a review of this topic Mathias and Williams (21) noted that:

> We, therefore, define SDS as a progressive neurodegenerative syndrome with features of primary autonomic failure that occur in combination with symptoms and signs indicating degeneration of other neurons, in particular the striatonigral and olivopontocerebellar systems. Clinically, one of these other systems may be predominantly involved. MSA symbolizes the constellation of symptoms and signs indicating degeneration of more than one neuronal system, although not necessarily implying autonomic involvement.

Multiple system atrophy typically begins during the fifth, sixth, or seventh decade (21,34). Autonomic symptoms predate motor system dysfunction (21) and manifest as urinary incontinence and impotence in men (21,24). Postural hypotension is also common (24).

Extrapyramidal symptoms are bilateral but usually asymmetrical as in PD (24). Unlike PD, postural instability develops early in the disease and progresses rapidly (24). Tremor, when present, is not the typical resting tremor of PD but an action tremor (21). Response to levodopa is usually poor. Good responses, when they occur, are typically transient, and dose escalation may be hampered by exacerbated postural hypotension (21,24).

Cerebellar symptoms in OPCA usually involve the trunk and legs, causing a gait disturbance that worsens steadily. Dysarthria and upper extremity dysmetria may also occur (5,24).

Cognitive function in MSA, even at its most advanced stages, is typically preserved. In one series of 150 patients with Shy-Drager/MSA, only 2 patients were demented (21).

In its fully advanced stages, patients with MSA exhibit what Quinn termed the "full house" scenario: "a non-demented patient who is impotent and incontinent with parkinsonism poorly responsive to levodopa and pyramidal and cerebellar signs" (24).

Workup of these patients includes magnetic resonance imaging (MRI), which may demonstrate cerebellar or brainstem atrophy (or both). Additionally, external sphincter electromyography may demonstrate loss of neurons in Onuf's nucleus (2). PET may also be useful. Putaminal ^{18}F-fluorodopa uptake correlates inversely with disease duration and locomotor function (3). Putaminal uptake is depressed in both MSA and PD, but uptake in the caudate is significantly worse with MSA (3). ^{18}F-Fluorodeoxyglucose utilization PET may also distinguish MSA from PD. DeVolder et al. (6) have demonstrated reduced putaminal and caudate glucose utilization in seven SND patients. Fulham et al. (12) demonstrated reduced cerebellar and frontal glucose utilization in those with OPCA. Eidelberg and co-workers (8) have demonstrated that FDG/PET can be used to distinguish SND from PD in most cases.

Pathological examination often reveals a normal-appearing cerebrum (21). The putamina are typically shrunken and have an orange-brown discoloration. Cell loss and gliosis are noted throughout the striatum, and the substantiae nigra are depigmented. In OPCA the cerebellum, pons, and protuberances of the olives are atrophied (5,21). There is atrophy of the basis pontis, cerebellum, and cerebellar peduncles. Examination of the medulla reveals atrophy of the dorsal motor nucleus of the vagus and, in OPCA, atrophy of the inferior olives. Finally, there is marked depletion of neurons from Onuf's nucleus, located in the second and third sacral segments of the spinal cord (31).

Medical treatment for MSA is disappointing. The disease progresses relentlessly, and median survival is 9.3 years (23).

Cortical-Basal Ganglionic Degeneration

Originally described as corticodentatonigral degeneration with neuronal achromasia by Reibeiz et al. in 1968 (27), Riley and co-workers (28) later coined the term currently used: cortical-basal ganglionic degeneration (CBGD). The hallmark of this degenerative disorder is a combination of extrapyramidal and cerebral cortical

dysfunction (19,27). The syndrome typically begins insidiously during the sixth decade of life and progresses to severe disability and death in 5 to 10 years (19). Disease onset is asymmetrical. Symptoms typically begin in one upper extremity and are limited to that extremity for 2 to 5 years before generalizing (19). Basal ganglia degeneration typically manifests as an akinetic-rigid syndrome. Initial symptoms often consist of action tremor, dystonic posturing of one hand, cortical sensory loss, or apraxia in the affected limb. In 60% the "alien limb phenomenon" is evident at some point in the course of the disease (19). Oculomotor and eye lid motor abnormalities can lead to a mistaken diagnosis of progressive supranuclear palsy. Dementia is a rare finding and, when present, occurs late in the course of the disease. Disease progression leads to postural instability and falls.

Magnetic resonance imaging reveals asymmetrical cerebral atrophy involving the frontoparietal region contralateral to the affected side (19). Regional cerebral oxygen utilization is reduced asymetrically in the frontoparietal region, most marked contralateral to the affected limb (3). FDG/PET reveals asymmetrical hypometabolism in the thalamus and inferior parietal lobule contralateral to the most severely affected side and the hippocampus ipsilateral to that side (3,19).^{18}F-Fluorodopa-binding PET reveals reduced precursor uptake contralateral to the more affected side, in contrast to the preserved fluorodopa uptake noted in patients with PD (3).

Gross examination of CBGD brains reveals marked cortical atrophy, which is most notable in the frontoparietal region and most severe contralateral to the more symptomatic side (19). Depigmentation of the substantia nigra is also observed. Histopathological examination reveals achromatic, swollen neurons, with eccentrically placed nuclei. The substantia nigra also demonstrates neuronal loss and gliosis without Lewy bodies.

PALLIDOTOMY FOR PARKINSON PLUS SYNDROMES

Little has been published on the results of pallidotomy, or any stereotactic procedure, in patients with Parkinson's plus syndromes (PPS). Fazzini et al. (11) published results from four PPS patients: two with SND and one each with OPCA and CBGD. One of the SND patients exhibited a mild, but transient, improvement following pallidotomy; only a modest improvement in gait was sustained 6 months after surgery. The other patients derived no benefit from surgery whatsoever. In the discussion section of that paper, the authors reported that three other PPS patients, two with SND and one with PSP, underwent pallidotomy at another institution, again without significant benefit. In our experience, lentiform hypometabolism on FDG/PET, which distinguishes PD from PPS, is a contraindication to performing pallidotomy in patients exhibiting parkinsonism (1); however, the need to use PET routinely for the preoperative evaluation of pallidotomy candidates is debatable.

PALLIDOTOMY FOR OTHER LEVODOPA-UNRESPONSIVE PARKINSONISM

Two cases have been reported in which levodopa-unresponsive parkinsonism improved after pallidotomy (14,18). Goto et al. reported excellent short-term improvement in motor function in a 45-year-old woman with medically resistant parkinsonism due to bilateral basal ganglia infarcts (14). The infarcts involved the putamen and globus pallidus externus bilaterally, which the authors theorize led to disinhibition of the subthalamic nuclei, which were spared. The internal segments of the globus pallidus, which were also spared, were therefore overstimulated by the STN, mimicking the parkinsonian state. Unfortunately, the authors make no mention of the neuronal activity recorded from the internal segments of the globus pallidus, though they state that microelectrode recording was performed.

Krauss et al. (18) similarly reported excellent results treating levodopa-unresponsive parkinsonism in a man who sustained a rotator cuff injury. The parkinsonism is said to have started following rotator cuff repair that failed to relieve the patient's shoulder pain. Microelectrode-guided pallidotomy generated marked improvement in motor function and provided total relief of the

patient's shoulder pain. The preoperative MRI was unremarkable. ^{18}F-Fluorodopa PET demonstrated mildly reduced fluorodopa binding in the putamen but normal uptake in the caudate.

CONCLUSIONS

Parkinson's plus syndromes are pathologically distinct disorders in which basal ganglionic degeneration occurs in conjunction with atrophy of other neurological systems. It is the symptomatology that occurs in addition to the akinetic/rigid parkinsonism that distinguishes these disorders from idiopathic Parkinson's disease and from each other. Though distinct entities, these syndromes share a number of attributes distinguishing them from PD.

All of these syndromes progress relentlessly and, unlike PD, shorten the life expectancy. Axial parkinsonism is common early in the disease. The response to levodopa is disappointing as would be expected based on pathological and PET evidence of D2 receptor loss in these patients. Finally, all exhibit lentiform hypometabolism on FDG/PET, in contrast to PD, in which the lentiform nucleus is hypermetabolic.

In most instances a detailed history and careful neurological examination by an experienced movement disorder specialist distinguish patients with PPS from those with idiopathic PD, although these syndromes are often misdiagnosed as PD even at experienced movement disorder clinics. Therefore when there is any doubt about a diagnosis of idiopathic PD in a medically refractory parkinsonian patient referred for surgery, it is our opinion that FDG/PET might be performed to clarify the issue. In those whose FDG/PET demonstrates lentiform hypometabolism, a diagnosis of Parkinson's plus syndrome should be considered, and surgery should not be recommended. Finally, in unusual circumstances where medically resistant parkinsonism results from a static insult, pallidal surgery may be offered as a last resort

REFERENCES

1. Alterman RL, Kelly P, Sterio D, et al. Selection criteria for unilateral posteroventral pallidotomy. *Acta Neurochir (Wien)* 1997;68 [suppl]:18–23.

2. Beck RO, Betts CD, Fowler CJ. Genitouinary dysfunction in multiple system atrophy: clinical features and treatment in 62 cases. *J Urol* 1994;151:1336–1341.

3. Brooks DJ. PET studies on the early and differential diagnosis of Parkinson's disease. *Neurology* 1993;43-[suppl 6]:S6–S16.

4. Cardoso F, Jankovic J. Progressive supranuclear palsy. In: Calne DB, ed. *Neurodegenerative diseases.* Philadelphia: WB Saunders, 1994:743–767.

5. Dejerine J, Thomas A. L'atrophie olivo-ponto-cerebelleuse. *Nouv Iconogr Salpetriere* 1900;13:330–370.

6. De Volder AG, Francard J, Laterre C, et al. Decreased glucose utilization in the striatum and frontal lobe in probable striatonigral degeneration. *Ann Neurol* 1989;26:239–247.

7. Eidelberg D, Moeller JR, Dhawa V, et al. The metabolic topography of parkinsonism. *J Cereb Blood Flow Metab* 1994;14:783–801.

8. Eidelberg D, Moeller JR, Ishikawa T, et al. Assessment of disease severity in parkinsonism with fluorine-18-fluorodeoxyglucose and PET. *J Nucl Med* 1995;36:378–383.

9. Eidelberg D, Moeller JR, Ishikawa T, et al. Early differential diagnosis of Parkinson's disease with ^{18}F-fluorodeoxyglucose and positron emission tomography. *Neurology* 1995;45:1995–2004.

10. Eidelberg D, Takikawa S, Moeller JR, et al. Striatal hypometabolism distinguishes striatonigral degeneration from Parkinson's disease. *Ann Neurol* 1993;33:518–527.

11. Fazzini E, Dogali M, Beric A, et al. The effects of unilateral ventral posterior medial pallidotomy in patients with Parkinson's disease and Parkinson's plus syndromes. In: Koller WC, Paulson G, eds. *Therapy of Parkinson's disease,* 2nd ed. New York: Marcel-Dekker, 1994:353–379.

12. Fulham MJ, Dubinsky RM, Polinsky RJ, et al. Computed tomography, magnetic resonance imaging, and positron emission tomography with [18F]-fluorodeoxyglucose in multiple system atrophy and pure autonomic failure. *Clin Auton Res* 1991;1:27–36.

13. Golbe LI, Davis PH, Schoenberg BS, Duvoisin RC. Prevalence and natural history of progressive supranuclear palsy. *Neurology* 1988;38:1031–1034.

14. Goto S, Kunitoku N, Soyama N, et al. Posteroventral pallidotomy in a patient with parkinsonism caused by hypoxic encephalopathy. *Neurology* 1997;49:707–710.

15. Graham JG, Oppenheimer DR. Orthostatic hypotension and nicotine sensitivity in a case of multiple system atrophy. *J Neurol Neurosurg Psychiatry* 1969;32:28–34.

16. Hoehn MM, Yahr MD. Parkinsonism: onset progression and mortality. *Neurology* 1967;17:427–442.

17. Jankovic J, Friedman DI, Pirozollo FJ, McCrary JA. Progressive supranuclear palsy: motor, neurobehavioral, and neuro-ophthalmic findings. *Adv Neurol* 1990;53:293–303.

18. Krauss JK, Jankovic J, Lai EC, et al. Posteroventral medial pallidotomy in levodopa-unresponsive parkinsonism. *Arch Neurol* 1997;54:1026–1029.

19. Lang AE, Riley DE, Bergeron C. Cortical-basal ganglionic degeneration. In: Calne DB, ed. *Neurodegenerative diseases.* Philadelphia: WB Saunders, 1994: 743–767.

20. Litvan I, Agid Y, Calne D, et al. Clinical research criteria for the diagnosis of progressive supranuclear palsy (Steele-Richardson-Olszewski syndrome): report of the NINDS-SPSP international workshop. *Neurology* 1996; 47:1–9.

21. Mathias CJ, Williams AC. The Shy-Drager syndrome (and multiple system atrophy). In: Calne DB, ed. *Neurodegenerative diseases.* Philadelphia: WB Saunders, 1994:743–767.

22. Pfaffenbach DD, Layton DD, Kearns TP. Ocular manifestations in progressive supranuclear palsy. *Am J Ophthalmol* 1972;74:1179–1184.

23. Quinn N. Multiple system atrophy-the nature of the beast. *J Neurol Neurosurg Psychiatry* 1989[suppl]:78-89.

24. Quinn N. Parkinsonism-recognition and differential diagnosis. *BMJ* 1995;310:447–452.

25. Quinn N, Wenning G. Multiple system atrophy. *Curr Opin Neurol* 1995;8:323–326.

26. Rajput AH, Rozdilsky B, Rajput A: Accuracy of clinical diagnosis in parkinsonism—a prospective study. Can J Neurol Sci 1991; 18:275–278.

27. Reibeiz JJ, Kolodny EH, Richardson EP. Corticodentatonigral degeneration with neuronal achromasia. *Arch Neurol* 1968; 18:20–33.

28. Riley DE, Lang AE, Lewis A, et al. Cortical-basal ganglionic degeneration. *Neurology* 1990; 40:1203–1212.

29. Spokes EG, Bannister R, Oppenheimer DR. Multiple system atrophy with autonomic failure. *J Neurol Sci* 1979;43:59–82.

30. Steele JC, Richardson JC, Olszewski J. Progressive supranuclear palsy. *Arch Neurol* 1964;10:333–359.

31. Sung HH, Mastri AR, Segal E. Pathology of Shy-Drager syndrome. *J Neuropathol Exp Neurol* 1979;38: 358–363

32. Tolosa E, Valldeoriola F, Marti MJ. Clinical diagnosis and diagnostic criteria of progressive supranuclear palsy (Steele-Richardson-Olszewski syndrome). *J Neural Transm* 1994;42[suppl]:15–31.

33. Van der Eecken H, Adams RD, van Bogaert L. Striopallidal-nigral degeneration: an hitherto undescribed lesion in paralysis agitans. *J Neuropathol Exp Neurol* 1960; 19:159–161.

34. Wenning GK, Shlomo YB, Magalhaes M, Daniel SE, Quinn NP. Clinical features and natural history of multiple system atrophy: an analysis of 100 cases. *Brain* 1994;117:835–845.

Pallidal Surgery for the Treatment of Parkinson's Disease and Movement Disorders, edited by J. K. Krauss, R. G. Grossman, and J. Jankovic. Lippincott-Raven Publishers, Philadelphia © 1998.

19

Pallidal Surgery: A New Option for Surgical Treatment of Dystonia

Jerrold L. Vitek and *Frederick A. Lenz

*Department of Neurology, Emory University, Atlanta, Georgia 30322, USA; and *Department of Neurosurgery, Johns Hopkins University, Baltimore, Maryland 21205, USA*

Dystonia is a movement disorder characterized by sustained or intermittent muscle activity leading to altered voluntary movement and abnormal postures (37). Dystonia is both a symptom and a disease. Primary dystonia is generally considered a hereditary disorder, but it also occurs sporadically. Secondary dystonia generally presents as a symptom of an underlying disorder or disease. Both primary and secondary dystonia may present in generalized and focal forms. The observation that dystonia may occur as a presenting symptom of Parkinson's disease (PD) prior to treatment with L-dopa or during periods when drug levels are low (39) has led to speculation that dystonia may be similar pathophysiologically to PD. However, dystonia also appears in PD patients as a complication of treatment with L-dopa, suggesting that at least some forms of dystonia resemble a hyperkinetic disorder.

When medical therapy fails to alleviate dystonia (16), thalamotomy generally has been considered the surgical therapy of choice (1,10,44). There has, however, been growing interest in pallidotomy for the treatment of dystonia (22–24, 50–52), predominantly as a result of observations in patients undergoing pallidotomy for PD (2,14, 34), in which almost complete amelioration of drug-induced, or "off," dystonia has been observed. This chapter compares the results of thalamotomy studies with the preliminary results of pallidotomy for the treatment of dystonia.

THALAMOTOMY

Indications

Studies of thalamotomy for dystonia suggest that patients with some clinical features are better candidates for this procedure than others. Tasker et al. noted better outcomes with symptomatic hemidystonia, particularly in patients with involvement of two or fewer limbs, without involvement of the trunk or neck, and without progressive disease (44). The greatest improvement was thought to occur in distal portions of the upper extremity. Among patients with primary dystonia, the absence of progressive disease and the absence of involvement of the neck or trunk were associated with better outcomes (44). Similarly, Cooper noted his best results in patients with predominant involvement of the limbs and his worst results in patients with truncal or midline dystonia (10). Non-Jewish patients with a positive family history were thought to have worse outcomes compared to Jewish patients with a positive family history. Finally, Andrew and co-workers noted that all patients with symptomatic hemidystonia had significant improvement after surgery; the results were less rewarding in those with primary dystonia (1). These findings suggest that the best candidates for thalamotomy to alleviate dystonia are those with stable symptomatic hemidystonia or focal dystonia predominantly involving the extremities, without involvement of the trunk or neck.

Techniques

The technique of thalamotomy is as previously described (5). The initial targeting is obtained from imaging the patient's brain in the stereotactic frame. The introduction of high-resolution magnetic resonance imaging (MRI) and MR-compatible stereotactic frames have allowed MRI-guided initial targeting. Computed tomography (CT) can accurately localize the anterior and posterior commissures, which can be used to locate targets in the thalamus and basal ganglia. Anatomical location may then be further defined by electrophysiological recording of neuronal activity. The response of neurons to light touch and passive and active movement, together with the sensory response to microstimulation (i.e., induction of paresthesias, the somatotopic localization of the elicited change in sensation, and the effect on the abnormal movement), may be employed for physiological localization. Stimulation in the thalamic principal sensory nucleus (ventralis-caudalis, Vc) evokes somatic sensations (32). When these sensations occur in the leg, the location is lateral in the Vc. The arm and face are found progressively more medial. Stimulation in the Vim may alter the ongoing movement disorder.

Cells responding to sensory stimulation in small, well defined receptive fields are found in the Vc (28). A mediolateral somatotopy has been described within the Vc (4,18,28,38) proceeding from the representation of oral structures medially to the leg laterally (28). Anterior to the Vc is the motor thalamus; Raeva has shown thalamic neuronal firing correlating with the response to commands to initiate movement, to the active phase of movement, and to the state of maximal muscle contraction during movement (41,42). She and others have demonstrated a large percentage of neuronal activity with significant statistical changes in firing rate related to voluntary movement (voluntary cells) (12,21, 29,41,42,46). It is suggested that movement-related activity of most cells in the motor thalamus is preferentially related to the execution of particular movements. Furthermore, some neurons anterior to the Vc, presumably within the Vim, respond to passive movements of a joint, with a somatotopy parallel to that of the sensory thalamus (29). A more detailed, albeit similar, somatotopy has been described in both the sensory and motor thalamus in the monkey (25,26,47,49). In patients with dystonia, there is a significant increase in cells with deep receptive fields and increased size of representative parts of the body undergoing dystonia (31). Similar changes in somatotopy have been observed in the sensory cortex of monkeys with "dystonic"? hand cramps as a result of overtraining (8,20).

Neuronal activity at the frequency of dystonic movements (31) has been observed in the motor thalamus in humans with dystonia. Many cells in the Vim and Vop are correlated with dystonic movement and electromyographic (EMG) activity in the dystonic limb (30). The lesion site in patients with dystonia is anterior to the Vc, where cells display activity related to the dystonic movement and where stimulation may evoke changes in the patient's dystonia. Two or more lesions are then made at the target defined by the above techniques (3,5). Lesions are made by radiofrequency coagulation using an electrode with a 1.1-mm outer diameter and a 3-mm exposed tip, with a thermistor at the tip of the electrode (TM electrode; Radionics, Burlington, MA). The temperature is held constant at 60°C over a 1-minute interval and then is increased at 1-minute intervals to a level of approximately 80°C. Neurological examinations stressing lemniscal sensory function, pyramidal function, cerebellar function, and speech are conducted before, during, and after each interval of the lesioning process. The coagulum of such a lesion approximates a cylinder with a diameter of 3 mm and a length of 5 mm (11,45).

Other series (15,31) suggest that lesions of the Vop and Vim can produce clear and immediate decreases in dystonia. The effect of thalamic lesions has been described previously, although the nuclei reportedly involved in these lesions is variable. The Vim and Vop have been lesioned in some studies (9,17,40,44), whereas the Vop and the ventral boundary of this nucleus was chosen in others (27). In still other studies the Vim, Vc, centrum medianum, and pulvinar were chosen as targets (1,10).

Clinical Results

A number of studies have documented relief from dystonia following thalamotomy (1,9,10,44). Decreased dystonia was noted in a proportion of patients in all reports, although some noted that improvement was sometimes delayed (9,10) and others reported that the dystonia sometimes returned over time (1,9,10,17,44).

In this section we focus on the results of four large thalamotomy series performed to relieve dystonia. In the earlier two studies (1,44) ventriculography and macrostimulation were employed for most of the patients. Tasker et al. targeted the Vim or Vop and reported that 68% of patients with secondary dystonia showed an improvement of between 25% and 100% in the scale they used to score dystonia (44). About one-third of those who benefited from the procedure experienced a degree of regression within 1 to 6 years afterward. About one-third of the patients who regressed were noted to have progressive disease prior to the surgery. Thus loss of benefit following thalamotomy could be due to disease progression. Among patients with primary dystonia, 46% showed significant (i.e., 25–100%) improvement in dystonia scores immediately postoperatively. More than 50% of these patients showed loss of improvement during the postoperative follow-up period, which could occur within months or years after the procedure.

Andrew and co-workers made lesions in the Vim, pulvinar, and centromedian nuclei and noted that all patients with secondary hemidystonia experienced immediate postoperative improvement (1). Improvement was sustained in all patients for whom follow-up data were available. One patient experienced some regression of the postoperative result but was still improved with respect to preoperative status. In contrast, immediate good results were obtained in 63% of patients with generalized dystonia, but only 37% retained any improvement at 1 year.

A number of significant complications were noted in these two studies. Hemiparesis of "some degree" was noted in 5% to 16%, and persistent ataxia of the hand was noted in 5% to 10% of cases (1,44). Dysarthria was noted in approximately 10% of patients undergoing unilateral pro-

cedures and in a higher percentage of those undergoing bilateral procedures. Other complications included dysphagia (with bilateral lesions) and hydrocephalus. The total number of patients with significant complications was approximately 20%, many of whom had bilateral procedures.

One study reported the results in 17 patients with primary and secondary dystonia treated by microelectrode- and CT-guided lesions directed at the pallidal relay nucleus, the Vop (9). Forty-seven percent (8/17) of patients had marked to moderate long-term improvement according to a global outcome score of 3 or 4 assessed by at least two of the authors. Overall ($n = 17$), six patients showed long-term deterioration in immediate postoperative benefit, and three patients showed delayed improvement in function. Long-term benefit was slightly greater in patients with secondary dystonia (50% moderately to markedly improved) than in those with primary dystonia (43%). One-third of patients developed complications immediately after surgery including confusion and contralateral weakness. The only persistent complications were contralateral weakness, dysarthria, and pseudobulbar palsy in one patient.

Another report detailed the long-term follow-up (mean 21 years) on 18 of 28 patients with dystonia on the basis of birth injury (43). One-half (9/18) had significant improvement in function and 72% (13/18) had improvement in hygiene, feeding, or dressing. The greatest benefit was seen in those with painful dystonic posturing or phasic "hyperkinetic" dystonic movements. Complications in the group of 28 included deterioration in speech, graded as severe in 2 (7%) and slight to moderate in 4 (14%); and hemiparesis was seen in 6 (21%).

PALLIDOTOMY

Indications

There is currently renewed interest in pallidotomy for dystonia. It is based, in part, on improved understanding of the functional organization of basal ganglia thalamocortical circuits and the demonstration of consistently significant amelioration of dystonia in patients with idiopathic PD following pallidotomy (54).

Observations of significant amelioration of dystonia in patients with primary or secondary generalized dystonia following lesions in the sensorimotor portion of the pallidum strongly suggest that pallidotomy offers an effective, reliable treatment to patients with medically intractable dystonia (24,35a,50,52). Whether it is similar to thalamotomy in its differential effect on various "types" of dystonia (i.e., primary versus secondary, segmental versus generalized) remains to be shown.

Techniques

The technique of single-cell recording, mapping, and lesioning is the same as that for pallidotomy for PD (35,36,55). This technique offers a reliable method for accurately identifying and defining the sensorimotor territory of the globus pallidus internus (GPi) prior to lesioning. Different patterns of neural activity in the striatum and external and internal segments of the globus pallidus (GPe and GPi) are identified together with nearby critical structures (i.e., optic tract and internal capsule). The optic tract can be identified in most patients by flashing a strobe light in the patient's eyes and listening for high-frequency modulation of the background audio signal coincident with the light stimulus. The optic tract can also be identified in most patients by microstimulation (5–50 µA, 300 Hz). Patients typically report seeing brief speckles or flashes of light of various colors in the contralateral visual field in a localized region that is most often lateral to or near the midline. The internal capsule can be identified by observing stimulation-induced (5–50 µA, 300 Hz) movement of the limbs or orofacial structures. The relative proximity of these structures (i.e., optic tract and internal capsule) can be ascertained by the stimulation threshold at which the patient reports seeing speckles or flashes of light, or muscle contraction occurs.

To determine the location of the sensorimotor territory of the GPi, the response of neurons in the GPi to passive manipulations and active movement of the extremities and orofacial structures is examined. There is a general somatotopic organization within the sensorimotor portion of the GPi, with the preponderance of cells representing the leg found medial and dorsal to those representing the arm and face (55). The location and boundaries of identified structures (i.e., striatum, GPe, and GPi), the presence and location of neuronal responses in the GPi to passive or active movement, and the relative location of the optic tract and internal capsule (noting the thresholds), are used to generate a topographical map of this subcortical region. This map is, in turn, used to guide lesion placement. The lesion site is the sensorimotor portion of the GPi and is the same for patients with dystonia as that for patients with PD.

Once the sensorimotor portion of the GPi and its borders are defined and the target is selected, the recording microelectrode is replaced with the lesioning electrode (1.1 mm diameter Radionics lesioning electrode with a 3-mm exposed tip identical to that used for thalamotomy). The lesioning electrode is advanced to the center of the GPi, based on the prior physiological recordings, and macrostimulation is carried out. At this point, the lesioning electrode is advanced to the ventral border of the GPi in 0.5- to 1.0-mm increments until stimulation-induced movements are observed at currents equal to or less than 0.5 mA at 300 Hz or visual responses are reported at currents less than or equal to 1.0 mA at 300 Hz. At the lesion site the lesioning probe is heated to 60°C for 60 seconds (all lesioning procedures are for 60 seconds), and the patient is examined repeatedly during this 1-minute interval for changes in strength (facial and limb), the development of visual field deficits, or speech difficulty. If changes are noted, lesioning is stopped and the electrode is moved dorsally 1.0 mm; the lesioning process is then repeated. If there are no motor or visual disturbances following the first lesion, the lesion probe is reheated in increments of 5° to 10°C to a higher temperature (75°C) at the same site. The probe is then moved 2 mm dorsally, and a second lesion is placed (75°–80°C). Based on the dorsal to ventral extent of the GPi, as determined from the physiological maps, a third lesion may be placed 1 to 2 mm above the second, generally at a slightly lower temperature (70°–75°C) to avoid extending the lesion into adjacent portions of the GPe dorsally and laterally.

Because the lesion is approximately 3.0 mm in diameter, the second lesion track is generally made 2.5 to 3.0 mm from the first in the same parasagittal plane. After the second lesion track is completed, a third lesion pass is generally made 2 to 3 mm medial or lateral to the initial plane. The choice of location for subsequent lesions is determined by the clinical picture, together with the physiological map. Our current strategy is to lesion as much as possible of the sensorimotor territory of the GPi while avoiding nearby critical structures, such as the GPe, the optic and corticospinal tracts, and the nucleus basalis.

During the mapping procedures in these patients neuronal activity in the GPe and GPi can be recorded and analyzed "off" line to determine the mean firing rates and assess patterns of neural activity and receptive field properties. Although there are no data from normal humans for comparison, the mean discharge rates of neurons in the GPe and GPi in patients with dystonia were reduced compared to those found in patients with PD but were similar to those found in a patient with hemiballismus (48,50). Patterns of neuronal activity in the GPe and GPi were also significantly different from those reported in normal animals. Unlike the tonic activity reported in normal primates, neuronal activity in the GPi displayed periods of irregularly grouped discharges interspersed with pauses. This pattern was observed in most of the cells in the GPe and GPi and was similar to that observed with hemiballismus (48,50,51). Receptive fields in the dystonic patients were also altered compared to those reported in normal animals. In normal animals, neurons respond to movement about one joint in one direction in the contralateral limb. In dystonic patients, neurons responded to movement of multiple joints, in multiple directions, and often to movement in the ipsilateral limb (13, 50). These data are consistent with the observations of broadened receptive fields in overtrained monkeys who develop occupational "dystonic"? hand cramps (8,19).

Clinical Results

Reports of pallidotomy for dystonia in the literature of the 1950s were generally in the form of case reports without well documented examinations. Although the anterodorsal portion of the pallidum was the common target at that time, the lesion location was generally unknown. Results were variable, with some patients having marked improvement and others receiving little benefit (10,20). In more recent reports, however, all patients, including those with primary or secondary dystonia, have been reported to benefit substantially from pallidotomy (6,22–24,35a,50,52,54). In one study, three patients with disabling, medically intractable primary generalized dystonia were evaluated at selected intervals pre- and postoperatively using the Fahn-Marsden Dystonia Movement (FMDRS-M) and Disability (FMDRS-D) Rating Scales (7,50, 52). In addition, the activity patterns of select muscle groups were studied with surface EMG during rest or by the execution of simple movements before and after pallidotomy. High-resolution MR images were used to reconstruct the lesions and confirm their location within the posterior (sensorimotor) portion of the GPi.

Contralateral dystonic symptoms were alleviated intraoperatively immediately following a unilateral lesion within the sensorimotor portion of the GPi. Postoperative clinical evaluations using the FMDRS-M and FMDRS-D revealed significant improvement immediately postoperatively, with movement and disability scores decreasing 80% and 72%, respectively. Coincident with the dramatic reduction in the movement and disability scores, each patient reported marked improvement in activities of daily living. The most severely affected patient with axial dystonia was able to achieve relief from his dystonia preoperatively only by lying on his right side. After pallidotomy he was able to sit, stand, and walk with minimal torsional movement. He could sit in a chair, go shopping, and perform fine motor tasks previously impossible for him.

Preoperatively, all three patients underwent systematic assessment of spontaneous muscle activity under different postures and during simple movements. All three patients demonstrated intermittent posturing of the limbs at rest or during sustained posture with arms held outstretched. It was associated with intermittent and often sustained EMG activity in agonist and antagonist muscle groups. During simple movements requiring reciprocal activation and inactivation of agonist–antagonist muscle groups, excessive and altered temporal patterning of muscle activity was routinely observed, with an "overflow" of activation into normally quiescent muscle groups. After pallidotomy, in accordance with the observed clinical benefit, there was a marked reduction of the resting EMG activity that had been present in the affected body regions preoperatively, and a more "normal" pattern of activation during movement with decreased coactivation of agonist–antagonist muscle groups.

Subsequent follow-up for more than a year has demonstrated continued amelioration of the dystonic symptoms on the side contralateral to the lesion in the two patients with appendicular dystonia. The patient with axial dystonia was followed for approximately 8 months, and although demonstrating significant improvement immediately postoperatively, experienced some return of dystonia (J.L. Vitek, unpublished observations). Although clearly improved from baseline, this patient continues to suffer from axial dystonic movements predominantly involving the lower trunk. Such patients, with predominantly axial dystonia, may require bilateral pallidotomy to obtain substantial functional benefit. Support for such a procedure in patients with generalized or axial dystonia is derived from reports in the early literature in which some patients demonstrated marked functional improvement sustained over years after bilateral pallidotomy (10).

There are more recent reports and unpublished observations concerning the effect of bilateral pallidotomy in three patients with generalized dystonia involving the axial musculature. These patients underwent bilateral pallidotomy, each at a different institution, and experienced significant improvement in both appendicular and axial dystonic movements (22,24,35a). Jankovic and co-workers (24) reported the results of pallidotomy in a 14-year-old girl who had a 7-year history of progressive generalized primary dystonia. Despite maximum medical therapy and repeated botulinum toxin treatments, her disability progressed and she became anarthric, required assistance with feeding and other activities of daily living; she was no longer able to ambulate, even with assistance. Within 5 days after bilateral pallidotomy, her dystonic condition had improved dramatically; she was able to feed and dress herself, she could walk in-

dependently, and her speech had become intelligible. Iacono et al. described a 17-year-old patient with severe truncal plus appendicular dystonia who underwent a bilateral pallidotomy with relief of dystonia and improvement in strength and coordination at follow-up of more than a year without evidence of loss of benefit (22). Lozano and Lang (35a) noted dramatic benefit during the early postoperative period in a 9-year-old boy with severe generalized dystonia. This patient is reported to show continued improvement over the subsequent postoperative period.

These observations suggest dramatic improvement in generalized dystonia including axial musculature following bilateral pallidotomy. Hypophonia was not reported to occur following any of those cases and may not occur to the degree or frequency reported in patients with PD. Experience with bilateral pallidotomy is limited, and it is not clear whether bilateral pallidotomy is associated with the same increased incidence of side effects as that reported for PD.

The need for bilateral procedures may depend on the distribution of the dystonia. Although patients with generalized dystonia may require bilateral pallidotomy to achieve optimal benefit, many may gain adequate relief following unilateral procedures. Jankovic and co-workers reported significant improvement in a patient with dystonia who underwent unilateral microelectrode-guided pallidotomy (24). The patient, a 57-year-old man, had a 17-year history of segmental dystonia involving chiefly his face, neck, and left arm. The patient became gradually disabled as a result of the progressive dystonia, which was unresponsive to a variety of medications and botulinum toxin treatments. Immediately after right pallidotomy, he experienced marked relief of the left arm and neck pain, which was accompanied by a robust reduction of the neck and arm spasms and improvement in function. He is now able to dress himself, drive, and play golf, which he could not do prior to the procedure. There are two additional reports regarding the effect of pallidotomy for dystonia (6,23). All of the patients in these preliminary reports, including those with primary or secondary dystonia, have been reported to benefit substantially from pallidotomy.

CONCLUSIONS

Thalamotomy produces significant long-term alleviation of appendicular dystonia in one-third to one-half of patients. Earlier studies reported significant persistent complications, including hemiparesis, ataxia, and dysarthria in approximately 20% of cases. Most of the cases of dysarthria occurred after bilateral procedures. One series, employing microelectrode localization, reported significant persistent complications of dysarthria, pseudobulbar palsy, and hemiparesis in 11% of cases. Concerning pallidotomy, preliminary data demonstrate significant improvement in virtually all patients with dystonia following inactivation of the sensorimotor portion of the GPi. Multiple case reports suggest that pallidotomy results in marked improvement in motor functioning and dystonic symptoms with a significant reduction in disability and no reported complications of ataxia, dysarthria, or hypophonia. The early results suggest that the benefit of pallidotomy may outweigh the long-term benefit of thalamotomy. However, long-term results of pallidotomy have not been reported for many patients in the modern era. Furthermore, imaging and electrophysiological techniques have advanced since most of the studies of thalamotomy were carried out. The variability in lesion location could account for the variable outcomes reported with thalamotomy, similar to earlier studies of pallidotomy for PD and dystonia. Thus a controlled clinical trial of these two therapies using standardized methods of clinical assessment should be conducted.

Acknowledgments. Some of the studies reviewed in this chapter were supported by grants to J.L.V. from the NIH (K08 NS1328, R29 NS30719, R01 NS 32047) and the Dystonia Medical Research Foundation and to F.A.L. from the Eli Lilly Corporation and the NIH (NS28598, K08 NS01384, P01 NS32386-Proj. 1).

REFERENCES

1. Andrew J, Fowler CJ, Harrison JG. Stereotaxic thalamotomy in 55 cases of dystonia. *Brain* 1983;106:981–1000.
2. Baron MS, Vitek JL, Bakay RAE, et al. Treatment of advanced Parkinson's disease with microelectrode-guided pallidotomy: 1-year pilot study results. *Ann Neurol* 1996;40:355–366.
3. Bakay RAE, Vitek JL, DeLong MR. Thalamotomy for tremor. In: Rengachary SS, Wilkins RH, eds. *Neuro-*

surgical operative atlas. Baltimore: Williams & Wilkins, 1992:299–312.
4. Bates JAV. Electrical recording from the thalamus in human subjects. In: Iggo A, ed. *Handbook of sensory physiology: somatosensory system.* Berlin: Springer-Verlag, 1972:561–578.
5. Bertrand CM, Lenz FA. Surgical treatment of dystonias. In: Tsui JKC, Calne DB, eds. *Handbook of dystonia.* New York: Marcel Dekker Inc., 1995:329–345.
6. Blount J, Kondoh T, Ebjner T. Pallidotomy for the treatment of dystonia. *Proc AANS* 1996;64:1906 (abst).
7. Burke RE, Fahn S, Marsden CD, Bressman SB, Moskowitz C, Friedman J. Validity and reliability of a rating scale for primary torsion dystonias. *Neurology* 1985;35:73–77.
8. Byl NN, Merzenich MM, Jenkins WM. A primate genesis model of focal dystonia and repetitive strain injury. I. Learning-induced dedifferentiation of the representation of the hand in the primary somatosensory cortex in adult monkeys. *Neurology* 1996;47:508–520.
9. Cardoso F, Jankovic J, Grossman RG, Hamilton W. Outcome after stereotactic thalamotomy for dystonia and hemiballismus. *Neurosurgery* 1995;36:501–508.
10. Cooper IS. 20-Year followup study of the neurosurgical treatment of dystonia musculorum deformans. *Adv Neurol* 1976;14:423–452.
11. Cosman ER, Cosman BJ. Methods of making nervous system lesions. In: Wilkins RH, Rengachary SS, eds. *Neurosurgery.* New York: McGraw-Hill, 1985:2490–2499.
12. Crowell RM, Perret E, Siegfried J. "Movement units" and "tremor phasic units" in the human thalamus. *Brain Res* 1968;11:481–488.
13. DeLong MR, Crutcher MD, Georgopoulos AP. Primate globus pallidus and subthalamic nucleus: functional organization. *J Neurophysiol* 1985;53:530–543.
14. Dogali M, Fazzini E, Kolodny E, et al. Stereotactic ventral pallidotomy for Parkinson's disease. *Neurology* 1995;45:753–761.
15. Evatt ML, Hashimoto T, Triche S, DeLong MR, Bakay R, Vitek JL. Thalamotomy for dystonia using electrophysiologic mapping. *Mov Disord* 1997;12:31 (abst).
16. Fahn S. Drug treatment of hyperkinetic movement disorders. *Semin Neurol* 1987;7:192–208.
17. Gros C, Frerebeau P, Perez-Dominquez E, Bazin M, Privat JM. Long term results of stereotaxic surgery for infantile dystonia and dyskinesia. *Neurochirurgia* 1976; 19:171–178.
18. Guiot G, Derome P, Arfel G, Walter SG. Electrophysiological recordings in stereotaxic thalamotomy for parkinsonism. In: Krayenbuehl H, Maspes PE, Sweet WH, eds. In: *Progress in neurological surgery.* Basel: Karger, 1973:189–221.
19. Hallett M. Physiology of basal ganglia disorders: an overview. *Can J Neurol Sci* 1993;20:177–183.
20. Hassler R, Riechert T, Mundinger F, Umbach W, Gangelberger JA. Physiological observations in stereotaxic operations in extrapyramidal motor disturbances. *Brain* 1960;83:337–350.
21. Hongell A, Wallin G, Hagbarth KE. Unit activity connected with movement initiation and arousal situations recorded from the ventrolateral nucleus of the human thalamus. *Acta Neurol Scand* 1973;49:681–698.
22. Iacono RP, Kuniyoshi SM, Lonser RR, Maeda G, Inae AM, Ashwal S. Simultaneous bilateral pallidoansotomy for idiopathic dystonia musculorum deformans. *Pediatr Neurol* 1996;14:145–148 (abst).

23. Iacono RP, Kuniyoshi S, Lonser R, Ashwal S, Mohamed A. Posteroventral pallidotomy in the treatment of primary and secondary dystonia. *Mov Disord* 1997;12:32 (abst).
24. Jankovic J, Ondo WO, Lai E, Grossman RG. Pallidotomy for dystonia. *Mov Disord* 1998 (in press).
25. Jones EG, Friedman GP. Projection pattern of functional components of thalamic ventrobasal complex on monkey somatosensory cortex. *J Neurophysiol* 1982;48:521–543.
26. Jones EG, Friedman DP, Hendry HC. Thalamic basis of place- and modality-specific columns in monkey somatosensory cortex: a correlative anatomical and physiological study. *J Neurophysiol* 1982;48:545–568.
27. Laitinen LV. Neurosurgery in cerebral palsy. *J Neurol Neurosurg Psychiatry* 1970;33:513–518.
28. Lenz FA, Dostrovsky JO, Tasker RR, Yamashiro K, Kwan HC, Murphy JT. Single-unit analysis of the human ventral thalamic nuclear group: somatosensory responses. *J Neurophysiol* 1988;59:299–316.
29. Lenz FA, Kwan H, Dostrovsky JO, Tasker RR, Murphy JT, Lenz YE. Single unit analysis of the human ventral thalamic nuclear group: activity correlated with movement. *Brain* 1990;113:1795–1821.
30. Lenz FA, Jaeger CJ, Seike M, et al. Cross-correlation analysis of thalamic neuronal and EMG signals in patients with dystonia. *Mov Disord* 1992;7:372 (abst).
31. Lenz FA, Seike M, Jaeger CJ, et al. Single unit analysis of thalamus in patients with dystonia. *Mov Disord* 1992;7:371 (abst).
32. Lenz FA, Seike M, Lin YC, Baker FH, Richardson RT, Gracely RH. Thermal and pain sensations evoked by microstimulation in the area of the human ventrocaudal nucleus (Vc). *J Neurophysiol* 1993;70:200–212.
33. Lenz FA, Dougherty PM, Reich SG. The effectiveness of thalamotomy for treatment of tremor and dystonia. *Mov Disord* 1996;11:18 (abst)
34. Lozano AM, Lang AE, Galvez-Jimenez N, et al. GPi pallidotomy improves motor function in patients with Parkinson's disease. *Lancet* 1995;346:1383–1386.
35. Lozano AM, Hutchinson W, Kiss Z, Tasker RR, Davis K, Dostrovsky JO. Methods for microelectrode guided posteroventral pallidotomy. *J Neurosurg* 1996;4:194–202.
35a. Lozano AM, Kumar R, Gross RE, et al. Globus pallidus internus pallidotomy for generalized dystonia. *Mov Disord* 1997;12:865–870.
36. Mandir AS, Rowland LH, Dougherty PM, Lenz FA. Microelectrode recording and stimulation techniques during stereotactic procedures in the thalamus and pallidum. *Adv Neurol* 1997;74:159–165.
37. Marsden CD, Fahn S. Surgical approaches to the dyskinesias: afterword. In: Marsden CD, Fahn S, eds. *Neurology 2: movement disorders.* London: Butterworth Scientific, 1982;345.
38. McComas AJ, Wilson P, Martin-Rodriguez J, Wallace C, Hankinson J. Properties of somatosensory neurons in the human thalamus. *J Neurol Neurosurg Psychiatry* 1970;33:716–717.

39. Muenter MD, Sharpless NS, Tyce GM, Darley FL. Patterns of dystonia ("I-D-I" and "D-I-D") in response to L-dopa therapy for Parkinson's disease. *Mayo Clin Proc* 1977;52:163–174.
40. Narabayashi H. Choreoathetosis and spasticity. In: Schaltenbrand G, Walker AE, eds. *Stereotaxy of the human brain.* Basel: Thieme Verlag, 1982:532–543.
41. Raeva SN. Unit activity of some deep nuclear structures of the human brain during voluntary movements. In: Somjen G, ed. *Neurophysiology studied in man.* Amsterdam: Excerpta Medica, 1972:64–78.
42. Raeva SN. Localization in human thalamus of units triggered during "verbal commands," voluntary movements and tremor. *Electroencephalgr Clin Neurophysiol* 1986; 63:160–173.
43. Speelman JD, Van Manen J. Cerebral palsy and stereotactic neurosurgery: long term results. *J Neurol Neurosurg Psychiatry* 1997;52:23–30.
44. Tasker RR, Doorly T, Yamashiro K. Thalamotomy in generalized dystonia. *Adv Neurol* 1988;50:615–631.
45. Tasker RR, Yamashiro K, Lenz FA, Dostrovsky JO. Thalamotomy in Parkinson's disease: microelectrode techniques. In: Lundsford D, ed. *Modern stereotactic neurosurgery.* Boston: Martinus Nijhoff Publishing, 1988:297–313.
46. Umbach W, Ehrhardt KJ. Micro-electrode recording in the basal ganglia during stereotaxic operations. *Confin Neurol* 1965;26:315–317.
47. Vitek JL, Ashe J, DeLong MR, Alexander GE. Physiologic properties and somatotopic organization of the primate motor thalamus. *J Neurophysiol* 1994;71: 1498–1513.
48. Vitek JL, Kaneoke Y, Hashimoto T, Bakay RAE, DeLong MR. Neuronal activity in the pallidum of a patient with hemiballismus. *Neurology* 1995;38:296 (abst).
49. Vitek JL, Ashe J, DeLong MR, Kaneoke Y. Microstimulation of primate motor thalamus: somatotopic organization and differential distribution of evoked motor responses among subnuclei. *J Neurophysiol* 1996;75: 2486–2495.
50. Vitek JL, Zhang J, Evatt M, et al. GPi pallidotomy for dystonia: clinical outcome and neuronal activity. In: Fahn S, ed. *Dystonia 3.* 1998 (in press).
51. Vitek JL, Zhang J, DeLong MR, Mewes K, Bakay RAE. Neuronal activity in the pallidum in patients with medically intractable dystonia. *Mov Disord* 1997;12(3):9 (abst).
52. Vitek JL, Evatt M, Zhang J, et al. Pallidotomy is an effective treatment for patients with medically intractable dystonia. *Mov Disord* 1997;12:31 (abst).
53. Vitek JL, Bakay RAE, Hashimoto T, et al. Microelectrode-guided pallidotomy: technical approach and application for treatment of medically intractable Parkinson's disease. *J Neurosurg* 1997;88:1027–1043.
54. Vitek JL, Bakay RAE. Pallidotomy for Parkinson's disease and dystonia. *Curr Opin Neurol* 1997;10: 332–339.

Pallidal Surgery for the Treatment of Parkinson's Disease and Movement Disorders, edited by J. K. Krauss, R. G. Grossman, and J. Jankovic. Lippincott-Raven Publishers, Philadelphia © 1998..

20A

Optimal Target of Pallidotomy: A Controversy

Roy A. E. Bakay and Philip A. Starr

Department of Neurological Surgery, Emory University School of Medicine, Atlanta, Georgia 30322, USA

Parkinson's disease (PD) is a progressive, degenerative disease involving loss of dopamine in the striatum and in other basal ganglia nuclei due to loss of the dopaminergic cells of the substantia nigra, pars compacta (SNc) (21,24,30). The cardinal clinical signs of PD are resting tremor, rigidity, akinesia, and postural instability. First described by James Parkinson in 1817 (48), the diagnostic characteristics have changed as the pathophysiology has become better understood (3). The diagnosis is strictly clinical. Accurate diagnosis of idiopathic PD requires ruling out other causes of Parkinson-like diseases, which can be secondarily induced by drugs, systemic diseases, trauma, or other neurodegenerative disorders. Autopsy findings have revealed that 20% to 30% of patients diagnosed clinically as having idiopathic PD cannot be confirmed pathologically because they do not demonstrate the degeneration of SNc neurons and the presence of Lewy bodies (31,41,49).

The symptoms are progressive. Levodopa therapy greatly enhances symptomatic improvement and life expectancy. Unfortunately, with time, most patients lose their response to levodopa and develop severe fluctuations and dyskinesias (44). Most patients, in addition to exhibiting the cardinal motor signs of PD (akinesia/bradykinesia, rigidity, tremor, and gait disorder/postural instability) also may experience drug-induced dyskinesias, motor fluctuations, dystonia, pain, and freezing episodes. Because of the complexity regarding diagnosis and responsiveness to pharma-

cotherapy, there is a need for evaluation and treatment by a movement disorder specialist. Patients with idiopathic PD who initially demonstrated a good response to levodopa but subsequently develop an unsatisfactory clinical response to optimal medical management are considered candidates for pallidotomy.

Pallidotomy is the surgical destruction of portions of the globus pallidus (GP). Throughout its 50-year history the practice of pallidotomy has varied greatly with respect to the selection of patients, lesion location, surgical techniques, lesioning techniques, and outcome assessment. These differences must be considered to interpret the wide variation in reported clinical results. As is often true in functional neurosurgery, a number of controversies have surrounded this procedure (35). The attempt here is to discuss surgical techniques from a clinical perspective based on a scientific rationale and evidence-based clinical practice. The focus is on answering a basic question: Where is the optimal target? First we review the literature, then discuss the experimental findings in relation to the clinical results, and finally synthesize the clinical and research data.

HISTORICAL REVIEW

The literature on pallidotomy for PD can be divided into the historical literature, dating from the 1930s to the introduction of L-dopa during the 1960s, and the contemporary literature, which begins with the reports of Burzaco and Laitinen et al. on the clinical results of posterolateral pallidotomy (7,37). It was Russell Meyers who in the 1940s first described surgery in the region of the GP for PD (45). His pioneering studies demonstrated that lesions of the GP or of its outflow tracts could reduce rigidity and tremor without causing paresis. During the 1950s and 1960s, several others confirmed this finding using a variety of techniques, including open surgical intervention (28), anterior choroidal artery ligation (9,50), closed free-hand procedures (10), and stereotactically guided procedures (58–60,63).

The clinical results of pallidotomy during the 1950s were unpredictable and were not reported in terms of objective, standardized rating scales (60). Akinesia/bradykinesia and rigidity were frequently confused, and it was not until the advent of stereotactic surgery for PD that these symptoms could be unequivocally distinguished (3). The stereotactic target coordinates were reported as 0 to 5 mm behind the anterior commissure and 15 to 17 mm lateral to the midline, which would have placed lesions in the anterodorsal globus pallidus, internal segment (GPi) (58). A small number of autopsy reports from the pre-L-dopa era show that location of the lesion within the pallidum was highly variable but did confirm that most lesions involved the anterodorsal portion of the GPi and that collateral damage was frequent (26,57,67). The major exception is the series by Leksell who systematically varied the target in the GPi from the anterodorsal region to the posterolateral region (63). Additional confirmation of the value of the posterior target was provided by Spiegel et al. (60). They reported five patients in whom early tremor recurrences following pallidal lesions 0 to 3 mm behind the AC were abolished (1–5 years of follow-up) by enlarging the lesion to 6 to 9 mm behind the AC.

CONTEMPORARY SERIES

During the decades following the introduction of levodopa, neurologists began recognizing that long-term medical therapy for PD is often unsatisfactory, with most patients eventually developing drug-induced dyskinesias, motor fluctuations, and variable responses to medications (44). At the same time, surgical techniques improved (22,25,35), and the theoretical and experimental basis for surgical interventions, including pallidotomy, were developed (1,2,5,11,12). It was in this setting that Laitinen et al. published a seminal paper describing the results of posterolateral GPi pallidotomy in 38 patients (37). They confirmed Leksell's earlier findings that all four cardinal disease signs can be relieved by this procedure (63). Dramatic benefit for drug-induced dyskinesias was also reported. Pallidotomy has thus reemerged as the preferred surgical procedure for medically uncontrolled PD. Interest in thalamotomy has also increased but only for the treatment of tremor. Although thalamotomy can relieve tremor, rigidity, and drug-induced dys- kinesias (47), its ineffectiveness for treating akinesia causes pallidotomy to be favored (35).

It is important to note the differences between pallidotomy during the 1990s and pallidotomy of the 1950s (17,46,65). Unlike the anterodorsal GPI lesions of most older series, the target for pallidotomy is now considered by most to be the posterolateral portion of the GPi.

The clinical effectiveness of pallidotomy can be assessed reliably only from contemporary studies. To quantify the clinical results of contemporary pallidotomy objectively, patients must be assessed before and after the procedure using standard rating scales of motor function and disability by movement disorder specialists in an unbiased manner. The Unified Parkinson's Disease Rating Scale (UPDRS) is the most commonly used rating scale for PD (15). Because motor signs in PD patients typically fluctuate widely between the "on" and "off" state, clinical ratings must be performed at multiple times in both states. Other standard evaluations include Hoehn and Yahr staging, the dyskinesia rating scale, and timed motor tests (40). An additional scale commonly used to measure overall disability in PD is the Schwab and England (S&E) Activities of Daily Living (ADL) score (54).

Until early 1997 only four groups had reported results of unilateral pallidotomy using standard rating scales in both the "on" and "off" periods that could be used for evidence-based clinical evaluation (4,13,39,42,43,62,66). These results form the core of this review. UPDRS total and motor scores improved in three of the standardized studies (all using microelectrodes), and only one study (without using microelectrodes) failed to demonstrate improvement. In the Toronto study, UPDRS rating was performed by blinded investigators based on videotaped examinations (43). At the 6-month follow-up, total UPDRS scores in the "off" state had improved 25%, and UPDRS motor subscale scores in the "off" state had improved 30%. "On" state motor scores did not change significantly. The Emory UPDRS results were similar to those of the Toronto study (4). At 2 years the Emory study continued to demonstrate significant improvements in UPDRS subscale motor scores over baseline, but the changes were quantitatively less than at the 1-year evaluations (66). The New York University (NYU) study, with a 1-year follow-up, showed an improvement in UPDRS subscale motor scores in the "off" state of 60% and UPDRS motor subscale score improvement in the "on" state (13). These improvements were sustained for 4 years (18). Scales that measure overall functional disability, such as the S&E scores and the UPDRS ADL subscores, also showed significant improvement in most reports, varying from 28% to 55% (4,13,43).

These centers reported that pallidotomy consistently alleviated contralateral tremor, rigidity, and bradykinesia in the "off" state (4,13,43). In the Emory series, tremor was nearly eliminated in 7 of 8 (85%) patients who had significant tremor preoperatively (4). Similar effects on tremor have been observed by others (13,43). Blinded evaluations of bradykinesia have shown contralateral improvements of 37% (timed motor tasks) in the NYU study (13) and 26% (UPDRS akinesia score) in the Toronto study (43). Multiple reports agree that there is a modest ipsilateral benefit of pallidotomy on bradykinesia (4,13,43). In the Toronto series, UPDRS contralateral rigidity scores improved 30% (43). Improvements in axial symptoms (gait, posture, falling, and freezing) have been observed (13) but in some studies failed to reach statistical significance at the longest evaluation times (4,43). Pallidotomy is reported to increase the amount of time spent in the "on" state (4) and to decrease motor fluctuations (4). Virtu-

ally all groups have reported dramatic and sustained amelioration of peak dose levodopa-induced dyskinesias on the contralateral side and in some cases ipsilateral improvements (4,43). At 2-year evaluations, the Toronto group report a significant 22% decrease in dopaminergic drug use (4). In most studies where this was examined, intake of levodopa did not change significantly (4,13,43).

Only the USC group (62) reported no improvement following pallidotomy. None of the five patients with advanced PD showed a significant reduction in the total score or subscores of the UPDRS 2 months postoperatively. Improvement in dyskinesias was the only positive result. Factors contributing to the lack of significant improvement may have been the relatively high mean age of the patients, symptom profiles, and possibly lesion location. Microelectrode recording was not used for localization. Although good outcomes have been reported without the use of microelectrode localization, the microelectrode documents the physiological location and abnormal function of the sensorimotor areas in the GPi that should improve the probability of including the sensorimotor area in this lesion.

PALLIDOTOMY FOR PARKINSON'S DISEASE: THEORETICAL BASIS

The basal ganglia–thalamocortical motor circuit plays a key role in regulating motor behavior (1,5,11,12). The pathophysiology of PD and the many effects of pallidotomy on PD are interpretable in terms of interruption of this circuit. A current model of the basal ganglia-thalamocortical motor circuit is illustrated in Fig. 20A-1A (1). The basal ganglia structures that participate in this circuit include portions of the striatum, the internal and external segments of the globus pallidus (GPi and GPe), the subthalamic nucleus (STN), and the substantia nigra, pars reticulata (SNr). Only a portion of these nuclei participate in the motor circuit, and this sensorimotor area is identifiable by neurons whose discharge rates are modulated by passive or active movements (or both) (1). Sensorimotor regions are anatomically separate from the regions that regulate nonmotor functions. Therefore it is possible to

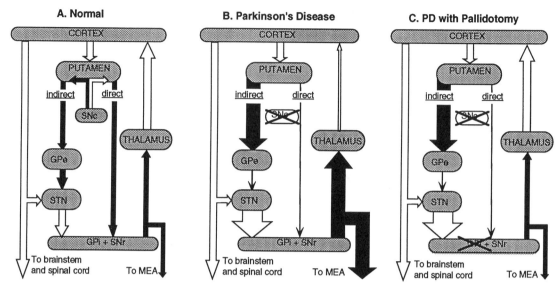

FIG. 20A-1. Basal ganglia-thalamocortical motor circuit in the normal state, in Parkinson's disease, and following GPi pallidotomy. *SNc,* substantia nigra, pars compacta; *SNr,* substantia nigra, pars reticulata; *GPe,* globus pallidus, external segment; *GPi,* globus pallidus, internal segment; *STN,* subthalamic nucleus; *MEA,* midbrain extrapyramidal area; *PD,* Parkinson's disease. *Open arrows,* excitatory connections; *filled arrows,* inhibitory connections. Changes in the widths of the arrows between (A), (B), and (C) indicate changes in the activity of the pathway represented. *Wide lines* indicate increased activity; *narrow lines* indicate decreased activity. **A:** Normal. **B:** Parkinson's disease. **C:** Parkinson's disease, showing the effect of pallidotomy on basal ganglia output and thalamocortical activity in comparison with normal. (Modified from ref. 11, with permission.)

design surgical interventions that alter function in the motor circuit without affecting nonmotor circuits.

Efferent projections from primary motor, premotor, and somatosensory cortex enter the basal ganglia via the striatum. The major basal ganglia output nuclei are the GPi and SNr, which project to subdivisions of the motor thalamus, the ventralis oralis anterior (Voa) nucleus, and the ventralis oralis (Vop) nucleus (Hassler terminology). Collaterals from the pallidothalamic and nigrothalamic pathways also innervate the midbrain extrapyramidal area (MEA) or pedunculopontine nucleus (PPN) (53,69). MEA is a motor area that may be involved in locomotion and posture. Within the basal ganglia, motor function is thought to be regulated by two major pathways, the "direct" and "indirect" pathways, both of which are modulated by striatal dopamine. The direct pathway is a monosynaptic projection from the putamen to the GPi/SNr. The indirect path-

way is multisynaptic through which the putamen affects the GPi/SNr via intermediate nuclei, the GPe, and the STN. Dopaminergic innervation of the putamen by the SNc is inhibitory to striatopallidal neurons via D2 receptors in the indirect pathway but excitatory to striatopallidal neurons via D1 receptors in the direct pathway. Most projections between the basal ganglia nuclei are γ-aminobutyric acid (GABA) ergic (inhibitory), except for the projection from the STN to the GPi/SNR, which is glutamatergic (excitatory).

Thus the indirect pathway provides negative feedback to cortical regions, and the direct pathway provides positive feedback. Balance between the direct and indirect pathways is considered critical for maintaining the appropriate modulation of neuronal activity within the cortical regions concerned with motor control. In PD the loss of dopaminergic modulation results in alterations in the basal ganglia–thalamocortical motor circuit, shown in Fig. 20A-1B(11). Loss of striatal dopamine inhibits the excitatory direct pathway and disinhibits the inhibitory indirect pathway, which leads to increased activity in the output nuclei (GPi and SNR), which in turn leads to excessive inhibition of the thalamocortical pathway. The reduction in cortical excitation is thought to be manifested by the hypokinetic motor signs of parkinsonism. This model of PD is supported by metabolic and electrophysiological studies of the basal ganglia of the *N*-methyl-4-phenyl-1,2,3,6-tetrahydropyridine (MPTP)-treated parkinsonian monkey. In this model, metabolic activity and neuronal discharge frequencies in GPi and STN are increased compared with those in normals (5,19,20,55).

Lesioning the GPi or STN ameliorates the motor signs of PD. The theoretical basis for the effectiveness of GPi pallidotomy in PD is illustrated in Fig. 20A-1C. Lesions in the motor-controlling region of the GPi should decrease the inhibitory influence of basal ganglia output nuclei on the motor thalamus and restore thalamocortical activity. Normalization of thalamocortical activity should lead to amelioration of the motor signs associated with parkinsonism. In support of this theory, pallidotomy in PD patients is associated with increased activation of cortical motor areas, as determined by positron emission tomography (PET) (8,14,27). The model illustrates how lesioning certain parts of the circuit can compensate for the effects of dopamine loss on cortical activity, even though lesioning clearly does not restore dopaminergic function.

The model is clearly incomplete. Alterations in mean discharge rates in the basal ganglia–thalamocortical motor circuit cannot explain all signs of PD or all effects of GPi pallidotomy. For example, the reason for the reduction of levodopa-induced dyskinesias following pallidotomy is unclear. In the pathophysiology of movement disorders, alterations in the patterns, rather than just the mean rates, of action potential firing may be important. As understanding of these altered patterns is gained, the role of thalamocortical pathways in mediating different types of movement disorders may be clarified. In addition, projections from the basal ganglia output nuclei to the MEA may be important in movement disorders. The projections from the GPi to the MEA

are interrupted by posterior ventral pallidotomy (53). Thus some effects of pallidotomy may be mediated via this descending connection to the brainstem rather than by thalamocortical pathways. Furthermore, although inhibition of thalamocortical projections is proposed as the primary cause of hypokinetic motor signs associated with PD, lesions within the motor thalamus do not exacerbate or induce parkinsonian motor signs, as might be predicted by the model, but alleviate or abolish parkinsonian tremor, rigidity, and drug-induced dyskinesias (22,25,35,47). This suggests that a decrease in activity of thalamic neurons cannot by itself account for the development of parkinsonian motor signs. Alternatively, these motor signs may occur, in part, because of an altered pattern of neuronal activity that disrupts the normal operation of corticocortical circuits involved in motor control.

SYNTHESIZING THEORY AND CLINICAL OBSERVATIONS

The appropriate target location within the GPi was originally discovered by trial and error. During the 1950s Leksell systematically varied the target in the GPi from the anterodorsal region to the posterolateral region, with improved symptom control in the latter target location (63). This posterolateral target has been repopularized by Laitinen et al. (37). Electrophysiological studies have justified the choice of posterolateral GPi as the appropriate pallidotomy target, as in both humans (4,13,32,43,44,61,64,65) and nonhuman primates (12,19,20) the posterolateral part of GPi is the part containing neurons whose discharge is modulated by joint movements. The posterolateral GPi is the sensorimotor part and is therefore the subdivision of the nucleus participating in the basal ganglia–thalamocortical motor circuit. Lesions in other, nonmotor parts of the GPi should primarily affect nonmotor functions. Lesions outside the motor territory of the GPi may temporarily relieve parkinsonian motor signs, presumably by partial lesioning or extension of edema into the motor territory, but the benefit of such lesions may be transient (65,66).

The optimal target site remains to be scientifically determined. There is general agreement within contemporary neurosurgery that the lesion must be posterior in the GPi to be effective. Theoretically, the lesion should include the entire sensorimotor territory of the GPi, including the neurons that give rise to the ansa lenticularis and fasciculus lenticularis. This lesion would eliminate both direct and indirect pathways and is the basis of most of the surgical approaches (4,13,16,34,42,43,50,64–66). Making a lesion too large in this area has the potential for increasing complications, and so careful placement and shaping of the lesion is required. Vitek et al., at Emory University, evaluated 11 patients from their pilot study and subdivided them into two groups based on lesion location determined on thin-section, volumetrically acquired postoperative magnetic resonance imaging (MRI) scans (65). Patients with lesions clearly centered in the posterolateral (sensorimotor) portion of the GPi had sustained improvement in UPDRS scores at 18 months. Patients with lesions that involved only a portion of this area or that encroached substantially on the GPe, sustained significantly less benefit. One of their early patients presented following a pallidotomy elsewhere, with a lesion anterior to the sensorimotor part of the GPi. Immediately postoperatively from the first lesion the patient reported resolution of all parkinsonian motor signs, but she experienced a gradual return of symptoms after 2 weeks. Repeat pallidotomy with lesion placement posterior to the first lesion has provided sustained benefit at 3 years (65). Although anecdotal, this case points out that accurate placement of a lesion in the GPi is essential for good results.

The safety and efficacy of stereotactic surgery for PD had been enhanced by electrophysiological verification of the target (2,25,35). With thalamotomy macroelectrode stimulation helps identify the target, but with pallidotomy the main purpose is to avoid complications by identifying the optic and corticospinal tracts. Some form of physiological localization is used for nearly all pallidotomies (16). Lesioning has been reported without electrophysiological localization by radiosurgical pallidotomy for PD, using the Leksell gamma knife (23,51,68). In two small series, symptomatic improvement was minimal, with only four of eight (51) and one of four (23) pa-

tients, respectively, experiencing relief. Young et al. (68), in a series of 15 PD patients, reported that gamma knife pallidotomy was effective treatment for drug-induced dyskinesias in all patients and for bradykinesia and rigidity in 77%. Patient assessment by a standardized PD rating scale was not performed, so it is impossible to compare these results with those of radiofrequency pallidotomy. No complications were reported initially, but later follow-up demonstrated problems with radiation necrosis (personal communication).

The sensorimotor region in the GPi is somatotopically arranged in a complex pattern (29,61,64). The boundaries between various somatotopic subdivisions of the GPi are less well demarcated than in the thalamus or motor cortex. The Emory Center has observed medial to lateral somatotopy in the GPi that may be important, as we have observed that small, single lesions based laterally tend to improve hand function more than leg function, whereas those placed more medially tend to improve leg function more than that in the hand (65). As a result, we have modified the surgical approach to making both lateral and medial lesions that encompass both regions. A triangular pattern of lesioning is currently used that matches the shape of the posterior GPi in an attempt to maximize the benefit from a posterior pallidotomy.

Not all groups agree that the entire posterior GPi is the optimal target. Another school of thought is that a pure ansotomy is sufficient for good clinical effect (33,56). The analysis of these reports is difficult because they are not reported in a standardized unbiased rating method and therefore not directly comparable to other studies. The ansa lenticularis is a thin, broad-based curvilinear structure that would be impossible to destroy completely by a small lesion. Ansotomy eliminates much of the inhibitory output from the GPi to the thalamus. However, a considerable amount of pallidothalamic output goes through the fascicul=aris lenticularis, which would not be affected by a small ansa lesion. In addition, isolated ansotomy should interrupt the output from the GPe to the STN, potentially leading to further disinhibition of the STN and further excitation of any remaining GPi cells with pallidothalamic fibers through the fascicularis lenticularis. Thus a pure ansa lesion may well improve a number of parkinsonian signs but may not be the optimal area for lesioning. Groups that perform ansa lesions also report minimal complications with bilateral lesioning (33,56). The data must be of higher quality before the results can be used to validate this target.

A final school of thought suggests that the optimal target would include the GPe (38). Laitinen and Horiz reported that by shifting to a more lateral target that included the GPe they achieved good results with fewer complications. The results are reported without standardized, unbiased rating scales and are therefore not directly comparable to those from other studies. The theoretical basis is to eliminate the striatopallidal and pallidosubthalamic pathways so as to release the "normal function of the medial pallidum" (38). The concept here is that both the direct and indirect pathways have been lesioned, and so stimulation and inhibition of the GPi is somehow again balanced. The problems with such a concept are that the direct striatopallidal pathway is diffuse and therefore difficult to lesion completely. Also, because of the deficiency in striatal dopamine, it is already functioning minimally. The indirect pathway through the STN is excitatory, and decreasing the pallidosubthalamic inhibition to the STN may produce an effect opposite to that which is desired. Although this type of lesion is described as a GPe lesion, all of the available information about lesions made in this area indicates that it must incorporate the posterior elements of the GPi and parts of the ansa (36,38). It is not clear whether inclusion of the GPe enhances or detracts from the effect of the GPi lesion. In the MPTP-treated primate model of PD, pure GPe lesions do not relieve L-dopa-induced dyskinesias (6), whereas the dyskinesias in Laitinen's patients were clearly relieved (36,38), suggesting that the therapeutic benefits from the lesion are derived from the GPi component of the lesion.

We have had the opportunity to examine 18 patients with failed pallidotomies performed at other institutes. After careful evaluation we determined that four of the patients did not have idiopathic PD, four had lesions placed too anteriorly, and ten had lesions placed too laterally. When five of these patients were reoperated with microelectrode localization, they all had abnormal activity in the GPi, obliteration of which has produced dramatic improvement (unpublished observations). Moving the target laterally to include the GPe may add safety but appears to decrease the efficacy of the procedure.

CONCLUSIONS

The choice of the posterolateral GPi as the target is supported experimentally and clinically. Anatomically segregated subregions of the GPi that mediate different functions, including motor, limbic, and associative functions, have now been defined. Electrophysiological studies in humans and nonhuman primates have shown that the posterolateral part of the GPi contains the portion of the nucleus that participates in motor function. Thus lesions in this area are likely to be more efficacious for treating motor signs than lesions in other, nonmotor parts of the GPi. This concept is supported by Leksell's series and contemporary studies in which the clinical results of posterolateral lesions were superior to those gained with anterodorsal lesions. The precise role of the GPe in lesioning remains to be determined. The size and location for optimal clinical results can only be determined in a systematic study with a large number of highly characterized PD patients using standardized testing, determining the lesion size and location by both true three-dimensional thin-section MRI studies and autopsy correlations.

REFERENCES

1. Alexander GE, Crutcher MD, DeLong MR. Basal ganglia-thalamocortical circuits: parallel substrates for motor, oculomotor, "prefrontal" and "limbic" functions. *Prog Brain Res* 1990;85:119–146.
2. Bakay R, DeLong M, Vitek J. Posteroventral pallidotomy for Parkinson's disease. *J Neurosurg* 1992;77: 487–488.
3. Barbeau A. Parkinson's disease: clinical features and etiopathology. In: Vinken PJ, Bruyn GW, Kiawans HL, eds. *Handbook of clinical neurology*, vol 5(49). Amsterdam: Elsevier Science, 1986;87–152.
4. Baron MS, Vitek JL, Bakay, RAE, et al. Treatment of advanced Parkinson's disease by posterior GPi pallidotomy: 1-year results of a pilot study. *Ann Neurol* 1996; 40:355–366.

5. Bergman H, Wichmann T, DeLong MR. Reversal of experimental parkinsonism by lesions of the subthalamic nucleus. *Science* 1990;249:1436–1438.

6. Blancet PJ, Boucher R, Bedard PJ. Excitotoxic lateral pallidotomy does not relieve L-dopa induced dyskinesia in MPTP parkinsonian monkeys. *Brain Res* 1994;650: 32–39.

7. Burzaco J. Stereotactic pallidotomy in extrapyramidal disorders. *Appl Neurophysiol* 1985;48:283–287.

8. Ceballos-Baumann AO, Obeso JA, Vitek JL, et al. Restoration of thalamocortical activity after posteroventral pallidotomy in Parkinson's disease. *Lancet* 1994; 344:814.

9. Cooper IS. Ligation of the anterior choroidal artery for involuntary movements of parkinsonism. *Arch Neurol* 1956;75:36–48.

10. Cooper IS, Bravo G. Chemopallidectomy and chemothalamectomy. *J Neurosurg* 1958;3:244–250.

11. DeLong MR. Primate models of movement disorders of basal ganglia origin. *Trends Neurosci* 1990;13:281–285.

12. DeLong MR, Crutcher MD, Georgopoulis AP. Primate globus pallidus and subthalamic nucleus: functional organization. *Neurophysiology* 1985;53:530–543.

13. Dogali M, Fazzini E, Kolodny E, et al. Stereotactic ventral pallidotomy for Parkinson's disease. *Neurology* 1995;45:753–761.

14. Eidelberg D, Moeller JR, Ishikawa T, et al. Regional metabolic correlates of surgical outcome following unilateral pallidotomy for Parkinson's disease. *Ann Neurol* 1996;39:450–459.

15. Fahn S, Elton RL, Members of the UPDRS Development Committee. Unified Parkinson's disease rating scale. In: Fahn S, Marsden CD, Goldstein M, Calne DB, eds. *Recent developments in Parkinson's disease.* New York: Macmillan, 1987.

16. Favre J, Taha JM, Hguyen TT, et al. Pallidotomy: a survey of current practice in North America. *Neurosurgery* 1996;39:883–890.

17. Fazzini E, Dogali M, Beric A, et al. Ventral pallidotomy operations in patients with Parkinson's plus syndrome. *Ann Neurol* 1993;34:266 (abst).

18. Fazzini E, Dogali M, Sterio D, Eidelberg D, Beric A. Stereotactic pallidotomy for Parkinson's disease: a longterm follow-up of unilateral pallidotomy. *Neurology* 1997;48:1273–1277.

19. Filion M, Tremblay L. Abnormal spontaneous activity of globus pallidus neurons in monkeys with MPTP-induced parkinsonism. *Brain Res* 1991;547:142–151.

20. Filion M, Tremblay L, Bedard PJ. Abnormal influences of passive limb movement on the activity of globus pallidus neurons in parkinsonian monkeys. *Brain Res* 1988;444:165–176.

21. Forno LS. Neuropathology of Parkinson's disease. *J Neuropathol Exp Neurol* 1996;55:259–272.

22. Fox MS, Ahlskog JE, Kelly PJ. Stereotactic ventrolateralis thalamotomy for medically refractory tremor in postlevodopa era Parkinson's disease patients. *J Neurosurg* 1991;75:723–730.

23. Freidman JH, Epstein M, Sanes JN, et al. Gamma knife pallidotomy in advanced Parkinson's disease. *Ann Neurol* 1996;39:535–538.

24. Gibb WR. The neuropathology of Parkinson disorders. In: Jankovic J, Tolosa E, eds. *Parkinson's disease and movement disorders.* Baltimore: Williams & Wilkins, 1993:205–233.

25. Gildenberg PL. The present role of stereotactic surgery in the management of Parkinson's disease. *Adv Neurol* 1984;40:447–452.

26. Gioino CG, Dierssen G, Cooper IS. The effect of subcortical lesions on production and alleviation of hemiballic or hemichoreic movements. *J Neurol Sci* 1966;3: 10–36.

27. Grafton AT, Waters C, Sutton J, et al. Pallidotomy increases activity of motor association cortex in Parkinson's disease: a positron emission tomographic study. *Ann Neurol* 1995;37:776–783.

28. Guiot G, Brion S. Traitement des mouvements anormaux par la coagulation pallidale: technique et resultats. *Rev Neurol (Paris)* 1953;89:578–580.

29. Hoover JE, Strick PL. Multiple output channels in the basal ganglia. *Science* 1993;259:819–821.

30. Hornykiewicz O, Kish SJ. Biochemical pathophysiology of Parkinson's disease. *Adv Neurol* 1986;45:19–34.

31. Hughes AJ, Daniel SE, Kilford L, Lees AJ. Accuracy of clinical diagnosis of idiopathic Parkinson's disease: a clinicopathological study of 100 cases. *J Neurol Neurosurg Psychiatry* 1992;55:181–184.

32. Hutchison WD, Lozano CA, David KD, et al. Differential neuronal activity in segments of globus pallidus in Parkinson's disease patients. *Neuroreport* 1994;5: 1533–1537.

33. Iacono RP, Shima F, Lonser RR, et al. The results, indications, and physiology of posteroventral pallidotomy for patients with Parkinson's disease. *Neurosurgery* 1995;36:1118–1127.

34. Johansson F, Malm J, Nordh E, et al. Usefulness of pallidotomy in advanced Parkinson's disease. *J Neurol Neurosurg Psychiatry* 1997;63:125–132.

35. Kelly PJ. Pallidotomy in Parkinson's disease: editorial comment. *Neurosurgery* 1995;36:1154–1157.

36. Laitinen LV. Pallidotomy for Parkinson's disease. *Neurosurg Clin North Am* 1995;6:105–112.

37. Laitinen LV, Bergenheim AT, Hariz MI. Leksell's posteroventral pallidotomy in the treatment of Parkinson's disease. *J Neurosurg* 1992;76:53–61.

38. Laitinen LV, Hariz MI. Movement disorders. In: Youmans JR, ed. *Neurological surgery.* Philadelphia: WB Saunders, 1996:3575–3609.

39. Lang AE, Lozano A, Galvez-Jimenez N, et al. Posteroventral-medial pallidotomy for late-stage Parkinson's disease: a 2-year followup. *Ann Neurol* 1996;40:538 (abstr).

40. Langston JW, Widner H, Goetz CG, et al. Core assessment program for intracerebral transplantations (CAPIT). *Mov Disord* 1992;7:2–13.

41. Larsen JP, Dupont E, Tandberg E. Clinical diagnosis of Parkinson's disease: proposal of diagnostic subgroups classified at different levels of confidence. *Acta Neurol Scand* 1994;89:242–251.

42. Lozano A, Hutchison W, Kiss Z, et al. Methods for microelectrode-guided posteroventral pallidotomy. *J Neurosurg* 1996;84:194–202.

43. Lozano AM, Lang AE, Galvez-Jimenez N, et al. Effects of GPi pallidotomy on motor function in Parkinson's disease. *Lancet* 1995;346:1383–1387.

44. Marsden CD. Late levodopa failure—pathophysiology and management. In: Poewe W, Lees AJ, eds. *20 years of madopar—new avenues.* Basel: Editiones Roche, 1993:65–76.

45. Meyers R. Surgical procedures for postencephalitic tremor with notes on the physiology of premotor fibers. *Arch Neurol Psychiatry* 1940;44:455–459.

46. Narabayashi H, Okuma T. Procaine oil blocking of the globus pallidus for the treatment of rigidity and tremor of parkinsonism. *Psychiatr Neurol Jpn* 1954;56:471–495.

47. Narabayashi H, Yokochi F, Nakajima Y. Levodopa-induced dyskinesias and thalamotomy. *J Neurol Neurosurg Psychiatry* 1984;47:831–839.

48. Parkinson J. *An essay on the shaking palsy.* London: Sherwood, Neely & Jones, 1817.

49. Rajput AH, Rozdilsky B, Rajput A. Accuracy of clinical diagnosis in parkinsonism: a prospective study. *Can J Neurol Sci* 1991;18:275–278.

50. Rand RW, Brown WJ, Stern WE. Surgical occlusion of anterior choroidal arteries in parkinsonism. *Neurology* 1956;6:390–401.

51. Rand RW, Jacques DB, Melbye RW, et al. Gamma knife thalamotomy and pallidotomy in patients with movement disorders: preliminary results. *Stereotact Funct Neurosurg* 1993;61[suppl]65–92.

52. Roberts-Warrior D, Overby AS, Orr D, et al. Postural control in patients with Parkinson's disease after pallidotomy. *Ann Neurol* 1996;40:534 (abst).

53. Rye DB, Turner RS, Vitek JL, et al. Anatomical investigations of the pallidotegmental pathway in monkey and man. In: Ohye C, ed. *The basal ganglia V.* New York: Plenum Press, 1996:59–75.

54. Schwab RS, England AC. Projection technique for evaluating surgery in Parkinson's disease. In: Gillingham FJ, Donaldson IML, eds. *Third symposium on Parkinson's disease.* Edinburgh: E&S Livingstone, 1969:152–157.

55. Schwartzman RJ, Alexander GM, Ferraro TN, Grothusen JR, Stahl SM. Cerebral metabolism of parkinsonian primates 21 days after MPTP. *Exp Neurol* 1988;102:307–313.

56. Shima F, Ishido K, Sun S, et al. Surgical control of akinesia in Parkinson's disease. *Eur Neurol* 1996;36 [suppl 1]:55–61.

57. Smith MC. Pathological findings subsequent to stereotactic lesions. *J Neurosurg* 1966;24:443–445.

58. Spiegel EA, Wycis HT. Ansotomy in paralysis agitans. *Arch Neurol Psychiatry* 1954;71:598–613.

59. Spiegel EA, Wycis HT. Thalamotomy and pallidotomy for treatment of choreic movements. *Acta Neurochir (Wien)* 1952;2:417–422.

60. Spiegel EA, Wycis HT, Baird HW. Long-range effects of electropallidoansotomy in extrapyramidal and convulsive disorders. *Neurology* 1958;8:734–740.

61. Stereo D, Beric A, Dogali M, et al. Neurophysiological properties of pallidal neurons in Parkinson's disease. *Ann Neurol* 1994;35:586–591.

62. Sutton JP, Couldwell WC, Lew MF, et al. Ventroposterior medial pallidotomy in patients with advanced Parkinson's disease. *Neurosurgery* 1995;36:1112–1117.

63. Svennilson E, Torvik A, Lowe R, et al. Treatment of parkinsonism by stereotactic thermolesions in the pallidal region: a clinical evaluation of 81 cases. *Acta Psychiatr Neurol Scand* 1960;35:358–377.

64. Vitek JL, Bakay RAE, DeLong MR. Microelectrode guided GPi pallidotomy for medically intractable Parkinson's disease. *Adv Neurol (in press).*

65. Vitek JL, Bakay RAE, Hashimoto T, et al. Microelectrode-guided pallidotomy: technical approach and application for medically intractable Parkinson's disease. *J Neurosurg* 1998;88:1027–1043.

66. Vitek JL, Baron M, Bakay RAE, et al. Pallidotomy for medically intractable Parkinson's disease: 2-year followup. *Ann Neurol* 1996;40:488 (abst).

67. White RJ, MacCarty CS, Bahn RC. Neuropathlic review of brain lesions and inherent dangers in chemopallidectomy. *AMA Arch Neurol* 1960;2:12–18.

68. Young, RF, Vermeulen SS, Grimm P, et al. Electrophysiological target localization is not required for the treatment of functional disorders. *Stereotact Func Neurosurg* 1997;66 (suppl 1):309–319.

69. Zweig RM, Jankel WR, Hedreen JC, et al. The pedunculopontine nucleus in Parkinson's disease. *Ann Neurol* 1989;26:41–46.

Pallidal Surgery for the Treatment of Parkinson's Disease and Movement Disorders, edited by
J. K. Krauss, R. G. Grossman, and J. Jankovic.
Lippincott-Raven Publishers, Philadelphia © 1998.

20B

Optimal Target of Pallidotomy: A Controversy

Lauri V. Laitinen

Sophiahemmet Hospital, S-114 86 Stockholm, Sweden

Ablative lesions in neurosurgery usually aim at interrupting neural pathways (spinal cordotomy for pain, anterior capsulotomy for obsessive-compulsive disorder) or destroying neurons [globus pallidus internus (GPi) pallidotomy, ventralis intermedius nucleus (Vim) thalamotomy]. A combination of the two may also occur. When I, together with Marwan Hariz and Tommy Bergenheim in 1985, began to test Leksell's pallidotomy, developed as early as in 1956 (15), our hypothesis was that lesions in the posteroventral pallidum might interrupt the direct γ-aminobutyric acid (GABA) ergic pathways between the posterior putamen and the medial pallidum and thus *release* the pars interna of the pallidum mediale (GPi) from inhibition caused by striatal dopamine deficiency (11). We thought that surgical lesions ought to lie so lateral that they also interrupt pallido (globus pallidus externus, or GPe)–subthalamic nucleus (STN) pathways and via the STN also favorably influence L-dopa-induced dyskinesias. Tsubokawa and Moriyasu had shown in 1975 that ventroposterolateral (VPL) pallidotomy had abolished hemiballism (16), which gave us reason to hope that Leksell's pallidotomy also would diminish or abolish the parkinsonian dyskinesias.

Leksell's pallidotomy target was mainly located in the posteroventral part of the globus pallidus (15). Its large laterality dimensions, 16 to 24 mm from the midline, were too inaccurate and unacceptable for modern stereotactic precision. The clinical effect of Leksell's pallidotomy had been good, however, and the complication rate had been low. In our study of 1992 we aimed at placing the lesion 20 mm from the midline of the third ventricle, corresponding to the average laterality of Leksell. The relative stereotactic inaccuracy caused our final laterality to vary from 18 to 21 mm when studied by postoperative computed tomography (CT). With this laterality there was a serious possibility of lesioning the optic tract. In fact, 14% of our patients had a contralateral lower central homonymous scotoma, which indicated that the dorsolateral part of the optic tract had been heated (11). We had used CT for targeting, in which the optic tract could not be visualized. As soon as our preliminary study had been completed, I began to investigate which laterality in fact was optimal. In 1994 I received a high-resolution magnetic resonance imaging (MRI) machine, which made it possible to visualize the pallidum in relation to the posterior limb of the internal capsule, the putamen, and the optic tract. Stereotactic MRI using Laitinen's Stereoadapter showed that the optic tract at the anteroposterior (Y) target level could reach as far as 21 mm lateral to the midline. To ensure that the optic tract would not be lesioned, the laterality of the target point had to be chosen as far as 24 to 27 mm from the midline. Such a lateral location corresponded to a distance of 3.5 mm medial to the posteroventral putamen.

LOGICAL ABLATIVE PALLIDOTOMY TARGET

As soon as neuroscientists in 1983 had the *N*-methyl-4-phenyl-1,2,3,6-tetrahydropyridine

(MPTP) model of PD for experimental animals (6), it was tested. Two findings were important: First, ablative surgical lesions in the STN reversed the akinesia, rigidity, and tremor produced by intracarotid injection of MPTP (3). Second, injections of excitatory amino acid antagonist (kynurenic acid) in the medial pallidum (GPi) also reversed the parkinsonian symptoms, whereas saline injection in the same target had no effect (5). As far as I know, no one has demonstrated in MPTP-treated animals that ablative lesions in the medial (GPi) pallidum are as effective as lesions in the STN. Nevertheless, probably due to misinterpretation of our paper of 1992, Mahlon DeLong and his colleagues of Emory University, believed that our target in the pallidum had been in the GPi (1). Because DeLong had an important position in American PD research, several other groups followed his line (2,7,13). Even when these groups reported positive results from unilateral pallidotomy, the real improvement seems to have been moderate, reaching a statistically significant improvement of various symptoms at a 5% probability level or close to it. The number of adverse effects of these GPi pallidotomies has been high, up to 50% (2). The effect of the GPi pallidotomy also seems to have a short-lasting effect on postural stability, freezing, and muscular pain (2). Their all-round results and the side effects seem to be similar to those seen with the medial pallidotomies of the 1950s, as reported by Claude Bertrand in 1958 (4), who, similar to all other neurosurgeons (Leksell excepted), abandoned pallidotomy and moved to thalamotomy. A similar risk for pallidotomy being questioned is discernible even today. There are alarming preliminary reports on unacceptable adverse effects after bilateral GPi pallidotomy (9).

Marsden and Obeso, in a review article on the functions of the basal ganglia in PD, were concerned about the evident discrepancy between the general concept of motor control at the pallidal level and the reported positive effects of GPi pallidotomy and VL thalamotomy (14). What they did not know was that the pallidotomy lesions reported by Laitinen et al. (11) in most patients had been lateral to the GPi. Nor did they know that successful thalamotomy prolongs the initiation and execution times of complicated

hand movements (12). Motor performance deteriorates also after bilateral GPi pallidotomy in MPTP-treated monkeys (8). Thus the early concept that intact pallidothalamocortical pathways are necessary for fast and controlled fine movements is still valid. Unilateral lesions in the GPi, ansa and fasciculus lenticularis, and ventrolateral thalamus can be tolerated by the brain relatively well; but bilateral lesions in these structures are always harmful.

These data indicate that pallidotomy lesions logically should not be placed in the GPi but in the lateralmost region of the posteroventral pallidum. Its role there would be, instead of destroying a group of neurons (GPi), to interrupt direct striatopallidal and indirect striatopallido (GPe)–subthalamic pathways and thus *release the GPi* in the same way as ablative lesions in the STN and kynurenic acid in the GPi.

VENTROPOSTEROLATERAL PALLIDOTOMY

To stress two important points, I call my approach ventroposterolateral (VPL) pallidotomy. First, the lesion ought to destroy about 4 to 6 mm of the posteroventral pallidum. It should extend to the pallidocapsular border and the base of the pallidum. Second, the lesion ought to lie as close as possible to the posteroventral putamen but not damage it. Thus I try to do everything I can to minimize damage to the GPi, and mainly interrupt striatopallidal and pallido (GPe) subthalamic pathways. This task may be difficult because the GPi and GPe seem to fuse in the posteroventral pallidum.

During 1994 to 1996 I carried out VPL pallidotomies in 200 PD patients. Fifty-one of them had staged bilateral surgeries, with a 3- to 36-month interval between the two approaches (Table 20B-1).

MRI Technique

The target is determined 1 day before surgery by stereotactic MRI using a Siemens 1-tesla Magnetom Expert machine with Laitinen's Stereoadapter (10) mounted on the patient's head. Axial

TABLE 20B-1. *Surgical results in 200 consecutive pallidotomy patients in 1994–1996*

Approach	Result (no.)			Adverse effects	Remarks
	Good	Fair	Poor		
Pallidotomy					
Right	67	8	2	—	
Left	56	2	6*	—	*One after adrenal transplantation; one dement; one MSA?
Bilateral	37*	13	1**	3***	*One side reoperation in 6 patients; **MSA? ***Brain abscess, dysphonia, impaired balance
Repallidotomy	4	2*	2	—	*One had two reoperations
Total	164 (82%)	25 (12.5%)	11 (5.5%)	3 (1.5%)	Total 264 pallidotomies

MSA, multiple systems atrophy.

scanning in 2 mm thick slices parallel to the transverse bars of the Stereoadapter with proton density parameters and coronary scanning perpendicular to the intercommissural line in a 4 mm thick slice 10 mm posterior to the anterior commissure with true inversion recovery parameters are used for visualizing the target. First, the laterality (X) and height (Z) coordinates of the target in relation to the Stereoadapter are measured from the coronary scan. The ventralmost target point lies at the bottom of the pallidum just lateral to the lateralmost extension of the disk-shaped optic tract, corresponding to a distance of 3 to 4 mm medial to the putamen (Fig. 20B-1A). Then the obtained laterality is placed on the axial scanning at the corresponding depth in relation to the midline of the third ventricle, at the corresponding anteroposterior level of the posterior margin of the ventral pallidum, which gives the anteroposterior Y coordinate of the target (Fig. 20B-1B).

Because the posterior border of the pallidum goes in an anteromedial to posterolateral direction, the Y coordinate of the target varies from 2 mm anterior to 2 mm posterior to the midcommissural point, the X coordinate from 21 to 27 mm lateral to the midline, and the Z coordinate 3 to 5 mm ventral to the intercommissural line.

Surgical Technique

Prior to surgery the patient is kept off medication for 12 hours. Stereotaxis is performed 1 day after MRI under local anesthesia with mild pain-reducing sedation. The Stereoadapter is remounted to the patient's head, and Laitinen's Stereoguide frame (10) is fixed around it on the skull. As soon as the MRI coordinates are transferred from the Stereoadapter to the frame, the former is detached. A burr hole 8 mm in diameter is placed 2.5 cm lateral to the midline, at the level of the coronary suture or just behind it. A 1.8 mm thick Laitinen-Wiksell RF electrode with an uninsulated tip 1.8 mm long is introduced toward the target under impedance monitoring. Before lesions are made, electrical stimulation of each lesion area is carried out with 6 and 60 Hz and 8 and 5 mA current, respectively. An individual lesion is produced in 1- to 2-mm steps until all parkinsonian symptoms disappear. Dyskinesias usually appear in the contralateral foot when the dorsalmost part of the target area is being lesioned and in the hand, arm, and neck when the lesion reaches the bottom of the pallidum. I believe it mandatory that the lesion reaches the base of the pallidum. The size of the lesion varies from 4 to 8 mm in dorsoventral length and 4 to 6 mm in diameter (Fig. 20B-1).

RESULTS AND ADVERSE EFFECTS

The results and side effects are shown in Table 20B-1. The assessment of the results is unconventional because my patients had been referred for surgery by several neurologists all over the world.

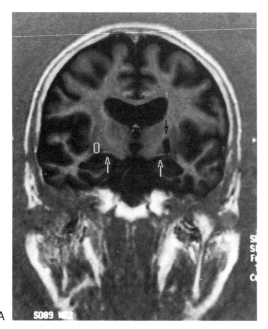
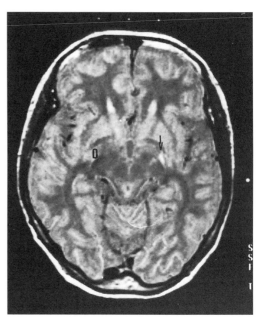

A   B

FIG. 20B-1. A. Coronary MRI scan with a large 1-year-old left pallidal lesion (*black arrow*), optic tracts (*white arrows*), and right pallidal target (*white ring*). **B.** Axial scan 4 mm below the intercommissural line with the same left pallidal lesion as in **A** (*black arrow*) and the new target for right VPL pallidotomy (*black ring*).

A "good" result means that the neurologist, the patient and family, and I all agreed that all or most parkinsonian symptoms and the activities of daily living (ADL) had remained well improved for 6 months at least. "Fair" means that the effect of surgery was positive albeit not as much as hoped (for instance, the freezings were still bothersome), and "poor" that the improvement was minimal or none. Thus 82% of the patients showed good result and 12.5% fair improvement. The akinesia, rigidity, and tremors reacted equally well to VPL pallidotomy, as did the dyskinesias and dystonias. In 5.5% the effect was poor. All 200 patients were able to leave the hospital within 24 hours after surgery. Complications were observed in three patients (1.5%). One of them developed a delayed postoperative brain abscess that was removed surgically. He then made a good general recovery with fair long-lasting alleviation of his parkinsonian symptoms. The increased dysphonia in the other patient with complications was noted several months after surgery and may have been due to the natural progression of the illness. One patient who had had a left GPi-pallido-ansotomy at Loma Linda 1 year earlier developed a severe balance disturbance 30 days after her right pallidotomy.

Repallidotomies were required quite often, usually because the first lesion lay too anterior (and dorsal) and did not reach the posteroventral border of the pallidum or because the lesion was smaller than planned. The reoperations were generally successful without increased morbidity. No patient had a visual field deficit.

CONCLUSIONS

The optimal pallidal lesion lies at the ventroposterolateral border of the globus pallidus. VPL pallidotomy is at least as effective as "Leksell's pallidotomy" in terms of relieving all parkinsonian symptoms and drug-induced dyskinesias. Adverse effects are rare. Even bilateral pallidotomy in this area can be done without marked risks.

The results indicate that VPL pallidotomy releases the medial pallidum without lesioning it (considerably). The approach can be recommended to neurosurgeons who are not satisfied with the GPi pallidotomy.

REFERENCES

1. Bakay RAE, DeLong MR, Vitek JL. Posteroventral pallidotomy for Parkinson's disease. *J Neurosurg* 1992; 77:487–488.
2. Baron MS, Vitek JL, Bakay RAE, et al. Treatment of advanced Parkinson's disease by posterior GPi pallidotomy: 1-year results of a pilot study. *Ann Neurol* 1996; 40:355–366.
3. Bergman H, Wichmann T, DeLong MR. Reversal of experimental parkinsonism by lesions of the subthalamic nucleus. *Science* 1990;249:1436–1438.
4. Bertrand CM. A pneumotaxic technique for producing localized cerebral lesions and its use in the treatment of Parkinson's disease. *J Neurosurg* 1958;15:251–264.
5. Brotchie JM, Mitchell IJ, Sambrook MA, et al. Alleviation of parkinsonism by antagonism of excitatory amino acid transmission in the medial segment of the globus pallidus in rat and primate. *Mov Disord* 1991;6: 133–138.
6. Burns RS, Chiueh CC, Markey SP, et al. A primate model of parkinsonism: selective destruction of DA neurons in the pars compacta of the substantia nigra by *n*-methyl-1,2,3,6-tetrahydropyridine. *Proc Natl Acad Sci USA* 1983;80:4546–4550.
7. Dogali M, Fazzini E, Kolodny E, et al. Stereotactic ventral pallidotomy for Parkinson's disease. *Neurology* 1995;45:753–761.
8. Guillén J, Luquin MR, Dominguez J, et al. Motor effects of posteroventral pallidotomy in MPTP-monkeys. *Mov Disord* 1996;11[suppl 1]:240.
9. Kim R, Alterman R, Kelly P, et al. Efficacy of bilateral pallidotomy. Presented at the 46th Annual Meeting of the Congress of Neurological Surgeons, Montreal, Sept. 28–Oct. 3, 1996.
10. Laitinen LV. The Laitinen system. In: Lunsford LD, ed. Modern stereotactic neurosurgery. Boston, Martinus Nijhoff, 1988:99–116.
11. Laitinen LV, Hariz MI, Bergenheim AT. Leksell's posteroventral pallidotomy in the treatment of Parkinson's disease. *J Neurosurg* 1992;76:53–61.
12. Laitinen L, Vilkki J. Measurement of parkinsonian hypokinesia with Purdue pegboard and motor reaction time tests. In: Siegfried J, ed. Parkinson's disease, vol 2. Berlin, Hans Huber, 1973;185–192.
13. Lozano A, Hutchison W, Kiss Z, et al. Methods for microelectrode-guided posteroventral pallidotomy. *J Neurosurg* 1996;84:194–202.
14. Marsden CD, Obeso JA. The functions of the basal ganglia and the paradox of stereotaxic surgery in Parkinson's disease. *Brain* 1994;117:877–897.
15. Svennilson E, Torvik A, Lowe R, Leksell L. Treatment of parkinsonism by stereotactic thermolesions in the pallidal region: a clinical evaluation of 81 cases. *Acta Psychiatr Neurol Scand* 1960;35:358–377.
16. Tsubokawa T, Moriyasu N. Lateral pallidotomy for relief of ballistic movement: its basic evidences and clinical application. *Confin Neurol* 1975;37:10–15.

Pallidal Surgery for the Treatment of Parkinson's Disease and Movement Disorders, edited by
J. K. Krauss, R. G. Grossman, and J. Jankovic.
Lippincott-Raven Publishers, Philadelphia © 1998.

20C

Optimal Target of Pallidotomy: A Controversy

*†Joachim K. Krauss and †Robert G. Grossman

*Department of Neurosurgery, Inselspital, University of Berne, 3010, Berne, Switzerland; and
†Department of Neurosurgery, Baylor College of Medicine, Houston, Texas 77030, USA

There is considerable debate as to which site within the pallidum is best suited to be lesioned by pallidotomy in patients with Parkinson's disease (PD). Should the lesion be directed primarily to abolish neuronal hyperactivity of the globus pallidus internus (GPi)? Should it involve the globus pallidus externus (GPe)? Or should it interrupt pallidal outflow? Furthermore, it is unclear whether there is one "best spot" that should be lesioned to alleviate all parkinsonian symptoms or there are different "best spots" for different parkinsonian symptoms (11). Considerations about this best spot must regard the amount of clinical benefit achieved as well as the expectation of adverse effects. The choice of a favored target is also guided by the interpretation of conceptual models of basal ganglia function and dysfunction. Recent studies have provided better understanding of the functional organization of the basal ganglia circuitry and the pathophysiological changes in PD (see Chapters 2 and 3). Nevertheless, the mechanisms by which pallidotomy improves parkinsonian symptoms and levodopa-induced dyskinesias are not fully understood (19). This scenario leaves room for different possible suggestions on the optimal target during pallidotomy.

There are several limitations to prove ultimately that one specific pallidal target is definitely better than another at this time, both with regard to the data available so far and with regard to contemporary operative and imaging techniques. With current lesioning techniques it appears not to be possible to place lesions exclusively (a) in distinct pallidal subterritories (or networks) such as the sensorimotor GPi without possible overlap with other territories and (b) in isolated pallidal pathways such as the ansa lenticularis. With regard to GPe pallidotomy, how far do the lesions extend into the lateral posteroventral GPi? How accurate are current imaging techniques such as magnetic resonance (MR) imaging for defining precisely the extension of a small lesion?

LOCATION AND SIZE OF PALLIDAL LESIONS IN PREVIOUS STUDIES

There is general agreement that pallidotomy should involve the posteroventral portion of the pallidum, among proponents of both GPi and GPe pallidotomy (1,10,11,17,22). Lesions located more anteriorly and dorsally are thought to be less effective for the treatment of the motor symptoms of PD. This notion appears to be supported by some clinical observations from early studies. Spiegel and colleagues, for example, achieved better control of tremor when they placed a second lesion more posteriorly in the pallidum in PD patients who had undergone anterodorsal lesioning previously (21). Leksell's group apparently achieved better clinical outcomes in PD patients when the lesion was placed more ventrally and more posteriorly (22). There is a paucity of pathoanatomical studies in patients who underwent pallidotomy. The evaluation of historical cases is limited, in particular with regard to clinicopathological correlations concerning pallidal subterritories. One postmortem study of a PD patient who underwent successful microelectrode-guided pallidotomy 7 months before his death demonstrated a radio-frequency lesion encompassing a large portion of the caudolateral GPi extending into the Gpe anterodorsally (4). So far, no comprehensive contemporary pathoanatomical studies on the correlation between the location of pallidal lesions and clinical outcome have been available. Precise delineation of the three-dimensional shape and extension of such a lesion within the complex anatomy of the pallidum might be difficult with conventional techniques.

There is also only limited information available on clinicopathological correlations with regard to the size and location of stereotactic pallidal lesions as assessed by contemporary imaging techniques. The size and site of the pallidal lesion did not correlate with clinical outcome in a completed tomography (CT) study of a small series of PD patients after pallidotomy (6).

We have investigated early (1–3 days) and late (6 months) postoperative MR findings and their correlation with clinical outcome in 36 PD patients after unilateral microelectrode-guided posteroventral lateral GPi pallidotomy (12). Microelectrode guidance was used to place the lesion at the ventral pallidal border but not for targeting movement-related cells specifically. All except two patients experienced moderate to marked clinical improvement at the 6-month follow-up. Clinical outcome was assessed with a prospective protocol including independent evaluation in defined "off" and "on" states according to the Unified Parkinson's Disease Rating Scale (UPDRS) (15). The mean motor UPDRS "off" score improved from 58.1 ± 13.8 preoperatively to 33.0 ± 9.8 ($p < 0.0001$), the mean UPDRS Activities of Daily Living (ADL) "off" score from 31.4 ± 6.1 to 18.2 ± 4.6 ($p < 0.0001$), the bradykinesia "off" score for contralateral extremities (Parts 23–26) from 11.6 ± 2.3 to 5.6 ± 2.5 ($p < 0.0001$), and the percentage of awake time with dyskinesias from 37.5 ± 21.4 to 18.1 ± 15.7 ($p < 0.0001$). No patient had a visual field defect, but one patient complained of "greenish" vision postoperatively. The early-phase lesions were composed of three concentric zones. The mean lesion volume was 262.2 ± 116.3 mm³. The lesion, as defined by the outer zone, involved the GPi in all cases. It was located

within the lateral portion of the GPi in immediate proximity to the posterior limb of the internal capsule. In 11 patients (32%) the lesion was completely within the GPi (Fig. 20C-1); in 16 patients (47%) the major portion of the lesion was located in the GPi but also involved the GPe to a minor extent; in 4 patients (12%) approximately half of the lesion was located in the GPi and the other half in the GPe; and in 2 patients (6%) the major portion of the lesion was located in the GPi but it also encroached on the internal capsule to a minor extent. In one patient the major part of the lesion involved the GPe. Commonly, the medial margin of the lesion was located just above the most lateral aspect of the optic tract or slightly lateral to it. The distance from the most inferior margin of the outer lesion zone to the optic tract or the choroidal fissure ranged between 0 and 1.5 mm in 27 cases (79%) (Fig. 20C-2) and between 2 and 5 mm in 6 cases (18%). Edema of the optic tract was noted in 11 cases.

Late-phase MR studies were available in 32 patients. Clearly discernible lesions were identified in 29 of those patients, whereas in 3 patients the lesion had disappeared. The lesion in all but one of the other patients was located in the posteroventral GPi. The mean volume of the late-phase lesions was 22 ± 28.8 mm³. The lesion was located completely in the GPi in 23 patients (79%); it was located mainly in the GPi but also involved the GPe in 2 patients (7%); and it extended slightly into the internal capsule in 3 patients (10%). In one patient it was confined to the GPe. This was the patient in whom the major portion of the early-phase lesion had already involved the GPe. The distance from the inferior border of the lesion to the optic tract or the choroidal fissure ranged from 0.5 to 2.0 mm in 22 patients (Fig. 20C-3) (76%) and from 3 to 5 mm in 6 patients (21%). One of the patients with only limited benefit was thought to have striatonigral degeneration in retrospect; and the other patient was the 49-year-old woman with typical PD, in whom the late-phase lesion was confined to the GPe. In the other patients, in general, there were no correlations between clinical outcome measures (subitems of the UPDRS) and lesion size or location, for example, lesion location in the GPi only versus lesion location in the GPi and GPe. Contralateral dyskinesias tended

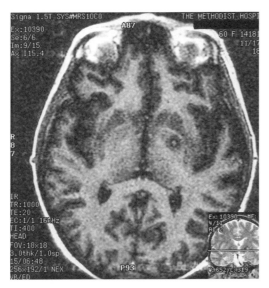

FIG. 20C-1. Axial inversion recovery (1000/20) MR image of a 60-year-old patient 1 day after a left-sided pallidotomy showing the pallidal lesion confined to the globus pallidus internus. (From ref. 12, with permission.)

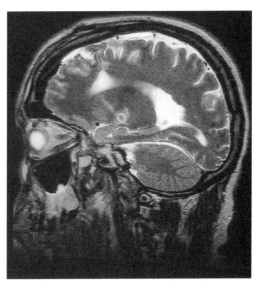

FIG. 20C-2. Sagittal T2-weighted MR image of a 40-year-old patient 2 days postoperatively demonstrating the proximity of the pallidal lesion to the optic tract. (From ref. 12, with permission.)

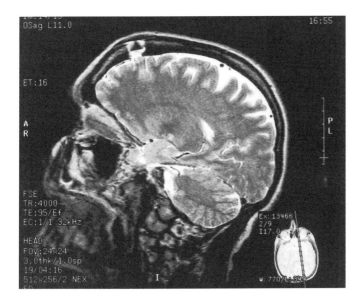

FIG. 20C-3. Sagittal T2-weighted MR image of a 51-year-old patient obtained 6 months after posteroventral lateral GPi pallidotomy showing the relation of the hyperintense lesion to the choroidal fissure and optic tract. (From ref. 12, with permission.)

to be more often abolished or almost abolished when the distance to the optic tract was less than 2 mm ($p = 0.11$).

The small range of variation in clinical outcomes and in the location of the core of the lesion may explain the lack of significant correlations between clinical outcome and lesion size and location in this study. On the other hand, these results indicate that when a lesion is precisely located at a strategic point its size may not be of primary relevance with regard to good clinical outcome. Remarkably, those three patients in whom no lesion was detectable at the 6-month follow-up had a good and stable clinical benefit that was comparable to that of the other patients. The location of the lesion in our series—in particular, the proximity to the optic tract and the choroidal fissure—indicates that in most patients the lesion also involved the ventral pallidal border zone or subpallidal region in addition to the posteroventral lateral GPi. Unfortunately, the spatial resolution of current MR technology does not allow us to determine precisely which pallidal pathways are affected and to which extent they are damaged by a small pallidal lesion.

A CASE FOR POSTEROVENTRAL LATERAL GPI PALLIDO-SUBPALLIDOTOMY

The optimal target for pallidotomy remains to be defined. We propose the choice of the posteroventral lateral GPi and the adjacent subpallidal region as the appropriate target site. Extension of the lesion to the subpallidal region may involve various pallidal pathways that are thought to be pivotal in the mediation of pathological activity in PD. Similar to lesioning the zona incerta or the fields of Forel in the subthalamic area (13,20), a small lesion in the subpallidal region affecting the tightly packed "motor" fibers might be as effective for ameliorating parkinsonian symptoms as a larger lesion located more dorsally affecting neurons distributed over a wider area.

With regard to anatomical studies lesions at the most ventral and posterior GPi can affect fibers from both pallidothalamic pathways: the ansa and the fasciculus lenticularis. Experimental studies in primates have shown that ventral lesions in the

caudal GPi produce degeneration in both projections (3). Subpallidal lesions might also affect pallidal outflow to the brainstem, in particular to the pedunculopontine nucleus. Another important aspect relates to pallidal inflow. Lesions in the posteroventral lateral GPi and the adjacent region could also involve the overactive excitatory pathway from the subthalamic nucleus to the GPi. Little is known about the detailed anatomy and its variations of this pathway in humans. In one study, high-frequency electrical stimulation of the STN appeared to have a slightly greater effect on parkinsonian motor symptoms than GPi stimulation (18). It is unclear whether this could be related to modifying the STN outflow to the substantia nigra pars reticulata. If not, lesioning of the STN–GPi pathway and the posteroventral pallidum might be an approach that could combine the advantages of targeting the STN and the GPi. The potential of increased dyskinesias secondary to reducing the activity of the STN–GPi outflow could be mitigated by concomitant reduction of GPi activity.

ANATOMICAL AND PHYSIOLOGICAL CONSIDERATIONS
Globus Pallidus Internus

Although most functional neurosurgeons would agree on the relevance of lesioning the posteroventral GPi, no consensus would be achieved on responding to the question how large the lesion should be and how far it should extend along the axis of the pallidum. The GPi is composed of two segments—an internal segment (GPi,i) and an external segment (GPi,e)—separated by a medullary lamina. According to microelectrode recording studies, these segments appear to have different neurophysiological properties (see Chapter 9). The firing rate and the degree of discharge of GPi,i neurons tend to be higher than those of GPi,e neurons. Furthermore, more "tremor cells" appear to be located in the ventral GPi. These findings suggest that lesioning the GPi,i may be more crucial. With this regard microelectrode recording is definitely helpful. Should the GPi,e also be included in the lesions? Most neurosurgeons use lesion-making electrodes with uninsulated tips of 2 or 3 mm length that create cylindrically shaped lesions. When a lesion is composed of multiple coagulations, with the most proximal coagulation made at 4 mm or even at 6 mm above the pallidal base, such a lesion inevitably includes the anterior and dorsal portions of the GPi. Another question yet to be answered is whether GPi lesions are more specific and more effective when they are targeted to the sensorimotor pallidum as identified by microelectrode recording. The concept of the sensorimotor GPi is based on the identification of neurons that change their activity upon active or passive movements of contralateral or ipsilateral joints. The rationale that it is beneficial to target such cells has been challenged (8). Indeed, movement-related cells may be found throughout the GPi that would require multiple small coagulations adding to a composite large lesion, which again would extend into the anterior and dorsal GPi regions. So far, it remains unclear whether there are more or less distinct pallidal domains serving sensorimotor, cognitive, or behavioral functions or whether these functions are mediated via interwoven parallel distributed neuronal networks. There is some support for the latter. Pallidal neurons that modulate their discharge activities upon mental activity have been found in GPi regions together with movement-responsive cells (7). Furthermore, we have observed that macrostimulation at a frequency of 100 Hz consistently elicits intense emotional responses—a feeling of fear and discomfort—in the posteroventral GPi. Clearly, further studies are needed for a better understanding of functional pallidal organization.

Globus Pallidus Externus

The posteroventral GPe has also been advocated as a target for pallidotomy (16,17). Clinical and experimental observations, however, raise some doubts whether the GPe alone or the GPe–STN pathway are suitable targets for the treatment of Parkinson's disease. Akinetic-rigid syndromes have been reported repeatedly to be associated with pallidal or pallidoputaminal lesions (9,14). So far, however, both the site of the lesion within the pallidum that might result in akinetic syndromes and the pathomechanisms have remained unclear.

The case of a 45-year-old woman with a hypokinetic-rigid parkinsonian syndrome due to hypoxic putaminopallidal lesions has been reported (5). Interestingly, MR studies showed that the GPe was involved bilaterally, but the GPi regions were largely spared. Parkinsonism improved markedly after bilateral GPi pallidotomy. It was suggested that parkinsonism in this patient was caused by (a) the GPe lesions leading to deafferentation of the STN from GABAergic inflow resulting in increased activity of the GPi, and (b) the putaminal lesions leading to decreased GABAergic transmission through the direct putamino–GPi pathway, resulting also in increased activity of the GPi.

Could GPe pallidotomy be beneficial for levodopa-induced dyskinesias? Such an effect might be more consistent with the current model of basal ganglia organization. Experimental animal studies, however, suggest that even the contrary might be the case. Excitotoxic GPe pallidotomy did not relieve levodopa-induced dyskinesias in MPTP-lesioned monkeys but, rather, exacerbated them (2). Remarkably, another MPTP parkinsonian levodopa-naive animal in whom the pallidotomy involved both the GPe and the GPi later developed ipsilateral but not contralateral levodopa-induced dyskinesias.

Pallidal Pathways

Theoretically, isolated lesioning of pallidal pathways might be an interesting alternative with regard to the considerations discussed earlier. This would be of special interest if altered pallidal firing patterns contribute more to the pathophysiology of PD than increased firing of GPi neurons per se. However, such lesions are barely possible with current techniques of lesioning. It has been shown that the pallidal base is not a sharp boundary between the globus pallidus and adjacent pathways (23). Attempts of "selective ansotomy" or subpallidotomy would be accompanied by a higher risk of lesioning the optic tract. Further studies on the microanatomy of the afferent and efferent pallidal pathways are needed, as knowledge about their three-dimensional relations is insufficient. Furthermore, it would be interesting to know the distribution of axons related to motor activity and to other functions within pallidal afferents and efferents.

PERSPECTIVES

There is a need for further clinical studies with adequate study designs to compare and evaluate clinical outcome with regard to different target sites in the pallidum. Technical improvements are necessary for more precise placement of the lesion and better postoperative imaging of the lesions and their relation to various pallidal subterritories and pathways.

REFERENCES

1. Baron MS, Vitek JL, Bakay RAE, et al. Treatment of advanced Parkinson's disease by posterior GPi pallidotomy: 1-year results of a pilot study. *Ann Neurol* 1996;40: 355–366.
2. Blanchet PJ, Boucher R, Bédard PJ. Excitotoxic lateral pallidotomy does not relieve L-dopa-induced dyskinesia in MPTP parkinsonian monkeys. *Brain Res* 1994;650: 32–39.
3. Carpenter MB. Anatomical organization of the corpus striatum and related nuclei. In: Yahr MD, ed. *The basal ganglia.* New York: Raven Press, 1976:1–36.
4. DeLong MR, Vitek JL, Rye D, et al. Comparison of physiological mapping, magnetic resonance imaging, and histologic lesion in a patient who underwent microelectrode-guided pallidotomy for Parkinson's disease. *Ann Neurol* 1995;38:298.
5. Goto S, Kunitoku N, Soyama N, et al. Posteroventral pallidotomy in a patient with parkinsonism caused by hypoxic encephalopathy. *Neurology* 1997;49:707–710.
6. Hariz MI. Correlation between clinical outcome and size and site of the lesion in computed tomography guided thalamotomy and pallidotomy. *Stereotact Funct Neurosurg* 1990;54/55:172–185.
7. Hutchison WD, Lozano AM, Taub E, et al. Cognitive modulation of human globus pallidus (GP) neurons. *Soc Neurosci* 1996;22:118.
8. Iacono RP. Stereotactic pallidotomy [Letter]. *J Neurosurg* 1996;85:987–988.
9. Jellinger K. Exogenous lesions of the pallidum. In: Vinken PJ, Bruyn GW, Klawans HL, eds. *Handbook of clinical neurology,* vol 5 (49). Amsterdam: Elsevier, 1986:465–492.
10. Johansson F, Malm J, Nordh E, Hariz M. Usefulness of pallidotomy in advanced Parkinson's disease. *J Neurol Neurosurg Psychiatry* 1997;62:125–132.
11. Kopyov O, Jacques D, Duma C, et al. Microelectrode-guided posteroventral medial radiofrequency pallidotomy for Parkinson's disease. *J Neurosurg* 1997;87:52–59.
12. Krauss JK, Desaloms JM, Lai EC, King DE, Jankovic J, Grossman RG. Microelectrode-guided posteroventral pallidotomy for treatment of Parkinson's disease: postoperative magnetic resonance imaging analysis. *J Neurosurg* 1997;87:358–367.
13. Krauss JK, Mohadjer M, Nobbe F, Mundinger F. The treatment of posttraumatic tremor by stereotactic surgery. *J Neurosurg* 1994;80:810–819.
14. Krauss JK, Mohadjer M, Wakhloo AK, Mundinger F. Dystonia and akinesia due to pallidoputaminal lesions after disulfiram intoxication. *Mov Disord* 1991;6: 166–170.
15. Lai EC, Jankovic J, Krauss JK, et al. Efficacy of unilateral microelectrode-guided posteroventral pallidotomy in the treatment of advanced Parkinson's disease (*submitted*).
16. Laitinen LV. Pallidotomy for Parkinson's disease. *Neurosurg Clin North Am* 1995:6:105–112.
17. Laitinen LV, Bergenheim AT, Hariz MI. Leksell's posteroventral pallidotomy in the treatment of Parkinson's disease. *J Neurosurg* 1992;76:53–61.
18. Limousin P, Greene J, Pollak P, Rothwell J, Benabid AL, Frackowiak R. Changes in cerebral activity pattern due to subthalamic nucleus or internal pallidum stimulation in Parkinson's disease. *Ann Neurol* 1997;42: 283–291.
19. Marsden CD, Obeso JA. The functions of the basal ganglia and the paradox of stereotaxic surgery in Parkinson's disease. *Brain* 1994;117:877–897.
20. Mundinger F. Stereotaxic interventions on the zona incerta area for treatment of extrapyramidal motor disturbances and their results. *Confin Neurol* 1965;26: 222–230.
21. Spiegel EA, Wycis HT, Baird HW. Long-range effects of electro-pallidoansotomy in extrapyramidal and convulsive disorders. *Neurology* 1958;8:734–740.
22. Svennilson E, Torvik A, Lowe R, Leksell L. Treatment of parkinsonism by stereotactic thermolesions in the pallidal region. *Acta Psychiatr Neurol Scand* 1960;35: 358–377.
23. Taha JM, Favre J, Baumann TK, Burchiel KJ. Functional anatomy of the pallidal base in Parkinson's disease. *Neurosurgery* 1996;39:1164–1168.

Pallidal Surgery for the Treatment of Parkinson's Disease and Movement Disorders, edited by J. K. Krauss, R. G. Grossman, and J. Jankovic. Lippincott-Raven, Philadelphia © 1998.

21

Neurosurgical Alternatives for Treatment of Parkinson's Disease

Richard D. Penn

Department of Neurosurgery, Rush-Presbyterian-St. Luke's Medical Center, Chicago, Illinois 60612, USA

Why would a book on pallidal surgery include a chapter on alternatives? The reason might be to list all the older, discarded stereotactic procedures so pallidotomy would clearly be shown to be the best currently available surgical approach, which it is. Another reason might be to show the obvious limitations the procedure has for treating the basic pathological processes that produce the symptoms of parkinsonism. Is there another surgical approach that deals with the progressive degeneration of neurons and the subsequent loss of autonomic, cognitive, and motor function? In this chapter, I address not the past failed surgical procedures but, rather, the new emerging ones that use cellular replacement and growth factors to deal with the basic disease process. Enough experience now exists to suggest that neural transplantation may be equal to pallidotomy in terms of results. If it were to become practical, it would be a serious alternative. The related approach of using growth factors is just beginning to be tested clinically but might become of great importance during the next decade.

The limitations of pallidotomy have been discussed in detail in early chapters. From a conceptual standpoint, it is difficult to understand how removing the major outflow of the basal ganglia is able to improve the patient's best motor function. Indeed, pallidotomy does not improve best performance, as no significant improvements are seen during the "on" periods when medicine is having its maximal effect. The major effect of pallidotomy during "on" periods is to decrease dopamine-induced dyskinesias. This is what one would predict from a destructive lesion that removes the abnormal output from the basal ganglia produced by a too high level of tonic dopaminergic stimulation. The failure of the "on" motor performance to improve is illustrated in Fig. 21-1 in which a simple motor task of moving the arm to a target as fast as possible is shown for normal subjects, those with mild Parkinson's disease, and before and after pallidotomy (Fig. 21-1) (16). Looking at Fig. 21-1, the profound effect that Parkinson's disease has on speed of movement is evident. Early Parkinson's patients are moderately impaired, and later-stage patients (Hoehn and Yahr stage III) are markedly impaired. This slowness remains after pallidotomy. Movements are smoother after pallidotomy, as they are not disrupted by dyskinesias, but they are not quicker. The point is that pallidotomy is a palliative procedure: It stops dyskinesias and improves "off"-period motor function, but it does not restore function beyond what dopamine can do. If it did, dopamine treatment could be reduced, but clinically this is not what happens. Most patients remain on the same or only slightly lower dopamine dosage.

An important unanswered question is whether pallidotomy slows the course of the disease. A study to answer this question is difficult to perform because unoperated controls would be needed, as would many patients and a long ob-

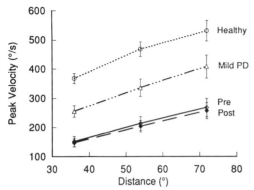

FIG. 21-1. Comparison of movement speeds to three target distances in age-matched normals and mild and severely affected parkinsonian patients (before and after pallidotomy). The postoperative pallidotomy patients remain markedly impaired. Peak velocity is not improved by a GPi lesion. Note that the patients are on optimal medications and are tested in the "on" state. (From ref. 16, with permission.)

servation time. Even if the rate of progression were slowed, the legitimate question could be raised: Is the degenerative process continuing but just not observed because the outflow from the basal ganglia has been disrupted? The most that can be said at the moment is that there is no obvious reason why a localized destructive lesion should stop or slow down a neurodegenerative process.

The desire to "fix" the problem rather than mask it is what has given the impetus to new therapies, namely neurotrophic factor infusion and transplantation. Medical treatments have been tried based on the antioxidant and free radical scavenger properties of deprenyl and vitamin E (18). Vitamin E had no effect on disease progression. Deprenyl did slow the time to treatment by L-dopa, suggesting an effect on progression. Unfortunately, the dopaminergic properties of deprenyl could cause a similar finding. On the other hand, medications may make the disease progress faster. Tissue culture and animal experiments demonstrate that L-dopa treatment in itself may cause striatal cell death.

Some neurologists argue that L-dopa therapy is so potentially toxic it should be delayed as long as clinically possible (5). The point is that much laboratory data and some clinical studies suggest that the rate of deterioration in Parkinson's disease can be changed for better or worse by treatment.

GLIAL-DERIVED NEUROTROPHIC FACTOR

It is within this context that the discovery, characterization, and production of a glial-derived neurotrophic factor (GDNF) was greeted with considerable excitement (20). GDNF has been found to be a potent neurotrophic factor that both protects dopaminergic neurons from neurotoxic damage (3) and potentiates dopaminergic function (11) (Fig. 21-2). It has little effect on serotoninergic or γ-aminobutyric acid (GABA)ergic cells. During postnatal development in rats, GDNF messenger RNA (mRNA) is expressed in the substantia nigra, so it is thought to have an important role in neurodevelopment (17). A high-affinity receptor system for GDNF has been identified, the GDNF receptor-alpha (9,19).

The potential for treating Parkinson's disease with GDNF has been suggested from the effects it produces in animal models. When GDNF is administered by injection into the striatum it protects the rat from 6-hydroxydopamine (6-OHDA)-induced substantia nigra damage (3). The mechanism for this protective action against a potent neurotoxic agent is not known. The most compelling data suggesting that GDNF can alleviate parkinsonian symptoms comes from monkey experiments on unilateral parkinsonian symptoms induced by carotid injection of the neurotoxin N-methyl-4-phenyl-1,2,3,6-tetrahydropyridine (MPTP) (7). If GDNF is injected into the substantia nigra in a hemiparkinsonian monkey, motor and behavioral deficits are relieved dramatically. These improvements begin a week after injection, reach a maximum at 2 to 3 weeks and then regress. Similar effects are seen with a single bolus in-

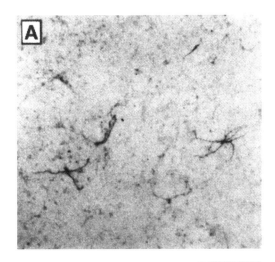

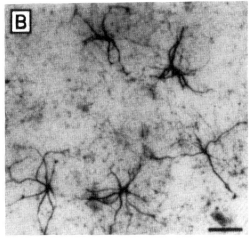

FIG. 21-2 A and B. Effect of GDNF on the morphology of TH+ neurons. (From ref. 20, with permission.)

traventricular injection. Figure 21-3A shows the time course of the change in symptoms after intraventricular injection, and Figure 21-3B shows the percentage change (7).

Where GDNF is acting and how it gets to the correct receptors have yet to be established. The presumption is that the nigral dose acts locally or indirectly on the striatum. How GDNF gets to the target tissue from cerebrospinal fluid (CSF) is a mystery. It is a large protein and is not expected to diffuse through neural tissue easily. Although the precise mechanism of action of GDNF on the MPTP hemiparkinsonian mon-

keys is not fully understood, the clinical effect is robust.

Recombinant techniques have allowed the manufacture of GDNF protein in large amounts for human clinical trials in Parkinson's disease. After appropriate toxicological and pharmacokinetic studies were performed on this formulation of GDNF, a trial was begun. Because this GDNF preparation is not stable in a drug pump and direct tissue perfusion is difficult, the intraventricular route using a reservoir system with a bacteriostatic filter was employed. Stereotactic placement is used to put a catheter in the lateral ventricle. Normal patterns of CSF flow then distribute GDNF throughout the ventricular system and eventually to the brainstem. This phase I study will look at dose response and side effects only. It will take several more years of clinical research to determine if GDNF has significant dopaminergic-stimulating effects, indicated by a reduced need for L-dopa, or slowing the rate of deterioration in Parkinson's disease.

The route of GDNF administration in the trial may not be optimal. Using the CSF flow to deliver a neurotrophic factor means that it is distributed throughout the neuraxis rather than to a particular target. When nerve growth factor (NGF) was given intraventricularly in a study on Alzheimer's disease, it caused severe dysesthetic pain (15), most likely due to stimulation of sympathetic fiber outgrowth around the dorsal area of the spinal cord (21). To avoid this effect, intraparenchymal delivery of NGF may be necessary. If GDNF has similar unwanted side effects, it also might have to be delivered into tissue, which would require precise stereotactic targeting, similar to that used for pallidotomy.

An important alternative to the use of a pump or catheter system to deliver neurotransmitter or neurotrophic agents into the brain is the use of encapsulated cells. Semipermeable membranes that allow only low- to moderate-molecular-weight compounds to reach the cells can protect xenografted cells from immunological detection and destruction (Fig. 21-4) (1). Experiments in animals and now humans have demonstrated

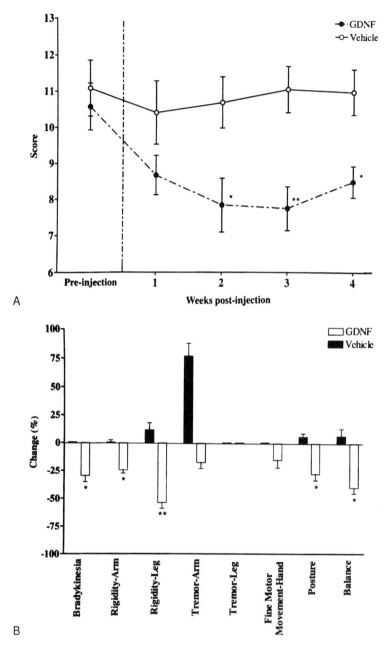

FIG. 21-3. A: Behavioral response to GDNF administration for the seven vehicle recipients. **B:** Significant alleviation of bradykinesia, rigidity, posture, and balance was seen in the GDNF recipients. (From ref. 7, with permission.)

that such protected cells can live for many months and produce neurotrophic factors (2). Because cells can be made to express more than one protein, multiple growth factors can be given by a single encapsulated system. The cap-

sule could be placed in CSF spaces or intraparenchymally depending on the target site and the diffusion of the neurotrophic factors. In animal models of Parkinson's disease, cells placed in the striatum that produce dopamine can re-

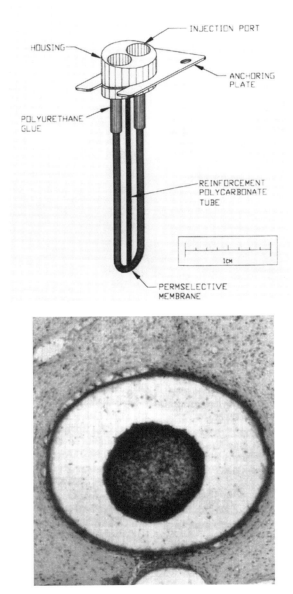

FIG. 21-4. U-Shaped device and the striatum of a hemiparkinsonian monkey. (From ref. 1, with permission.)

verse parkinsonian symptoms (1). In the quinolinic model of Huntington's disease, ciliary neurotrophic factor (CNTF) producing cells have a strong neuroprotective effect when placed in the striatum (4). The major disadvantage to these cellular systems is that the cells may not live long-term or express the programmed proteins.

Another problem is that, once implanted, the dose cannot be controlled. Devices that could be reloaded with cells on a periodic basis may solve some of these difficulties in the future.

Neither the infusion of neurotrophic factors by pump or by cellular systems is ready to replace ablative procedures for Parkinson's disease. Much work is needed before these techniques can be considered a possible alternative to pallidal surgery.

NEUROTRANSPLANTATION

Neurotransplantation using human fetal tissue is another alternative for treatment of Parkinson's disease. A book on pallidotomy is not the place to review the complex and controversial history of neurotransplantation for Parkinson's disease, so only the major implications of this work can be mentioned. The review of fetal transplants by Olanow et al. should be consulted for details (14).

What is becoming clear after considerable years of study is that the clinical results of human fetal transplantation are steadily improving as each of the technical problems has been addressed in the laboratory and the results applied to human implants. Table 21-1 shows this pattern, as benefits shift from none to mild to moderate in successive studies. Few or no routine effects were noted in the first transplant studies (12). In the last series by Freeman et al., all four patients had significant improvement in the total United Parkinson's Disease Rating Scale (UPDRS) and the Schwab and England disability during "off" periods, their percentage time "on" increased, and dyskinesias decreased (6). Equally impressive are the results of the Madrid transplant group on ten patients followed for a 5-year period (13). They employed an open operation, creating a cavity in the caudate for blocks of human fetal tissue. No improvement was seen for 6 months; then stepwise over the next 3 years the patients improved. In these patients the levodopa dose was decreased 64%, the "on" phase during the day went from 39% to 72%, and dyskinesias decreased. The peak improvement in the "off" UPDRS score was a striking 46%. During the last 2 years of the 5-year follow-up after implant, mild deterioration was seen. Figure 21-5 provides the patient averages for the UPDRS scores and percentage of time "on." The improvements are much greater than these same investigators found when adrenal medullary tissue alone or in combination with peripheral nerve tissue was used for the transplant.

Enough evidence now exists to state that transplanted human fetal tissue survives long term (Fig. 21-6) and is definitely beneficial to Parkinson's disease patients. Of course, many issues must be resolved to produce the most beneficial results. How old should the fetal tissue be, how should it be stored, should a solid graft or suspension be used, how many fetuses should be used, where should the tissue be placed in the striatum, and how should immunosuppression be managed? These factors are likely to be critical to optimum outcome; currently, they have been solved so that acceptable results are being seen in current implant patients.

A number of practical and ethical concerns may limit fetal transplantation. Harvesting enough appropriate tissue for transplant is a major logistical problem. This situation would be improved if fetal tissue can be safely preserved, and many laboratories are working on cellular preservation techniques. Ethical issues have been raised and strict guidelines established for experimentation in the United States and many other countries. However, these guidelines will never satisfy those who oppose abortion on religious grounds. How these views will limit the use of transplantation remains to be seen. Using xenograft tissue for transplant may be an alternative that avoids these ethical issues. However, the immunological response of the host to a xenograft in the brain has yet to be overcome, and the animal sources of fetal material must be proved to be of low risk for transmissible disease, especially retroviral infections (8).

PALLIDAL SURGERY VERSUS NEUROTRANSPLANTATION

The issue is which of the surgical approaches for Parkinson's disease can be improved the most. Does destroying a major output of the basal ganglia provide as much clinical gain as trying to improve basal ganglia function?

TABLE 21-1. Published outcomes of fetal transplantation

Study	No. of patients	Follow-up period (months)	CsA	Type of graft	Donor age (weeks PC)	No. of donors	Bilateral graft	Site	Benefit[a] None	Benefit[a] Mild	Benefit[a] Mod	Decreased levodopa (%)	FD uptake[b] (PET)
Lindvall et al.	2	6	Yes	Susp	7–9	4	No	Ant. P+C	0	2	0	0	−
Lindvall et al.	2	5, 14	Yes	Susp	6–7	4	No	P	0	0	2	0	+
Lindvall et al.	2	36	Yes	Susp	6–7	4	No	P	0	0	2	100	++
Freed et al.	2	12–33	4/7	Solid	5–6	1	No	C+P	1	0	1	39	NA
	5			Solid	5–6	1	Yes	P	0	2	3		
Spencer et al.	4	4–18	Yes	Solid	5–9	1	No	C	1	3	0	24	ND
Perchanski et al.	2	10, 17	Yes	Susp	6–8	2–3	No	C+P	0	0	2	0, 19	++
Widner et al.	2	12, 24	Yes	Susp	6–8	6–8	Yes	P/C+P	0	0	2	0–70	++
Freeman et al.	4	6	Yes	Solid	6.5–9	6–8	Yes	Post. P	0	0	4	0	++

[a] Estimates based on clinical reports.

[b] −, no benefit; +, increased uptake; ++, markedly increased uptake; ND, not done; NA, not available; ant. P, anterior putamen; C, caudate; CsA, cyclosporin A; FD, fluorodopa; Mod, moderate; P, putamen; post. P, posterior putamen; PC, post conception; PET, positron emission tomography; Susp, suspension.

From ref. 14, with permission.

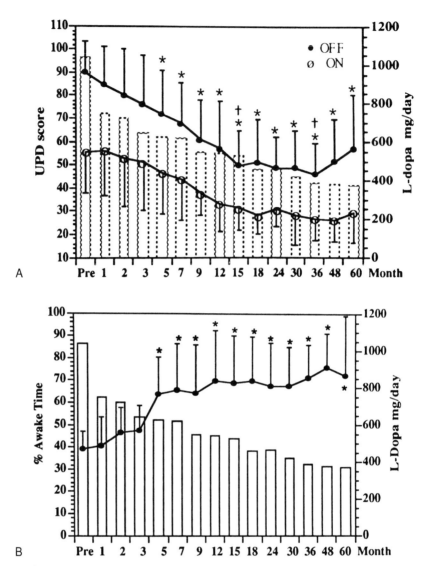

FIG. 21-5. A: Overall progress in parkinsonian symptomatology from presurgery to 60 months after surgery according to the UPDRS score. **B:** Mean percentage of awake time spent in the "on" phase. (From ref. 13, with permission.)

Another question is whether neurotransplantation truly slows the progress of the disease and provides new tissue to replace damaged tissue. Unfortunately, the mechanism by which fetal cells produce improvement in humans is not clear (14). The original concept was that the fetal cells would produce dopamine and create synapses thereby replacing dying host cells. Although some evidence from autopsy studies supports this view (10), it is still possi-

ble that the major effects are due to neurotrophic factor production or other modifications of the host brought about by the structural damage from implantation or inflammation. The increased dopamine metabolism seen on positron emission tomography scans in transplanted patients could be surviving and integrated fetal tissue or the host response to that tissue. Understanding how fetal tissue transplantation works will eventually lead to an ac-

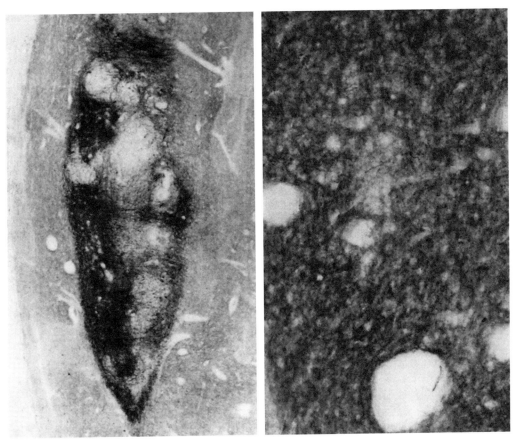

FIG. 21-6. Survival of a fetal nigral graft in a human brain. (From ref. 14, with permission.)

curate assessment of how much the technique can be improved. For the present, many more centers can do pallidal surgery than human fetal transplants or perform other novel techniques, so at least for a while pallidal surgery will remain the major surgical approach to Parkinson's disease. What the long term holds is uncertain.

REFERENCES

1. Aebischer P, Goddard M, Signore A, Timpson R. Functional recovery in hemiparkinsonian primates transplanted with polymer-encapsulated PC12 cells. *Exp Neurol* 1994;126:151–158.
2. Aebischer P, Schlup M, Déglon N, et al. Intrathecal delivery of CNTF using encapsulated genetically modified xenogeneic cells in amyotrophic lateral sclerosis patients. *Nat Med* 1996;2:696–699.
3. Choi-Lundberg D, Lin Q, Chang Y, et al. Dopaminergic neurons protected from degeneration by GDNF gene therapy. *Science* 1997;275:838–841.
4. Emerich D, Winn S, Hantraye P, et al. Protective effect of encapsulated cells producing neurotrophic factor CNTF in a monkey model of Huntington's disease. *Nature* 1997;386:395–399.
5. Fahn S, Bressman S. Should levodopa therapy for parkinsonism be started early or late? Evidence against early treatment. *Can J Neurol Sci* 1984;11 [suppl]: 200–205.
6. Freeman T, Olanow C, Hauser R, et al. Bilateral fetal nigral transplantation into the postcommissural putamen in Parkinson's disease. *Ann Neurol* 1995;38: 379–388.
7. Gash DM, Zhang Z, Ovadia A, et al. Functional recovery in parkinsonian monkeys treated with GDNF. *Nature* 1996;380:252–255.
8. Isacson O, Breakefield XO. Benefits and risks of hosting animal cells in the human brain. *Nat Med* 1997;3:964–969.
9. Jing S, Wen D, Yu Y, et al. GDNF-induced activation of the ret GDNFR, a novel receptor for GDNF. *Cell* 1996;85:1113–1124.

10. Kordower J, Freeman T, Snow B, et al. Neuropathological evidence of graft survival and striatal reinnervation after the transplantation of fetal mesencephalic tissue in a patient with Parkinson's disease. *N Engl J Med* 1995; 332:1118–1164.

11. Lin L. Doherty D, Lile J, Bektesh S, Collins F. GDNF: a glial cell line-derived neurotrophic factor for midbrain dopaminergic neurons. *Science* 1993;260: 1130–1132.

12. Lindvall O, Rehncrona S, Brundin P, et al. Human fetal dopamine neurons grafted into the striatum into patients with severe Parkinson's disease: a detailed account of methodology and a six-month follow-up. *Arch Neurol* 1989;46:615–631.

13. Lopez-Lozano J, Bravo G, Brera B, et al. Long-term improvement in patients with severe Parkinson's disease after implantation of fetal venal mesencephalic tissue in a cavity of the caudate nucleus: 5-year follow up in 10 patients. *J Neurosurg* 1997;86:931–942.

14. Olanow C, Kordower J, Freeman T. Fetal nigral transplantation as a therapy for Parkinson's disease. *TINS* 1996;19:102–109.

15. Olson L. NGF and the treatment of Alzheimer's disease. *Exp Neurol* 1993;124:5–15.

16. Pfann K, Penn R, Shannon K, Corcos D. The effect of pallidotomy on movement speed and trajectory variability in medicated patients with Parkinson's disease. *Neurology (in press)*.

17. Schaar D, Sieber B-A, Dreyfus C, Black I. Regional and cell-specific expression of GDNF in rat brain. *Exp Neurol* 1993;124:368–371.

18. Shoulson I, Group TPS. Effect of deprenyl on the progression of disability in early Parkinson's disease. *N Engl J Med* 1989;321:1364–1371.

19. Treanor J, Goodman L, Sauvage FD, et al. Characterization of a multicomponent receptor for GDNF. *Nature* 1996;382:80–83.

20. Weiss R. Promising protein for Parkinson's. *Science* 1993;260:1072–1073.

21. Winkler J, Ramirez G, Kuhn H, et al. Reversible Schwann cell hyperplasia and sprouting of sensory and sympathetic neurites after intraventricular administration of nerve growth factor. *Ann Neurol* 1997; 41:82–93.

Subject Index

SUBJECT INDEX